For — Mike Nettles
with best regards,
Jim Skinner

Mike —
It occurred to me after our
lunch that this history of U.T.
Memphis would help to supplement your familiarity with
our campus.
Jim

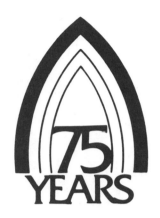

THE UNIVERSITY OF TENNESSEE, MEMPHIS 75th ANNIVERSARY— MEDICAL ACCOMPLISHMENTS

By

James Edward Hamner, III, D.D.S., Ph.D.

Assistant to the Chancellor, and
Professor, Department of Pathology
U.T. College of Medicine

Published by
The University of Tennessee, Memphis, 1986

The University of Tennessee, Memphis
62 South Dunlap, Suite 507
Memphis, Tennessee 38163

Design: John Halliburton

Library of Congress Cataloging-in-Publication Data

Hamner, James E.
   The University of Tennessee, Memphis, 75th anniversary.

   Includes bibliographies and index.
   1. University of Tennessee, Memphis—History.
2. Medical colleges—Tennessee—Memphis—History.
I. Title.   [DNLM: 1. University of Tennessee, Memphis.
2. Schools, Medical—history—Tennessee.]
R747.U6839H36   1986   610'.7'1176819   86-16170
ISBN 0-9616311-3-9

DEDICATED TO

*All of the faculty, alumni, and students
of the University of Tennessee, Memphis:
past, present, and future*

"Finally, although a bit of stoicism may be helpful, and the right view of life is important, what is ultimately essential to good health is to be a part of a community committed to health of body, mind, and spirit. We have need of doctors—doctors of the mind, body, and spirit—but we have a greater need to remember that the first responsibility for our health lies within ourselves."

The Reverend Canon Charles Martin
Washington Cathedral
Emeritus Headmaster,
St. Alban's School

Chancellor's Ad Hoc Advisory Group
on Medical Advances at U.T. Memphis

GROVER C. BOWLES, D.SC.
Professor, Department of Pharmacy Administration
U.T. College of Pharmacy

SIMON R. BRUESCH, M.D., Ph.D.
Emeritus Professor of Anatomy and
the History of Medicine
U.T. College of Medicine

LEMUEL W. DIGGS, M.D., F.C.A.P.
Emeritus Goodman Professor of Medicine
U.T. College of Medicine

JAMES N. ETTELDORF, M.D., F.A.A.P.
Emeritus Goodman Professor of Pediatrics
U.T. College of Medicine

RUTH NEIL MURRY, B.S.N., M.A.
Emeritus Dean
U.T. College of Nursing

RICHARD R. OVERMAN, Ph.D.
Emeritus University Distinguished Professor
U.T. College of Medicine

SAMUEL L. RAINES, M.D.
Emeritus Clinical Professor of Urology
U.T. College of Medicine

RICHARD J. REYNOLDS, D.D.S., F.A.C.D.
Past President, American College of Dentists

SAM HOUSTON SANDERS, M.D., F.A.C.S.
Emeritus Clinical Professor of Otolaryngology—
Head and Neck Surgery
U.T. College of Medicine

MARCUS J. STEWART, M.D., F.A.C.S.
Professor, Department of Orthopaedic Surgery
U.T. College of Medicine

TABLE OF CONTENTS

FOREWORD

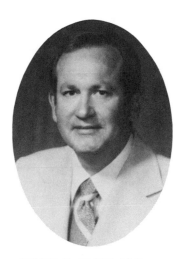

JAMES C. HUNT, M.D.
Chancellor The University of Tennessee, Memphis

AS we enter into the 75th Anniversary of the establishment of the University of Tennessee, Memphis, we have every reason to be justifiably proud of our distinguished past. We celebrate that heritage by examining where we stand at the present, and more importantly, how we shall move ahead into the future. Our best is yet to come. This University is composed of land, buildings, facilities, research laboratories, equipment, patient care, and educational programs—but most importantly, U.T. Memphis is made up of "people", our greatest asset.

It seems especially appropriate to commemorate this 75th Anniversary Year with the publication of a lasting memorial—a book, which describes so articulately those eventful 75 years, not merely by a dry recitation of dates and events, but by the enlivening of such a history by stimulating descriptions of the people and events, in the form of their medical contributions.

In writing such an authoritative history, a special sense of appreciation and commendation must be extended to the author, James E. Hamner, III, D.D.S., Ph.D., for his quality of writing and leadership that brought this extensive, interesting history to fruition. It is especially noteworthy that this accomplishment was achieved in a limited time frame, in which his many other responsibilities neither let up nor could be placed aside. He was fortunate to be advised and encouraged by such an outstanding array of distinguished Emeritus Faculty and Alumni, who are the treasure of any accomplished academic institution—the individuals who have lived so much of this colorful history and who continue to support us as we move into the future. I firmly believe that this book will be enjoyed by alumni, faculty, students, parents, and all friends of the University.

The University of Tennessee, Memphis belongs to and is a part of the lives of all of the people of Tennessee. It is the product of the people it strives to serve. As we head into the next 75 years of our future, we look forward to being a national leader, to setting the pace, and to forming productive new associations. With motivated alumni, faculty, and students, with exciting new educational programs, through advances in knowledge through research, and through close association with Tennessee's hospitals, educational institutions, and the health professional communities, we shall better serve the citizens of our State, region, and the nation. Such a vision and philosophy fulfill our mission and reason for existence—improving the quality of life tomorrow.

James C Hunt

P R E F A C E

I T is appropriate that the University of Tennessee, Memphis should notice in 1986 the completion of its 75th year in Memphis. James E. Hamner, III, D.D.S., Ph.D. has undertaken the demanding task of compiling and writing the history of the major events involving the development of the Health Sciences in Memphis to their current level. As the University of Tennessee, Memphis accelerates its progression towards excellence in research, service, and teaching, such an evaluation of past events will provide evidence as to the extent of fulfillment of its goals. Furthermore, such an evaluation will clarify its present status and assist in charting a path towards future development.

Dr. Hamner has summarized the first 60 years of the University of Tennessee Health Sciences Colleges (Medicine, Dentistry, and Pharmacy) in Nashville to assist the reader in integrating events of 75 years in Memphis into the 135 year existence of these Colleges. Although surviving the struggles of a time span of 135 years is worthy of note, the University of Tennessee, Memphis can also celebrate its achievement of excellence and is in a position to anticipate even greater progress in the future.

The early years of the University of Tennessee, Memphis, 1911 to about 1925, might be designated the infancy of the institution, the struggle for survival. The national trend towards elevation of standards of medical education resulted in a drastic reduction of medical schools in the United States. The University of Tennessee, Memphis survived because of success in its search for competent leadership, the recruitment of qualified students, and the securing of funding from the State and other sources beyond student tuition. It is clear from Dr. Hamner's discussion of these perils that the very existence of the institution was uncertain, but having survived its infancy, the next twenty years (through World War II), might be considered the period of its adolescence. There was still instability with some successes and discouraging failures, but each year brought some progress, and confidence developed in the face of uncertainty. Teaching and service were the main concerns of the faculty and administration. As there was little time or money for research, those of the staff who did research had to overcome severe obstacles. Maturity came in the period following World War II, bringing a great increase in the physical plant, the enlargement of the full-time clinical faculty, and, most notably, the increase in funding from

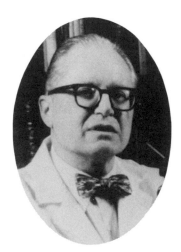

S. R. BRUESCH, M.D.,
Ph.D. *Emeritus Professor of
Anatomy and the History of
Medicine, The University
of Tennessee, Memphis*

Federal and State governments, as well as endowments from private sources. Because of the number and complexity of the developments in the mature phase, the narration of the post-war era has been, at times, condensed out of necessity in an effort to cover as many people and events as possible.

I believe Dr. Hamner's historical narrative will provide the reader with insight into the evolution and development of the Health Sciences in Memphis. This work is a fitting commemoration of the 75th Anniversary of the University of Tennessee, Memphis.

INTRODUCTION

$\mathcal{T}$HE genesis of this book was an initial request by our Chancellor, James C. Hunt, M.D., to chair an Ad Hoc Advisory Group (composed of notable Emeritus Faculty and Alumni), which would assist Mr. Michael Lollar (a writer for the Mid-South Magazine) with a brief listing of the medical accomplishments achieved in Memphis. Mr. Lollar's article appeared in the May 27, 1984 issue of the *Commercial Appeal* Mid-South Magazine, in conjunction with the opening of the Memphis Pink Palace Museum's $250,000 medical collection—"From Saddlebags to Science". In the process of collecting this material, it became readily apparent that only the tip of the iceberg was visible—a wealth of important historical information, concerning U.T. Memphis, lay buried in countless places. The University's early records were in a very chaotic state; some were lost, and others were kept in such a variety of sundry places that it often seemed impossible to locate them. With 1986 fast approaching and with it the 75th Anniversary of the University of Tennessee in Memphis, the next logical step suggested was to collect as much historical material as possible and arrange it into a commemorative book, featuring the medical contributions (clinical, educational, research, and administrative) of U.T. alumni and faculty. The term "medical contributions" is used here in the generic sense—it encompasses all of the health care professions.

Even though the task proved to be a Herculean one, I am extremely grateful to Chancellor Hunt for the opportunity of tackling it. Having first been a student here, then an alumnus, and now years later, a member of the College of Medicine faculty, I have a deep personal interest and feeling for the University of Tennessee, Memphis. This book has proven to be a tremendous learning experience, and one should never shun that opportunity.

An author never plunges into a task such as this one without the kindly assistance of many people. To all of the members of the Chancellor's Ad Hoc Advisory Group on Medical Advances at U.T. Memphis (Grover Bowles, D.Sc.; Simon R. Bruesch, M.D., Ph.D.; Lemuel W. Diggs, M.D.; James N. Etteldorf, M.D.; Emeritus Dean Ruth Neil Murry; Richard R. Overman, Ph.D.; Samuel L. Raines, M.D.; Richard J. Reynolds, D.D.S.; Sam H. Sanders, M.D.; and Marcus J. Stewart, M.D.), I owe a deep debt of gratitude for their assistance in data collection and their careful reviews of each chapter. Many of these fine gentlemen taught me as a student, and it should be borne in mind that any doctor is the sum total of all knowledge imparted by his academic regimen, the influence of professors and mentors, clinical maturity, and the special rapport with patients. These advisors possess accurate and tenacious memories, and they have made many valuable suggestions to these pages. I am under a lasting obligation to them for their unstinting time, meticulous review, and staunch encouragement to see the work through to a pleasing conclusion. The painstaking review of the numerous manuscript drafts for correct English grammar and punctuation and the proofing of all the galleys was accomplished by Catherine A. Clark in a supportive, cheerful exemplary manner. The arduous task of typing and proofing the manuscript on the word processor in final form with accuracy, outstanding quality, and dedication to high standards was performed in meritorious fashion, always with pleasantness and enthusiasm, by Mary F. Nelson.

The sources for the historical materials and photographs were quite varied. The Chancellor had the 75th Anniversary Book placed as an item on the Executive Committee's agenda. Next, each College Dean sent letters of exhortation regarding data collection to his Departmental Chairmen, who often, in turn, assigned the medical accomplishments collection to a senior member in the department. Written solicitations for materials, relating to history and medical accomplishments, were placed in each College's Alumni Magazine, as well as the "U.T. Record" newspaper. Even with all of this extensive effort, Murphy's Law will prevail, and sincere apologies are extended to all persons who may feel slighted that an accomplishment of theirs was somehow overlooked. Even after exhaustive readings by my long-suffering reviewers, many errors and omissions will still be found, for which I accept responsibility. Appreciation for many forms of assistance are owed to numerous people, because most of the historical facts, photographs, and many of the medical contributions had to be personally gleaned from a myriad of sources. Their willing endeavors were an immense aid: our fine librarians—Jess Martin, Wilma Lasslo, and Rose Williams; our pleasant and always efficient Registrar—Jean Melton and her "Keeper-of-the-records", Madge Huggins; our Alumni Affairs—Cathy Dernoncourt and June Montgomery for his special knowledge afforded by the "U.T. Center Grams"; our journalists on the "U.T. Record"—Claire Lowry and Adria Bernardi; Ruth Crenshaw and the Health Sciences Museum Foundation; our competent Photography Division—Jim Connelly, Thurman Hobson, and Jan Miller; and the cooperation and excellent book design by John Halliburton. When all other sources failed, inevitably I fell back on Dr. Simon Bruesch's extensive personal historical collection and expertise. His historical knowledge of Medicine in general and the University of Tennessee in particular, his abiding interest, and his deep love for this University are unsurpassed. I deeply treasure the valuable insights which I derived from our stimulating conversations and reminiscences.

Of the countless persons who have rendered advice and assistance in the compilation of the materials for this book, I wish particularly to thank: John Autian, Bridget Baldonado, Gloria Burness, Lynne Evans, Martin Hamner, Jimmy Hughes, Jim Johnson, Jim Kelly, Charles Kossmann, Patricia LaPointe,

Jim McKnight, Eric Muirhead, Bill Murrah, Bill Robinson, Bob Summitt, Jean Sweet, and Martha Jo Young.

This book is structured with an introductory portion which covers the history of medical education in Great Britain, Europe, and the United States, where the state of American medical education stood just prior to 1911, and what factors came into play in President Brown Ayres' decision to locate the medical branches of the University of Tennessee permanently in Memphis. Each succeeding chapter describes the historical events, leadership personalities, and construction of buildings, sprinkled with the medical contributions of alumni and faculty and permissible, humorous anecdotes about some of the more colorful cast of characters.

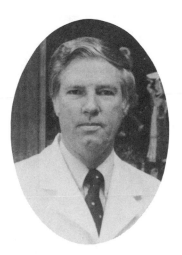

JAMES E. HAMNER, III, D.D.S., Ph.D.
Assistant to the Chancellor, and Professor, Department of Pathology U.T. College of Medicine

I was surprised to learn that there were no existing lists of previous Chancellors, Deans, etc. Therefore, with respect to purposefulness of direction, it seemed appropriate to chronicle them. Much useful information can be gleaned from these Appendices, and they speak for themselves. I would utter a strong plea for voluntary additions to the Wallace Collection (scientific books authored by U.T. Memphis Faculty or Alumni). Mr. Jess Martin, our astute Librarian, furnished the listing for this collection. Only authentic textbook contributions were selected—not study guides, chapters in books, etc. If the reader has published such a scientific book, and it is not listed in the Wallace Collection, then please contribute a copy to the University in order for it to be included in the future. Two hundred and forty illustrations, sixteen tables, and two maps are included to supplement the text. The 1872 map of Memphis depicts where the U.T. Memphis germinal seeds— Lindsley Hall, Eve Hall, and Rogers Hall—stood in the early years. The excellent 1986 map of the U.T. Memphis Campus, drawn in such fine, artistic detail by Fred Rawlinson, illustrates its mammoth size today.

Over its 75 years in Memphis, there have been many dedicated faculty members in the U.T. Memphis basic sciences and clinical specialties who are not emphasized in this account. Their contribution and lasting memorial are the fine health care professionals they have produced—the molding of enthusiastic young minds, arousing the inquiring curiosity of research, and instilling a sense of keen sensitivity and concern for what is in the best interest of the patient. The daily conduct of all U.T.-produced health care professionals in their daily practice of the pursuit of excellence composes countless "medical contributions", which remain unknown and unsung except by their benefiting patients.

I hope that this book will arouse fond memories for all U.T. Memphis Alumni—that it will cause each of us to pause and reflect on the past and the future. As disease often raises the sufferer, granting him an intimate vision of life and making it more precious by revealing a more direct route to his soul, so too, this history may give us glimpses into our own souls.

James Edward Hamner, III

CHAPTER ONE

Introductory History

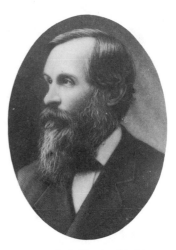

FIGURE 1. *J. Berrien Lindsley, M.D. (1822–1897)*

EFORE commencing to enumerate the medical achievements of the many individuals who have comprised the University of Tennessee, Memphis over its 75 years of existence, it is important and necessary to reflect on the history of its genesis and how matters truly stood, just prior to the publication of the famous Flexner Report of 1910. This document markedly influenced the future of health professional education in the United States.

Well-meaning efforts to establish both medical and dental education within the University of Tennessee had proven difficult in the mid-nineteenth century. the University of Tennessee was founded in Knoxville as "Blount College" in 1794. It was reorganized and renamed "East Tennessee College" in 1808. Later in 1840, the Tennessee General Assembly authorized its name to be changed to "East Tennessee University", and on March 10, 1879, it became "the University of Tennessee" by a legislative act and represented the entire State. The East Tennessee Medical Society had made several abortive attempts to establish a medical school in Knoxville, but the young, struggling University of Tennessee simply did not have the financial means to achieve this goal.[2,10,13]

The oldest school of the group of five medical schools, which eventually merged to form the University of Tennessee College of Medicine, was the University of Nashville Medical Department.[10,11,13] This school had its inception as Davidson Academy in 1785, became Cumberland College in 1806, and eventually evolved into the University of Nashville in 1826.[14] The Medical Department of the University of Nashville owed its origin on October 11, 1850 to the devoted leadership of Dr. J. Berrien Lindsley (Figure 1), Dr. William King Bowling (Figure 2), and Drs. A.H. Buchanan, Robert Porter, Charles K. Winston, and John M. Watson, who developed plans and comprised the original faculty.[11,12] Dr. Lindsley, while only 28 years old, was the motivating force to stimulate Nashville physicians to invest thousands of dollars in buildings and equipment for this school. While it was associated with the University of Nashville, the Medical School had complete financial autonomy. Figure 3 demonstrates how this Medical School appeared in 1897. During its nearly 60 years of existence, the University of Nashville Medical Department graduated approximately 5,000 physicians.[12]

Later, believing that a new medical school was needed in Nashville, this same group of men in 1876, under the leadership of Dr. Paul Fitzsimmons Eve, Sr. (Figure 4) and his son, Dr. Duncan Eve, organized the Nashville

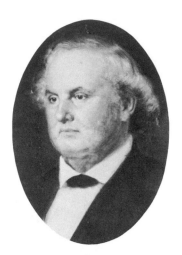

FIGURE 2. *William King Bowling, M.D. (1803–1885) Professor of Medicine & Dean University of Nashville Medical Department*

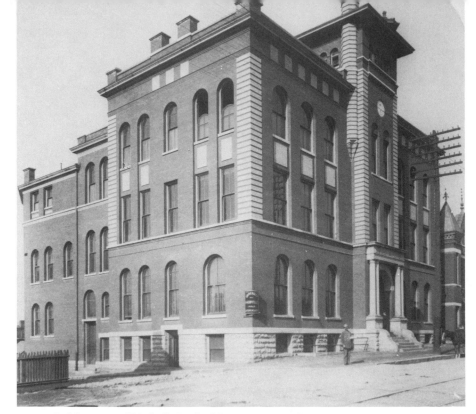

FIGURE 3. *University of Nashville Medical Department, 1897*

Medical College.[1,14] Earlier, in 1874, the University of Nashville had affiliated itself, without losing its own identity, with the newly created Vanderbilt University and its accompanying Medical School, causing some of the professors to break away in 1876 to form the Nashville Medical College.[14] This loosely related joint medical department arrangement lasted for 21 years, then terminated in 1895. The Vanderbilt University built separate buildings for its medical college.[13] Recognizing the advantages of having the University of Tennessee's name on their medical degrees, these enterprising men approached the Trustees of the University of Tennessee in Knoxville and proposed a merger.[1,10,11,12] The Trustees accepted this loosely constructed agreement, whereby the University of Tennessee assumed an affiliation, which existed in name only. In other words, it provided no funding, no management, and no control—they merely issued medical diplomas in the name of the University of Tennessee, and these were signed by its President.[6,7,11,12] Figure 5 illustrates the appearance of the University of Tennessee Medical Department in Nashville in 1897. The Medical Department was allowed to collect and use its fees for various operating costs and for the profit of its owners. If there was a loss, the Trustees for the University of Tennessee assumed no liability. It remained in Nashville, along with three other medical schools: the University of Nashville Medical Department, the Vanderbilt University Medical School, and Walden University, which subsequently became Meharry Medical College.[1,10]

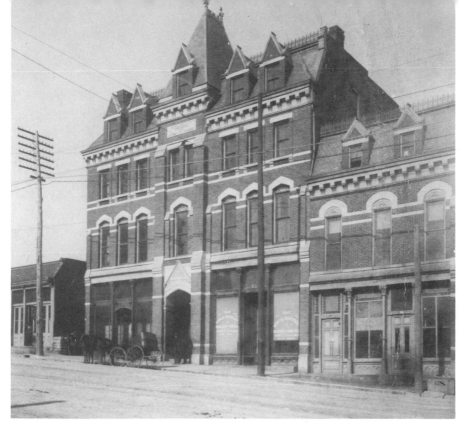

FIGURE 5. *University of Tennessee Medical Department in Nashville, 1897*

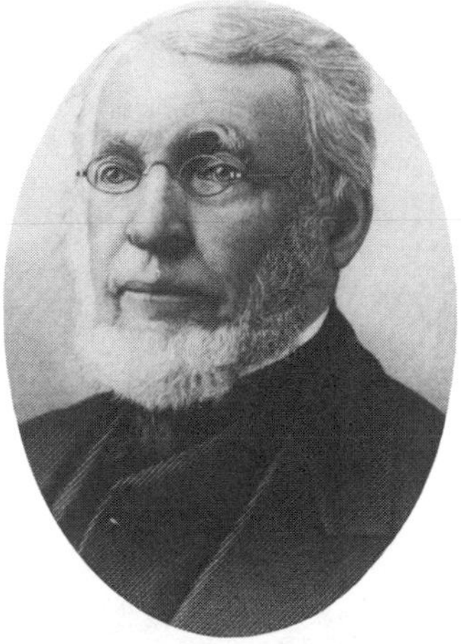

FIGURE 4. *Paul Fitzsimmons Eve, Sr., M.D. (1806–1877)*

Paul Fitzsimmons Eve, Sr., was a Renaissance individual who made tremendous contributions to medicine and medical education in Tennessee, after moving to Nashville from his native Georgia (Figure 4). He was born in 1806, received his M.D. degree from the University of Pennsylvania in 1828, was extremely active in medical education in Nashville from 1851 onwards, and died in 1877. His book on surgery, involving his most interesting cases, was published in 1857 and was used widely in the United States for teaching purposes. He published 436 scientific articles and served as President of the American Medical Association, as well as Professor of Surgery and Dean of the two Medical Schools, previously mentioned, which he nurtured in Nashville.[1,14]

Two of the five medical schools which merged to form the University of Tennessee College of Medicine were located in Memphis. Their development followed a circuitous route, evolving from two predecessor medical colleges. On January 21, 1846 during the 1845–46 Session of the Tennessee State Legislature, a charter was granted for the opening of the Memphis Medical College; on February 2, 1846 a second charter was granted to the Memphis Botanico-Medical College.[1,2,6,8] It is surprising that two medical colleges would commence on November 2, 1846 in such a small river town, whose total population was less than 7,000 persons—hardly enough to support one medical school, much less two.

Under the Deanship of Dr. Abner Hopton, who was also Professor of Chemistry, the Memphis Medical College conducted sessions for the years

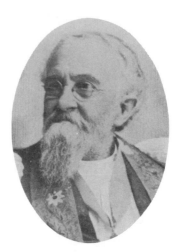

FIGURE 6. *Rt. Reverend Charles Todd Quintard, M.D. D.D., S.T.D., LL.D. Second Bishop of Tennessee*

1846–47, 1847–48, and 1848–49. Clinical instruction for this College was offered at the newly reorganized Memphis City Hospital, which was opened in November, 1841 on a ten-acre tract of land that now comprises Forrest Park in Memphis.[2,8] However, financial difficulties and in-fighting among the faculty made it impossible for the College to open its doors in 1849; a reorganization achieved this goal in November of 1852.

Dr. Lewis Shanks, a prominent Memphis physician, became Dean and Professor of Obstetrics and Diseases of Women and Children in 1851.[2,8] He assembled a distinguished faculty for its day, including Dr. Charles Todd Quintard, who was Professor of Physiology and Pathologic Anatomy.[2] This gentleman was born on December 22, 1824 in Stamford, Connecticut of French Huguenot extraction, attended Trinity School in New York City, studied medicine with Dr. James R. Wood and Dr. Valentine Mott, and received his M.D. degree from University Medical College (New York University) in 1847.[9] After an additional year of training at Bellevue Hospital, he moved South to Athens, Georgia to practice medicine and improve his health. Later, after becoming a member of the faculty of the Memphis Medical College, he also served as one of the editors of the *Memphis Medical Recorder*. His thorough reports on the health and mortality statistics of Memphis for the years 1852–53 earned him nationwide attention.[2] Dr. Quintard enjoyed rapid recognition from his medical colleagues and was well respected and liked by his medical students as an outstanding teacher. As a devoted member of the Episcopal Church, in 1854 he began to study for the ministry under the tutorship of Bishop James H. Otey. In 1855 he was ordained to the Diaconate, in 1856 to the Priesthood, and shortly afterwards became Rector of Calvary Church in Memphis. At that time he resigned his position on the faculty of the Memphis Medical College. At the outbreak of the War Between the States, he was elected Chaplain of the 1st Tennessee Infantry Regiment and served the Confederacy as both a Chaplain and as a Surgeon. In 1865 he was elected the second Bishop of Tennessee and was consecrated in Philadelphia. He became a national and international figure for his work within the Anglican Communion and received an LL.D. degree from Cambridge University. He is perhaps best remembered as the second founder of the University of the South at Sewanee after the War, for his continuing devotion to better undergraduate and medical education, and for his heroic efforts in raising relief funds during the terrible yellow fever epidemics of 1873, 1878, and 1879 in Memphis. Dr. Quintard appears in his vestments as a Bishop in Figure 6.[9] In 1954, St. Mary's Cathedral would establish the "Quintard House" for Episcopal students at the University of Tennessee Medical Units, named for this famous physician and bishop.

During the years from 1851 through 1861, the Memphis Medical College offered a session each year. Medical education came to a near standstill throughout much of the South during the War Between the States; however, even though Federal troops occupied the school buildings for a hospital and barracks, Dr. Lindsley and his staff at the University of Nashville Medical

Department continued to give medical instructions to a greatly reduced student body.[8] With its suspension after 1861, the Memphis Medical College faced an uncertain future. Efforts were made to revive it, but only the 1871–72 session was conducted with 20 graduates receiving the M.D. degree.[2] Personal losses and financial hard times, caused by the War Between the States and the aftermath of Reconstruction, dealt this school a death blow. Thus, its existence ceased in 1872 after having graduated almost 240 physicians.[2,8]

The Botanico-Medical College, which emphasized plant remedies, "water cures", and steam vapor in its treatment of diseases, also commenced its existence on November 2, 1846.[8] It attracted 93 students during the 1846–47 session and awarded 27 M.D. degrees.[2] Yet, by 1851 it had only 15 students enrolled. Salvation efforts for this school were enhanced by a new building facility on the north side of Beale Street, near the corner of Beale and Lauderdale. It conducted annual sessions until the outbreak of the War Between the States in 1861, which caused it to cease to exist thereafter as a school.[2,8] Thus ended the two predecessor medical schools in Memphis, which remained without any medical school from 1872 until 1880.

By 1877, there was an increased national demand for medical services, and under the inspired leadership of Dr. William E. Rogers (1826–1885), a new school named the Memphis Hospital Medical College was organized in 1877.[2,6,7] Plans called for the inaugural school term to commence in the autumn of 1878, but the severe yellow fever epidemics of 1878 and 1879 postponed its opening until 1880.[2] Perhaps the best accounting of the yellow fever epidemic of 1878, the worst of the three to afflict Memphis, is given by J. M. Keating in his book for the Howard Association entitled, *The Yellow Fever Epidemic of 1878 in Memphis, Tennessee.* A brief summary of this tragic time in the history of Memphis reveals that 17,600 cases and 5,150 deaths attributable to yellow fever occurred between August 2 and December 12, 1878.[2] In the midst of this severe health calamity, there were many examples of extreme heroism and devotion to duty, exhibited by members of the Howard Association (businessmen who were organized to aid victims of yellow fever and procure relief funding); the 111 Howard Association physicians, of whom five contracted Memphis physicians and 28 outside volunteer physicians died, while 20 others suffered from yellow fever and recovered (24 non-Howard Memphis and Shelby County physicians died); numerous valiant nurses, who served with remarkable zeal, caring devotion, and efficiency in this crisis; and members of religious orders (38 nuns and 23 priests from Episcopal and Roman Catholic orders died in the epidemic, serving the sick).[2,8] John H. Erskine, M.D., the Memphis Health Officer and a veteran of the Confederate Army Medical Corps (Figure 7) and Sister Constance, Mother Superior of St. Mary's Episcopal Convent (Figure 8), were among the many dedicated individuals who remained in Memphis to care for the needs of the stricken yellow fever victims and who paid the supreme price.

From this devastating chapter in Memphis' history, which left it deci-

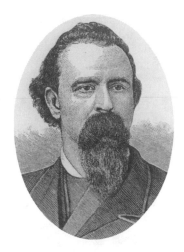

FIGURE 7. *John H. Erskine, M.D. Memphis Health Officer during the Yellow Fever Epidemic of 1878*

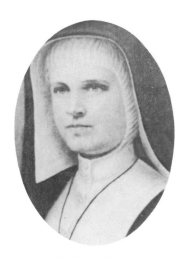

FIGURE 8. *Sister Constance Mother Superior of St. Mary's Episcopal Convent Memphis, Tennessee, 1878*

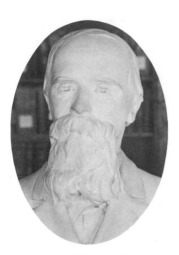

FIGURE 9. *William E. Rogers, M.D. (1826–1885) Founding Dean (1880–1884) Memphis Hospital Medical College*

mated in population and in financial ruins with its city charter abolished, Memphis emerged from the chaotic 1870's into the 1880's as a revitalized city, founded on the sound principles of good public health and proper sanitation.

On Union Avenue opposite the old Memphis City Hospital (opened in 1841), the Memphis Hospital Medical College erected a new three story brick and stone building in 1880. Dr. William E. Rogers (Figure 9) served as the first Dean until 1884 when he resigned due to ill health, dying the following year. The new facility had an amphitheatre for lectures, a dissecting room for anatomy, a museum for medical specimens, a small clinical laboratory, and a small dispensary; it controlled 40 charity beds in the Memphis City Hospital for teaching purposes.[8] This medical school's first faculty included Dr. William B. Rogers, the son of the founder, and Drs. D. D. Saunders, S. C. Maddox, F. L. Sim, W. J. Armstrong, Heber Jones, W. W. Hall, Julius Fahlen, A. G. Sinclair, and B. G. Henning.[2] Enrollment grew slowly at first with 60 medical students in the first session, then more rapidly, reaching 752 students matriculating in 1899–1900. After attaining this peak, a steady decline commenced, falling to 380 by 1911.[2] In 1885 Dr. A. G. Sinclair, who was Professor of Ophthalmology and Otology, was elected Dean. Drs. T. J. Crofford, Alexander Erskine, Richard Brooke Maury, and E. M. Willett were distinguished additions to the faculty, which is illustrated as it was in the 1898 graduation in Figure 10.[2] The school's facilities were enhanced by the completion of the new Memphis City Hospital, which was a brick building located on the north side of Madison Avenue, just east of Dunlap Street. This building was patterned after the famous Johns Hopkins Hospital in Baltimore, Maryland and is depicted in Figure 11.

With increased enrollment, the main medical school building was enlarged in 1890, and in 1893 laboratories were added for pathology, histology, and bacteriology. Dr. William Krauss, who was Memphis' most famous pioneer clinical pathologist, had graduated from the Memphis Hospital Medical College's two-year program in 1889. He returned to his native Germany for postgraduate work under many of the famous German medical scientists such as Ehrlich, Esmark, Fleming, and Koch. Upon his return to Memphis, he assumed the lead as a demonstrator of pathology to introduce microscopy and laboratory pathology techniques to his medical students, being the first physician in Memphis to use an oil immersion microscope in 1897.[2,8] In 1902 this medical school erected a new building at 718 Union Avenue near Marshall Street which was later named Rogers Hall, after the founder and first Dean. Figure 12 demonstrates its appearance in 1913 when it was converted to the College of Dentistry with the University of Tennessee merger. Dr. William Boddie Rogers (1856–1915), the son of Dr. William E. Rogers and Professor of Surgery, became Dean in 1894 and served in this capacity until this school merged with the University of Tennessee College of Medicine in 1913 (Figure 13). By the year 1911, the Memphis Hospital Medical College had awarded 2,625 M.D. degrees.[2,6,8]

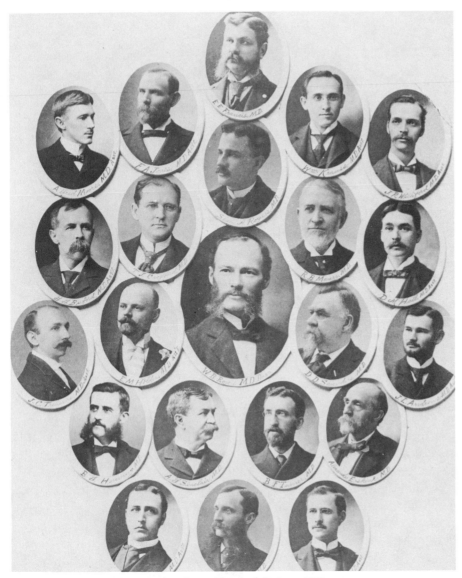

FIGURE 10. *Faculty of the Memphis Hospital Medical College, 1898*

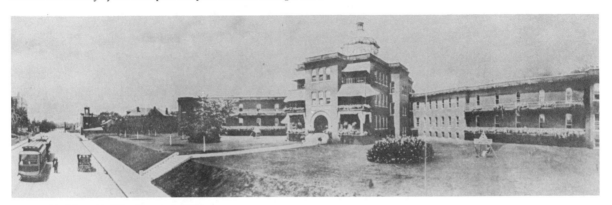

FIGURE 11. *Memphis City Hospital, 1898*

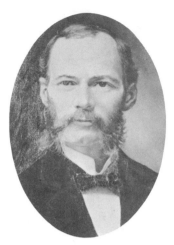

FIGURE 13. *William Boddie Rogers, M.D. (1856–1915) Professor of Surgery & Dean Memphis Hospital Medical College*

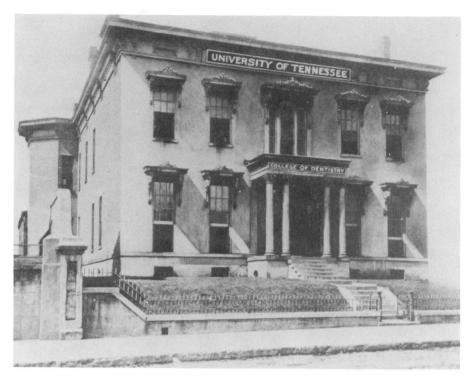

FIGURE 12. *Memphis Hospital Medical College, 1902 (renamed Rogers Hall—College of Dentistry—1913)*

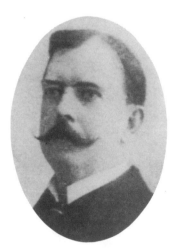

FIGURE 14. *Heber Wheat Jones, M.D. (1848–1916) Professor of Clinical Medicine & Dean The College of Physicians and Surgeons*

The second Memphis Medical School, which formed a part of the 1911 merger into the University of Tennessee College of Medicine, was the College of Physicians and Surgeons. It was founded in 1905 by a group of prominent Memphis physicians, who erected a new building in 1906 and began the first formal session in the fall of 1906. Among the original faculty members were: Drs. G. G. Buford, W. C. Campbell, J. A. Crisler, E. C. Ellett, M. Goltman, Marcus Haase, A. G. Jacobs, Heber Jones, Louis Leroy, George R. Livermore, J. M. Maury, J. L. Mclean, Edward C. Mitchell, O. S. McGown, Richmond McKinney, W. T. Pride, and Percy W. Toombs.[1,2] The first Dean was Heber Jones, M.D. (Figure 14), who had obtained his medical degree from the University of Virginia. The Building Committee was composed of Drs. G. G. Bufford, E. C. Ellett, and M. Goltman.

This school occupied an excellent new building at 879 Madison Avenue, which was well located since it faced the newly completed Memphis City Hospital (1898), and the founders gave a building site adjacent to its east side to Baptist Memorial Hospital.[11] Thus, it was in close proximity to two major hospitals with easy access to their charity wards for teaching.

The College of Physicians and Surgeons was among the first of the medical schools in the South to offer a four-year, graded curriculum to its students.[2,8] Although its newly constructed building provided an excellent modern facility, its general laboratory equipment was inadequate. There

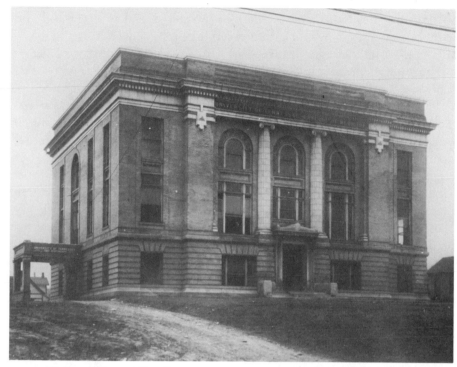

FIGURE 15. *The College of Physicians & Surgeons, 1906 (renamed Lindsley Hall—College of Medicine—1911)*

were few scientific medical books, no medical museum, and no instructional charts.[3] In 1909 in an unsuccessful attempt to provide undergraduate as well as medical education, the College of Physicians and Surgeons joined in a loosely constructed relationship as the Medical Department of the University of Memphis. This ambiguous effort was labeled by Abraham Flexner in his 1909 visit as "a fictitious affair".[3] With its merger into the University of Tennessee in 1911, the College of Physicians and Surgeons was renamed Lindsley Hall in honor of J. Berrien Lindsley, M.D., the principal organizer of the University of Nashville Medical Department. Figure 15 depicts its appearance in 1912.

In its brief existence of only five years (1906–1910 classes), it did attain the achievement of graduating more knowledgeable physicians to the Mid-South area. Its most distinguished medical graduate was August Hermsmeier Wittenborg, M.D., who graduated in 1910 (Figure 16). Dr. Wittenborg's many fine contributions to the University of Tennessee will be discussed in detail in subsequent chapters. Perhaps a more typical example of the student of that day would be Otus Preston Gaston, M.D. (Figure 17). He had been born and reared in the small rural town of Vaiden, Mississippi, took two sessions at the University of Nashville Medical Department, worked in the intervening times as a preceptor for several Mississippi physicians, transferred to the College of Physicians and Surgeons in Memphis, and graduated in 1909. Similar to most young medical graduates

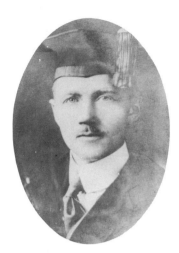

FIGURE 16. *August Hermsmeier Wittenborg, M.D. (1883–1941) (1910 graduation photograph from the College of Physicians & Surgeons)*

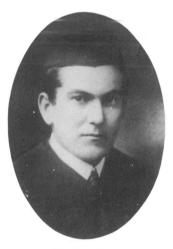

FIGURE 17. *Otus Preston Gaston, M.D. (1909 graduation photograph from the College of Physicians & Surgeons)*

of that time, he immediately went into private general practice and also operated a drug store. While faithfully serving his patients during the severe international influenza epidemic of 1918, he died in Washington, D.C.

The fifth medical school, which merged to form the University of Tennessee College of Medicine, was the Lincoln Memorial University Medical Department in Knoxville, Tennessee.[10,11] Following the War Between the States, Northerners established in 1897 the Lincoln Memorial University in Harrogate, Tennessee, which is situated in the beautiful mountainous region of the Cumberland Gap, where the three states of Virginia, Tennessee, and Kentucky meet.

Desiring expansion as a university, this school entered into a nominal relationship with the Tennessee Medical College, a typical proprietary medical school, which was already located in Knoxville. It was an arrangement similar to the one that existed earlier between the Nashville Medical College and the University of Tennessee in Knoxville, whereby the University of Tennessee issued M.D. degrees in name only, with no actual control or responsibility for the Nashville Medical College. On July 15, 1905 the name of the Tennessee Medical College was changed to Lincoln Memorial University Medical Department, and thereafter Lincoln Memorial University issued the M.D. degrees in its name.[2,3,10] The Tennessee Medical College held its first session in 1889–90 and was located originally on the corner of Gay and Main Streets (Figure 18). Although it underwent several moves, the Tennessee Medical College held continuous annual sessions until its merger with the University of Tennessee College of Medicine in 1914.

When the Tennessee Medical College settled at Cleveland Place and Dameron Avenue, it expanded by building an adjoining hospital, which in actuality was the private hospital of the faculty for which medical student fees helped to pay its expenses and cost of construction.[3] It had an average of 40 in-patient beds, but there were no charity wards for teaching. According to the Flexner Report, clinical instruction was very sparse and poor.[3] Figure 19 illustrates how the Tennessee Medical College and Hospital appeared in 1901, prior to its change in name in 1905 to the Lincoln Memorial University Medical Department. From 1889–1905 the original school awarded 179 M.D. degrees. Under the name of Lincoln Memorial University Medical Department, it awarded an additional 261 medical degrees from 1905–1914 for a total of 440 M.D. degrees.[2] In 1914 the Trustees of Lincoln Memorial University decided to cease operations, and they transferred the majority of their students to Memphis in the final merger forming the University of Tennessee College of Medicine.

Before describing the final amalgamation of these five medical schools into the University of Tennessee College of Medicine and the genesis of the University of Tennessee College of Dentistry and School of Pharmacy, it is important to pause and briefly review the general conditions of medical education, especially in America. Flexner categorized the origin

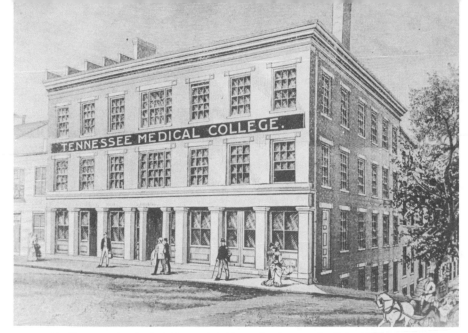

FIGURE 18. *Tennessee Medical College, 1889 Knoxville, Tennessee*

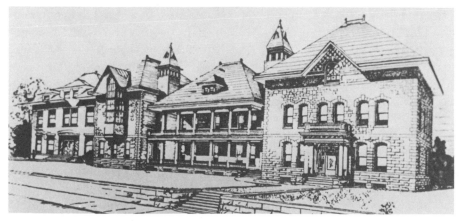

FIGURE 19. *Tennessee Medical College and Hospital, 1901 (renamed Lincoln Memorial University Medical Department, 1905)*

and development of medical schools into three types: (A) the clinical type, (B) the university type, and (C) the proprietary type.[5]

The clinical type developed in France and Great Britain as pathological-clinical schools. Other than basic anatomy, all of the other various subjects were learned in the hospital, as the apprentice medical student followed his master physician from bed to bed. At first he merely watched, then later assisted, while absorbing the words of learning that fell from the physician's lips. Thus, the medical student in this setting was not so much an actual university student as he was the disciple of the physician or surgeon whom he followed.[4,5] The basic objective of the clinical type of medical school was to train doctors by practical methods. The French variety was in name a university faculty, while the British variety of medical school was practically independent. At Oxford and Cambridge Universities, beginning medical

11

schools were established for training in the basic sciences and for research; then the student progressed to the hospital clinical school portion. This route was an exception, not the rule. [4,5]

The university type of medical school originated and developed in Germany, Scandinavia, the Netherlands, and German-speaking Switzerland. The German University in the 19th century stressed research as much as teaching, and eminence in research became the accepted basis for promotion within the university. [4,5] Prolonged training in scholarship and science produced the great masters of German medicine, such as Rudolf Virchow and Paul Ehrlich. The accomplishments of original work in pathology, anatomy, bacteriology, or medicine lent itself to recognition, promotion, and honors. The university type of medical school's philosophy was that chemistry, physiology, and pathology were not simply subjects to be taught to medical students, but they were vast domains to be probed, explored, and conquered.

The third type of medical school was the proprietary type and was indigenous to North America.

In American colonial days young men, who were interested in medicine, served an apprenticeship under physicians who had been trained either in Great Britain or in Europe and who had emigrated to North America. The young man would literally indenture himself to a reputable practitioner of medicine, to whom his service was successively menial, pharmaceutical, and professional. His tasks were many, from running errands, fetching materials, washing medicine bottles, mixing drugs and medications, spreading the plasters, and gradually learning by clinical experience the art of medicine from the daily practice of his preceptor. It is easy to see that under such a method the quality of training would vary, largely within the limits of the capacity and conscientiousness of the preceptor physician. After serving such an apprenticeship in America, a few of these young men would then journey to the famous hospitals and medical lecture halls of London, Edinburgh, Paris, Berlin, and Leyden.

The complete study of medicine, within the confines of America, most likely began in 1762 with Dr. William Shippen in Philadelphia. After spending five years of medical study abroad in Great Britain, he returned to Philadelphia and began a course of lectures on midwifery. The following year he commenced a series of anatomical lectures for young men who did not have the financial means to attend the more famous schools in Great Britain and Europe. In 1765 the first professorship in the theory and practice of medicine was established by the College of Philadelphia in conjunction with the Pennsylvania Hospital. From this emerged the University of Pennsylvania College of Medicine in 1766. These Colleges of Medicine were an integral part of the university to which they belonged. In 1768 the Medical Department of King's College, which became Columbia University, was established in New York. By 1814 it had united with the College of Physicians and Surgeons in New York. The Harvard College Medical Department was established in 1783, followed by the Dartmouth College

Medical Department in 1798. The last of these five major schools was the Yale College Medical Department, which was founded in 1810. These first medical students in America emulated the famous British and European schools in all respects. Unfortunately, the sound beginnings of the original medical schools in the United States were not long maintained, and their scholarly ideals were first compromised, then totally forgotten. Early in the 19th century, the first proprietary medical school arose at the University of Maryland.

The original American colleges of medicine had been a vital branch of emerging universities. Had the proprietary movement not originated, medical education would have remained a part of the entire national education movement forward, not an exception to it. Between 1810 and 1840 there were 26 new medical schools established in the United States. Between 1840 and 1876, 47 more medical schools had sprung up. By 1908, 457 medical schools had arisen in the United States and Canada, of which number, 155 survived and were functioning in 1910.[3]

The loss of university standards among these proprietary schools was unfortunate. Their physical facilities were notoriously poor. The educational process, except for a little anatomy demonstration, was wholly didactic, with lectures often being given in large, insufficiently lighted amphitheatres. These "schools" were primarily stock companies that were developed as private ventures and were run strictly for profit. They usually were a good financial investment, since there was little monetary investment in books and equipment, and the return on money invested by physicians was excellent. Most teaching was done on a part-time basis over brief six-week terms. Each school set its own requirements and often accepted anyone who paid the fees and signed his name. Student fee income was split among the various lecturers, who reaped a rich harvest in the larger schools. It is easy to see why "Chairs" became a valuable commodity in such schools, because a chairmanship meant a larger share of the income.[2,3] However, many such schools lost money and went bankrupt.

In some states the state medical society initially issued licenses to practice medicine. However, with the laissez-faire doctrine in economic affairs gaining dominance in the early 1800's, all licensure laws were repealed. Then, there were no state board examinations, much less national board examinations. Any medical school degree from a "diploma mill" was in itself a license to practice medicine. Until 1889 there was no medical licensure in Tennessee; dental licensure came in 1891. There were no written examinations, only brief oral exams given by the faculty—few students were ever failed.[3] Therefore, the student who formally registered and paid his tuition to the bursar was virtually assured of his M.D. degree, whether he attended lectures or not.

The preceptorial system, which had begun in the United States, was originally a mixture of the apprentice and university systems. The aspiring student of medicine registered himself with his preceptor physician and literally followed him, learning by practical experience as has been men-

"Nothing that was worthy in the past departs; no truth or goodness ever dies or can die."

Thomas Carlyle

13

tioned earlier. At the end of several years, he applied to medical school, which required a letter of certification from a reputable preceptor physician in order to be admitted. Medical subjects were taken over a two-year period—the usual medical school year was in the winter, consisting of two "courses" or "sessions" of four months each of assorted lectures (November-Mid-March). In the interim period from this formal lecture training, the student would return to his preceptor physician.[2,3,5] This system produced a surprising number of good, dedicated physicians and was a necessity in an emerging nation.

The later wave of commercial exploitation, caused by the proprietary medical school system, continued as an irresponsible condition into the 1890's. It became common practice for a student to register with a preceptor physician in name only and then never to see him again. An active apprenticeship of valuable clinical lessons at the patient's bedside became a thing of the past. All the training that a young physician received was procured within the proprietary medical school. It was not a supplement or refinement to a preceptorship system; it had become everything. With little clinical exposure in school (students often "looked on" in surgery, medicine, and obstetrics) and didactic lectures, the vital personal contact between professor and student and between student and patient was lost. As time passed, the school sessions were lengthened to two sessions of 16–20 weeks each, but the second session lectures were identical to those subjects covered in the first session, thus the student heard the same lectures twice.[2,3,5]

In November of 1908, the Trustees of the Carnegie Foundation for the Advancement of Teaching authorized a study and report on the schools of medicine and law in the United States. They commissioned Mr. Abraham Flexner, a distinguished educator of the time, to visit the medical schools in every state and prepare a report. For the purposes in this book, I wish briefly to cite a few medical educational statistics for the State of Tennessee in 1909, quote Mr. Flexner directly on his "general considerations" for Tennessee, and summarize the significant facts of his important study and report.

Tennessee in 1909 had a population of 2,248,404 persons. With 3,303 physicians, this calculation yields a ratio of one physician to every 681 citizens. At that time Tennessee had ten medical schools: Chattanooga Medical College in Chattanooga, Tennessee Medical College in Knoxville, Knoxville Medical College in Knoxville, the College of Physicians and Surgeons in Memphis, the Memphis Hospital Medical College in Memphis, the University of West Tennessee Medical Department in Memphis, Vanderbilt University Medical Department in Nashville, the University of Nashville Medical Department in Nashville, the University of Tennessee Medical Department in Nashville, and Meharry Medical College in Nashville. There was a total medical student enrollment of 1,458 in these ten schools.[3]

The following direct quote registers Mr. Flexner's impressions of medical education in Tennessee and his recommendations:

"The State of Tennessee protects at this date more low-grade medical schools than any other Southern state. It would be unfair and futile to criticize this situation without full recognition of local conditions. A standpoint that is entirely in order in dealing with Cincinnati, Chicago, or St. Louis is here irrelevant. The ideals held up must indeed be the same; but their attainment is much further in the future. The amount of money available for medical education is small; the preliminary requirement must be relatively low. Practically all that can be asked of Tennessee is that it should do the best possible under the circumstances.

This it does not do. The six white schools value their separate survival beyond all other considerations. A single school could furnish all the doctors the state needs and do something to supply the needs of adjoining states as well. Low as the entrance standard must be, it has been made lower in order to gather in students for six schools where one would suffice. The medical schools solicit and accept students who have not yet made the best of the limited educational opportunities their homes provide; and to this extent, not only injure the public health, but depress and demoralize the general education situation.

The same is true in reference to laboratories and clinics. However small the sums applicable to building and equipping laboratories, conditions are needlessly aggravated when six plants are equipped instead of one. These that ought now to be used in providing better teaching are still paying for the expensive buildings in Memphis and Nashville. The city hospitals of both places, small at best, are divided between two schools, though they do not furnish enough material for one.

Those who deal with medical education in Tennessee are therefore making the worst, not the best, of their limited possibilities. Their medical schools, treated on their merits commonly, would speedily reduce to one; the utterly wretched establishments at Chattanooga and Knoxville would be wiped out; the more showy but quite mercenary, concerns at Memphis would be liquidated. The University of Tennessee, with an annual income that does not yet suffice for the legitimate needs of its own plant at Knoxville should abandon for the present the effort to develop at Nashville a school that it can neither control nor support. The time may come when there will be a call for the State University to enter the field. But that time is not now. For the present it is dividing its own forces and hindering the most effective use of such resources as Nashville affords. The whole field is strangely confused; Lincoln Memorial University (which is an industrial school, not a university) at Cumberland Gap shelters a medical school in Knoxville; the University of Tennessee at Knoxville shelters an entirely superfluous school at Nashville.

If our analysis is correct, the institution to which the responsibility for medical education in Tennessee should just now be left is Vanderbilt University; for it is the only institution in position at this juncture to deal with this subject effectively. This does not mean that Vanderbilt has now any large sums of money available or that it should inaugurate impossible entrance standards. It can do neither, for the general situation countenances neither. The suggestion merely recognizes the facts that one school can do the work; that Vanderbilt occupies as in Nashville the point of vantage; that, in the public interests, the field should be left to the institution best situated to handle it.

On the other hand, any such arrangement imposes upon Vanderbilt a very distinct responsibility. It would have to nurse its enrollment; having to determine just how large a school local needs require, it must fix and enforce the strictest entrance requirements compatible therewith. At the present time this standard

"Medicine, to produce health, has to examine disease."

Plutarch

15

would be less than four-year high school graduation; but whatever it be, if only it is real and definite, it will operate to brace up general conditions. Improved teaching should compensate student effects. To this end, every effort should be made to secure endowment specifically applicable to the Medical Department; in the interval, these must be employed not to wipe out old obligations, however incurred, but to improve the school. The contract between Vanderbilt University and its medical department should be cancelled. The practitioner teachers must make good their ambition to advance medical education by being content with the indirect advantages accruing from school connections. If the entire fee income is used to equip the laboratories, to employ full-time teachers in the fundamental branches, to fit out and organize a good dispensary, there will still remain defects and make-shifts enough; but the school will wear a different aspect than is presented by any institution in the state today.

Let it be said ungrudgingly that these suggestions are offered in no spirit of unkindness. The State University and Vanderbilt have had their hands full. They have worked valiantly amidst conditions that might well appall the strongest heart. They deserve no blame for the past, providing only they unselfishly and vigorously cooperate in forgetting it. In the last few years right courses of action in medical education have for the first time been defined. A decade hence it will be fair to look back and ask if the universities of the state have followed them."

The five major significant facts that appeared to be nationwide in Flexner's study of medical school education in 1909 are summarized as follows:

(1) In the 35 year period between 1875–1910, there was an overproduction of poorly educated and ill-trained medical practitioners in the United States without any serious thought of the best interests of the public. At that time in the United States there were four to five times as many physicians in ratio to the general population as in older countries such as Germany and Great Britain.

(2) The overproduction of such ill-trained physicians was due chiefly to the existence of the huge number of commercial, proprietary medical schools.

(3) Many universities, desirous of parent educational completeness as a university, annexed or entered into loose agreements with medical schools without making themselves either responsible for the standards of these professional schools or for their financial support. Thus, universities had failed during this time span to appreciate the tremendous advances in medicine, the need for better thorough medical education along university lines, and the increased cost of teaching modern medicine at that time.

(4) The argument that many of these unnecessary and inadequate medical schools were necessary for the "poor boy" was proven indefensible and insincere because it was acknowledged that the poor boy had no right to enter any profession for which he was not willing to obtain adequate preparation.

(5) Medical schools and their accompanying hospitals should have been under complete educational control, as is best afforded in a university setting. Universities and hospitals were urged to secure sufficient funds to

ceeded in scuttling the joint University of Tennessee—University of Nashville agreement of 1909 by lobbying against its final approval by the Tennessee State Legislature. So, at the conclusion of the 1910–11 session, the Board of Trustees of the University of Nashville formally transferred all of the books and equipment of their Medical Department to the University of Tennessee Board of Trustees. They also transferred their goodwill and authority to the University of Tennessee to operate the Medical Department in a singular fashion.[7,10,12]

Although bids to attract the Medical Department came from Knoxville and Chattanooga, as well as Memphis, the latter city was chosen because its proposal was the most appealing. The powerful Memphis Business Men's Club was strongly supportive of the Memphis location, and Memphis offered a much better numerical advantage for accruing patients, being the largest city in the State. President Ayres and the University of Tennessee Board of Trustees met in Memphis with the proprietors of the College of Physicians and Surgeons and the proprietors of the College of Dentistry, both of whom belonged to the loosely knit paper organization under the name of the University of Memphis.[2,6,9] The University of Tennessee Trustees agreed "to take over all the property, goodwill, and equipment of the College of Physicians and Surgeons of Memphis, Tennessee, and to establish the same as the Medical Department of the University of Tennessee."[9,12] Under the terms of this contract, the new Medical Department would operate as any other University department, and the faculty of the College of Physicians and Surgeons was assured that it would be retained for at least five years at their current salaries. The University of Tennessee thus obtained title to the buildings and other property of the College of Physicians and Surgeons, assumed its current indebtedness, and made arrangements to handle the preferred stock of this proprietary school.[1,7,12]

On a typical, hot, humid August day in Memphis, five railroad freight cars arrived within the city carrying 100,000 pounds of medical and hospital equipment from the previous Medical Departments of the University of Nashville and the University of Tennessee in Nashville . With a tremendous effort, the move into the new facilities of the previous College of Physicians and Surgeons, now renamed Lindsley Hall, was accomplished, and classes commenced in the fall of 1911 as the University of Tennessee Medical Department.[1,7]

In 1912, at a cost of about $50,000 the University of Tennessee erected a four-story laboratory building on the same grounds as the previous College of Physicians and Surgeons.[1] The right end of that building, named Eve Hall for the famous Dr. Paul Fitzsimmons Eve who had aided in establishing the original Medical Schools in Nashville, can be seen in a 1962 photograph (Figure 20); Lindsley Hall is seen in the foreground and the Physicians and Surgeons Office Building of the Baptist Memorial Hospital appears on the left in Figure 20.

The University of Tennessee Trustees had rejected the Memphis Hospital Medical College's bid to join the merger of 1911 because that school had an employ men as teachers who were devoted to clinical science and who could provide quality education.

By the turn of the 20th century, new influences were beginning to stir in medical education across the United States. The American Medical Association, which was founded on May 5, 1847, at the Academy of Natural Sciences in Philadelphia, Pennsylvania, was concerned about the deficiencies and abuses in proprietary medical education. President John A. Wyeth appointed the A.M.A. Council on Medical Education and Hospitals in 1902, and it gave its first report at the A.M.A.'s annual meeting the next year in New Orleans. Since it was given the responsibility and authority to grade medical schools for approval or disapproval, it could exert pressure to elevate standards, improve facilities, and upgrade equipment.[9] Also exerting an influence at this time was the Association of American Medical Colleges, which was founded in 1876 in Evanston, Illinois. Later, in 1942 the Council of the Association of American Medical Colleges and the A.M.A. Council on Medical Education would unite to form the Liaison Committee for Medical Education which is the body that now accredits American medical schools. From this external pressure and internal concern, President Brown Ayres of the University of Tennessee entered into negotiations in 1908 with Chancellor James D. Porter of the University of Nashville and Chancellor James H. Kirkland of Vanderbilt University in an effort to consolidate their three Medical Departments in Nashville into a single school, sponsored by all three universities. Difficulties naturally arose with Vanderbilt University over the blending of a private institution with a State one. However, during the winter and spring of 1908–09, an agreement between the respective Boards of Trustees of the University of Tennessee and the University of Nashville was reached, and the result of this reorganization agreement was the joint Medical Department of the University of Nashville and the University of Tennessee.[7,9,12] A joint committee from the two Boards of Trustees was formed to administer the new united Medical Department, and Dr. Ayres was elected as its chairman.[12]

In 1910, the famous Flexner Report (Bulletin No. 4—Carnegie Foundation for the Advancement of Teaching) was published for general consumption, making public the news and facts of medical education's shortcomings. Abraham Flexner had completed his undergraduate degree in two years at the Johns Hopkins University in Baltimore, and his brother, Simon, had graduated from its medical school. Both events undoubtedly influenced his opinions. Johns Hopkins University was in the forefront of medical education at this time, and general opinion did reach a consensus that its program was the best one to train physicians. This curriculum called for definite acceptance criteria for premedical students, plus two full years of basic sciences and two full years of clinical practice at an institution which was an integral part of a reputable university.[3,5,9] Of the approximately 160 medical schools functioning in 1907, only 80 remained operational by 1927.[9]

Representatives from the Medical Units of Vanderbilt University suc-

"Hippocrat(
the first kn
all those w
both physic
philosopher
as he was t
recognize w
effects."

Galen

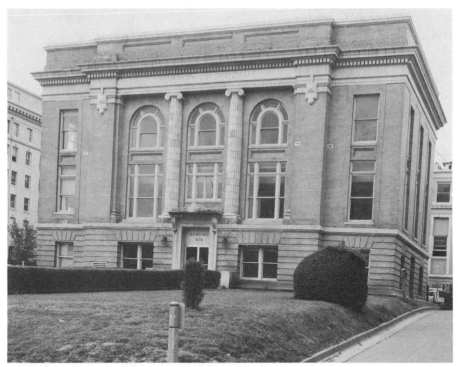

FIGURE 20. *Lindsley Hall and Eve Hall, University of Tennessee Medical Units (photo taken in 1962 when it was the U.T. College of Nursing)*

indebtedness of nearly $135,000. By 1913, their indebtedness had been reduced to approximately $50,000, and the University of Tennessee Trustees voted to consolidate the Memphis Hospital Medical College with the other three merged Medical Units in Memphis as the University of Tennessee College of Medicine.[1,7,9] In 1914, the last of the five schools to join the University of Tennessee College of Medicine merger was the Lincoln University Medical Department in Knoxville. Their Trustees elected to cease operations in medical education and transfer the majority of their students to the University of Tennessee in Memphis. This decision, which was approved by the A.M.A. Council on Medical Education, formed the final act in the creation of the University of Tennessee College of Medicine as we know it today. In commenting on the merger, President Ayres stated:

"One year ago last summer I started out with the avowed purpose of combining four Medical Schools—the Medical Department of the University of Nashville, the Medical Department of the University of Tennessee, the College of Physicians and Surgeons, and the Memphis Hospital Medical College, both at Memphis. As a result of the recent action, all four schools have been consolidated in Memphis leaving the entire field at Nashville open to Vanderbilt, and leaving the University of Tennessee the whole field at Memphis."[9]

The oldest dental college in the United States was the Baltimore College of Dental Surgery, which became the University of Maryland College of Dentistry in later years. It was established by the Maryland State Assembly

19

on February 1, 1840 through the pioneering educational efforts of Dr. Horace H. Hayden and Dr. Chapin A. Harris. Prior to the establishment of the Baltimore College of Dental Surgery, prospective dentists customarily followed the apprenticeship route of training under the guidance of an established dental practitioner. Some of these students would also attend a session or two of a proprietary medical school, while others would obtain an M.D. degree and specialize in dentistry. In the 1820's and the 1830's the sale of dental equipment and supplies to practicing physicians and even lay persons was a common practice. In the sparsely populated areas of the rural South, dental care was rendered either by physicians or by itinerant dentists, who traveled from place to place. I. T. Gilmer, M.D., advertised himself in the June, 1836 Memphis Enquirer as an operative dentist with offices in the Henley Hotel, and thus appears to be one of the earliest dentists in Memphis. By 1840, Memphis had locally established dentists with permanent offices.[8]

The oldest dental college in the South and one of the oldest in the nation was the University of Tennessee Dental Department, founded in 1878 in conjunction with the establishment of the University of Tennessee Medical Department in Nashville, which had been derived from the Nashville Medical College, founded in 1876 by Drs. Paul F. Eve and Duncan Eve.[1,9] The deficiencies of dental education in the United States were similar to those of medical education. In addition, there was an overemphasis on the technical, mechanical aspects of the dental profession at the expense of adequate instruction in the basic medical sciences. The University of Tennessee Dental Department in Nashville had also been formed as a proprietary stock company whose main purpose was to make money for its dentist investors, not to strive for excellence in education.

Dentistry had made significant advancements in the South during the War Between the States, as documented in H. H. Cunningham's book, *Doctors in Gray*. There were about 500 dentists practicing in the South in 1861, and the Confederate Government wisely enlisted them to provide dental care for thousands of Confederate soldiers. Maxillofacial surgery made tremendous gains due to the many facial war injuries. Dr. James Bean of Atlanta is believed to be the first dentist to utilize interdental wiring to stabilize maxillary and mandibular fractures. Another historical contribution that dentistry made to alleviate pain and suffering was the successful use of nitrous oxide by Dr. Horace Wells, a Connecticut dentist, for the painless extraction of teeth. Dr. Crawford Long had used ether as a surgical anesthetic as early as 1842, but it was not publicized until Dr. William Morton demonstrated ether anesthesia at the Massachusetts General Hospital in Boston on October 16, 1846.[8]

The American Dental Association was organized August 3, 1859 in Niagara Falls, New York. Organized dentistry began in Tennessee on July 26, 1867 when the Tennessee State Dental Association was formed in Nashville. Dr. William T. Arrington, who had studied both medicine and dentistry and obtained his D.D.S. from the Philadelphia College of Dental

Surgery in 1856, was the motivating force for this organization and was elected as the recording secretary (Figure 21). In 1869 he helped to found the Southern Dental Association and served as its first President.[8] Another important contributor to early Tennessee dentistry was Dr. Joseph Lemuel Mewburn (Figure 22), who received his D.D.S. from the New York College of Dental Surgery in 1871 and came to Memphis. As President of the Tennessee State Dental Association in 1891, he played a vital role in securing legislation to control the practice of dentistry and in setting up the first State Board of Dental Examiners, which was appointed by Governor Buchanan on April 21, 1891. He served on this Board from 1891 through 1904.[8] The first Tennessee dentist to become President of the American Dental Association was Dr. Llewwellyn Garnet Noel in 1902–03 (Figure 23). He had obtained his M.D. degree from the University of Nashville Medical Department in 1871 and his D.D.S. from the Philadelphia College of Dental Surgery in 1872. Among his many professional accomplishments was appointment as Professor of Operative Dentistry at the University of Tennessee Dental Department in Nashville.

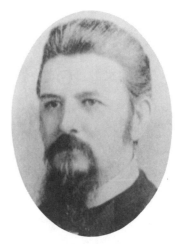

FIGURE 21. *William T. Arrington, D.D.S. (1836–1900) First President of the Southern Dental Association*

Robert Russell, M.D., D.D.S. was the first Dean of the University of Tennessee Dental Department in Nashville, which became operational in connection with the new Nashville Medical College in 1878. Some of the most prominent men in the dental profession in Tennessee formed its first faculty; the school was located on Market Street near the Public Square. After the end of the first session, both the dental and medical schools were incorporated into the University of Tennessee as the Dental and Medical Departments, respectively. However, each school retained its own independent proprietary status. The following individuals composed the original faculty of the University of Tennessee Dental Department: Dr. Robert Russell, Dean, Professor of Operative Dentistry; Dr. L. C. Chisholm, Professor of Mechanical and Corrective Dentistry; Dr. Frank Glenn, Professor of Anatomy; Dr. Duncan Eve, Professor of Surgery and Microscopy; Dr. William Vertrees, Professor of Materia Medica and Therapeutics; Dr. Charles E. Ristine, Professor of Physiology; Dr. George S. Blackey, Professor of Chemistry and Toxicology; Dr. W. L. Dismukes, Dr. J. Y. Crawford, Dr. Gillington Chisholm, demonstrators of Operative and Mechanical Departments; and Dr. Rogers, demonstrator of Anatomy.

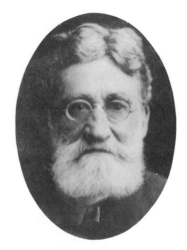

FIGURE 22. *Joseph Lemuel Mewburn, D.D.S. (1838–1917) Chairman of the first Tennessee Board of Dental Examiners in 1891*

Dr. Russell's tenure as Dean lasted six years. The classes at that time were very small, and the quarters occupied by the Dental Department were in keeping with the size and requirements of the classes. After Dr. Russell's resignation, he was succeeded by Dr. J. Y. Crawford, who remained as Dean for another six years. Dr. Crawford, in turn, was succeeded by Dr. Lees who in 1896 also resigned, and Dr. Gray was chosen to succeed him as Dean. One of the outstanding members of the faculty, Dr. Llewwellyn G. Noel, was elected to the Chair of Operative Dentistry and Pathology. Dr. Robert Boyd Bogle was the Professor of Orthodontia and Anesthesia. The classes remained small at this time, comprising only about 35 students in number by 1896.

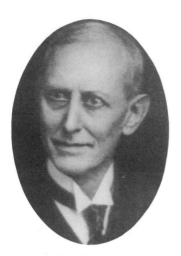

FIGURE 23. *Llewwellyn Garnet Noel, M.D., D.D.S. (1852–1927) President of the American Dental Association 1902–03*

In the summer of 1905, Drs. J. P. Gray, Llewwellyn G. Noel, and Robert Boyd Bogle, who were the major owners of the University of Tennessee Dental Department in Nashville, sold their interests to Vanderbilt University and were immediately appointed to the Vanderbilt University Dental School faculty.[9] In early July of 1905, Chancellor James H. Kirkland of Vanderbilt University abruptly wrote President Ayres of the University of Tennessee in Knoxville the following statement:

"I write to acquaint you with the fact that negotiations are on foot between me and Professors Gray, Noel, and Bogle . . . whereby there may be what we might call a consolidation of the facilities of the Department of Dentistry here in Nashville. We have all felt for years that there was not room in Nashville for two successful dental schools. There ought not to be more than one dental school in Nashville."[9]

Naturally, President Ayres was distressed and disgusted with this development and attempted to hold the dental professors to their contract agreement with the University of Tennessee. When this action failed, the University of Tennessee Trustees accepted resignations, appointed a new faculty staff, and decided to attempt to continue their Nashville affiliation. Dr. Joseph T. Meadors (Figure 24) and six other dentists agreed to serve on the faculty and operate the University of Tennessee Dental Department at Nashville with the same loose agreement between them And the University of Tennessee in Knoxville. In other words, the property title remained as before, in the hands of these private dentists, who would continue to issue D.D.S. degrees in the name of the University of Tennessee with President Ayres' signature on them.[1,9] Student enrollment declined to only 33 dental students for the 1905–06 session at the University of Tennessee in Nashville, but the class enrollment had increased to 115 at the time of the 1911 merger and move to Memphis.

When President Ayres and the University of Tennessee Trustees selected Memphis as the site for its 1911–14 mergers for the future of State medical education, it was logical to move the University of Tennessee Dental Department in Nashville to Memphis and consolidate it with the nominal Dental College of the University of Memphis, which had been founded by Dr. Justin Towner and Dr. Max Goltman. Both "colleges" were private stock companies and were amenable to such a merger. In 1911–12, the University of Tennessee paid $5,000 each to the Memphis Dental College and to the Joseph Thompson Meadors group of U.T. in Nashville for all of their equipment. Thus, the University acquired both of these enterprises and relocated all of its dental education in Memphis as the University of Tennessee College of Dentistry. The Memphis Business Men's Club guaranteed $10,000 capital to underwrite the venture. The original Dental School was housed in the Y.M.C.A. building, but when the Memphis Hospital Medical College was accepted and integrated into the University of Tennessee College of Medicine in 1913, its facility of Rogers Hall (Figure 12) was designated as the University of Tennessee College of Dentistry.[1,6,9]

The American Pharmaceutical Association was founded in 1852. It is believed that the first drugstore in Memphis was opened in 1827 by Nathaniel Ragland.[8] Other drugstores commenced business in the 1830's in Memphis, often operated by physicians or dentists as a sideline. Many of these early doctors compounded their medicines within their offices. More frequently, however, early pioneers in the rural regions of the United States sought medicinal relief from "patent medicines". These bogus remedies usually promised cures for every ailment. In the South there was a widespread sale of patent medicines to cure or protect one from the various local Southern fevers. These concoctions often contained a large amount of alcohol, which was mixed with quinine, vegetable ingredients, and flavoring agents.

In 1860 the city of Memphis had established charity dispensaries in which the poor population of the city could have prescriptions filled free. Dr. Daniel F. Wright, who was a demonstrator of anatomy at the early Memphis Medical College, advocated distinction between the practices of medicine and pharmacy. During the severe Yellow Fever Epidemic of 1878, all of the wholesale drug companies in Memphis and most of the retail drugstores were closed, due to absence, illness, or death of the owners. The supply of medicines became a crucial factor in this dilemma, and both national and local responses aided in alleviating this scarcity. The Howard Association pharmacists were: C. L. Clay from Florida, R. G. Hotchkiss from Georgia, S. W. Hunter from Virginia, O. G. Rollman from Cincinnati, Ohio, and Albert Dieck from Cincinnati, Ohio, who died from yellow fever.[8]

The first Pharmacology Institute was the one that originated in Strasbourg, France in 1872. There was a School of Pharmacy that was organized in 1881 in connection with the Memphis Hospital Medical College. It graduated four pharmacists in 1882. During the 1890's the Memphis physicians strongly advocated legislation to establish standardized drugs and prevent the sale of narcotics except by a physician's prescription. Dr. William Krauss was a leading figure in this struggle for drug standardization. On September 1, 1905, the U.S. Pharmacopoeia of 1900 did become by law the official standard for all drugs in the United States. President Theodore Roosevelt pressured Congress to pass the Pure Food and Drug Act of 1906. And in 1909, it was noted that an apothecary shop had opened in Memphis with the pledge not to sell any patent medicines and to dispense only pharmaceuticals ordered by a physician's prescription.[6,8]

The University of Tennessee in Knoxville had a strong faculty in both biology and chemistry, so President Dabney decided in 1898 to develop a Department of Pharmacy on the Knoxville campus.[10] The first pharmacy degrees were conferred by the University in 1900. By the time of the 1909–10 school year, the Department of Pharmacy had only attracted six students for that year. So, with the medical and dental school moves from Nashville occurring in 1911, the University of Tennessee Trustees decided to move the Department of Pharmacy from Knoxville to the Memphis campus as a part of the University of Tennessee College of Medicine structure.[1,9,10]

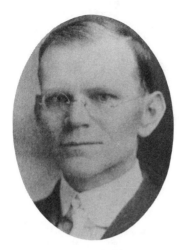

FIGURE 24. *Joseph Thompson Meadors, D.D.S. (1875–1948) Dean, University of Tennessee Dental Department in Nashville*

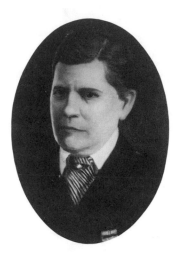

FIGURE 25. *Lena Angevine Warner (1869–1948) President of the Tennessee Nurses Association from 1905–1918*

Florence Nightingale is universally regarded as the founder of trained nursing as a profession. She was born May 12, 1820 as a British subject, and in 1850 she trained as a nurse in Kaiserswerth, Germany. In 1853 she was appointed Superintendent of the Institution for Care of Sick Gentle Women in London. Miss Nightingale is best known for her tremendous efforts in the Crimean War which began in 1854. Taking three nurses with her, she established the first nursing care for wartime wounded on a professional basis. With political influence, she later had a much larger number of British nurses sent to the Crimean area, and she was placed in charge of all nursing in the British military hospitals in Turkey. Later, her nurses were involved in caring for the wounded in the Crimea in Russia. For many years student nurses received their caps at a special capping ceremony, in which they held a small lighted lamp as they recited the "Florence Nightingale Pledge", which embodies nursing ethics.

Nursing care for the ill and injured had been carried out in various settings in the Memphis area since its earliest days as a small hamlet on the Mississippi. During the War Between the States both female and male nurses served in Confederate and Federal Hospitals, tending the wounded. As it has been mentioned earlier, both Episcopal and Roman Catholic nuns devoted themselves to caring for the sick and dying during the terrible Yellow Fever Epidemics in Memphis during the 1870's.

In 1885, Dr. Robert Wood Mitchell and Dr. Richard Brooke Maury, who had been appointed as Professor of Gynecology at the Memphis Hospital Medical College in 1888, had opened their Infirmary for the Diseases of Women at 73 Court Avenue in Memphis. Two years later (1887) they began the first professionally sponsored training program for nurses with Miss Winifred M. Hatch, a graduate of the Cook County Hospital School of Nursing in Chicago, as the first Superintendent of Nurses.[2,8] This school graduated four young ladies as nurses on June 22, 1889; among these young nurses was Lena Angevine, who was to become the dominant figure in professional nursing education on both the Memphis and State levels.[8]

The new Memphis City Hospital was completed in 1898, and the medical staff petitioned the Mayor to appoint Mrs. Lena Angevine Warner (Figure 25) as the first Superintendent of the Memphis City Hospital Training School for Nurses. After her graduation from the Maury-Mitchell Infirmary School of Nursing in 1889, she had taken further nursing training at the Cook County Hospital in Chicago under Isabel Hampton, who was a nationally recognized leader in American nursing. Miss Angevine returned to the Maury-Mitchell Infirmary to serve as the Head Surgical Nurse. After five years, she married Edward Charles Warner of St. Louis, who unfortunately died four months later. Mrs. Warner again returned to Memphis to work with Dr. Maury.

The earlier founded Maury-Mitchell Infirmary Training School for Nurses was also transferred to the Memphis City Hospital Nurses Program in 1898. Mrs. Warner had established a well-conducted, creditable, two-year training program for nurses. In 1900 this school was granted a charter by the

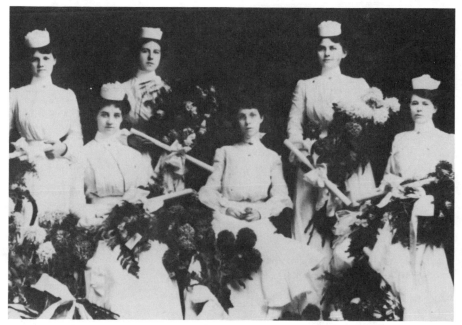

FIGURE 26. *The 1903 Graduating Class of the Memphis City Hospital Training School for Nurses (courtesy of Dean Ruth N. Murry)*

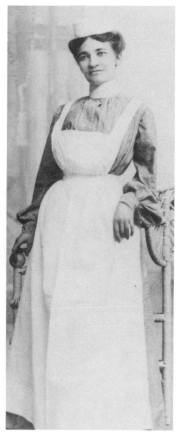

FIGURE 27. *Minnie Lee Nail Memphis City Hospital Training School for Nurses (1906) (courtesy of Dean Ruth N. Murry)*

State of Tennessee, and in June of 1900 it graduated its first eight nurses. Figure 26 depicts the 1903 graduating class of the Memphis City Hospital Training School for Nurses. The nursing uniform is illustrated by Minnie Lee Nail in 1906 (Figure 27). This school was developed in step with other schools of the pioneering era of nursing, and it became recognized as a sound diploma program from which many outstanding nurses graduated and played important roles in both civilian and military health care. Twenty-eight years later in 1926, a contract was arranged with the University of Tennessee, and this school became a Division of the U.T. College of Medicine.

At the end of fifteen months, Mrs. Lena Warner resigned and volunteered for service in the Spanish-American War. She was posted to Cuba to supervise the Yellow Fever Isolation Camp and to work with the Walter Reed Expedition. Mrs. Warner was elected President of the Tennessee Nurses Association from 1905 through 1918 and was a leading advocate for legislation to regulate the practice of nursing through a uniform curriculum. From 1900 through 1921, a number of Memphis hospitals established various schools of nursing: Lucy Brinkley Hospital, 1900; Presbyterian Home Hospital, 1901; Jane Terrell Memorial Hospital, 1909; Gartly-Ramsay Hospital, 1910; Baptist Memorial Hospital, 1912; St. Joseph Hospital, 1918; and Methodist Hospital, which absorbed the Lucy Brinkley Nursing School, 1921.[8]

REFERENCES

1. Alden, Roland H.: "The History of the University of Tennessee Center for the Health Sciences", (An Oral Taped Interview by Dr. Howard E. Sandberg), 1979.

2. Bruesch, Simon R.: Chapters on "City of Memphis Hospitals" and "Medical Education" in *History of Medicine in Memphis*, editors—Stewart, Marcus J. and Black, William T., Jr., (McCowat-Mercer Press, Inc.: Jackson, TN.), 1971.

3. Flexner, Abraham: *Medical Education in the United States and Canada*, (The Merrymount Press: Boston, MA.), 1910.

4. Flexner, Abraham: *Medical Education in Europe*, (The Merrymount Press: Boston, MA.), 1912.

5. Flexner, Abraham: *Medical Education: A Comparative Study*, (The Macmillan Co.: New York, NY.), 1925.

6. Hyman, Orren W.: "U.T. Health Branch is Medical Center of National Importance" in *The Commercial Appeal*, Sunday Magazine Section, June 18, 1933.

7. Hyman, Orren W.: *Early Development of the Medical Units, University of Tennessee* (Private Typed Manuscript Bound by Miss Kate A. Stanley, Registrar, University of Tennessee Medical Units: Memphis, TN.), 1970.

8. LaPointe, Patricia M.: *From Saddlebags to Science*, (The Health Sciences Museum Foundation: Memphis, TN.), 1984.

9. Malone, Dumas: *Directory of American Biography*, vol. 15:313–14 (Charles Scribner's Sons: New York, NY.), 1935.

10. Montgomery, J.R. Folmsbee, S.J., and Greene, L.S.: *To Foster Knowledge: A History of the University of Tennessee 1794-1970*, (The University of Tennessee Press: Knoxville, TN.), 1984.

11. Morse, Charles R.: "History of the University of Tennessee", *University of Tennessee Magazine*, vol. 50:352–357, 1920.

12. Register: University of Tennessee (1911–1912), Vol. 15, No. 1 (University of Tennessee Press: Knoxville, TN.), 1912.

13. Turner, Eugene F.: "The College of Medicine of the University of Tennessee: A Brief History", *U.T. Record*, vol. 18, #5: p. 37–45, 1915.

14. Wittenborg, August H.: "The University of Tennessee Health Services Departments at Memphis", (Private Papers), 1933.

CHAPTER TWO
1911–1919

$\mathcal{T}$HE various medical school mergers by President Brown Ayres, described in the previous chapter, made 1911 a landmark year because they established the University of Tennessee's presence in West Tennessee. This action was a milestone since for the first time the University of Tennessee became truly a statewide institution. The entire University of Tennessee, Memphis was located in two buildings in 1911. The College of Medicine (including the School of Pharmacy) was located in Lindsley Hall, the former main building of the College of Physicians and Surgeons. The College of Dentistry was located at 177 Union Avenue in a building which was originally the Y.M.C.A. Building, and which later housed the University of Memphis Dental College.[8,9,10]

In 1912, Eve Hall was built just behind Lindsley Hall. On the first floor of this building was located the Outpatient Department of the College of Medicine. The second floor was occupied by the Department of Physiology and Pharmacology with Professor Warr in charge. The third and fourth floors were taken up by the Departments of Pathology and Bacteriology, which fell under the jurisdiction of Professor Brooks. By the absorption of the Memphis Hospital Medical College in 1913, the University of Tennessee acquired Rogers Hall, which was remodeled. Its large amphitheatre was divided in such a manner, that only the part on the first floor and basement remained as it had been. Part of the second floor was developed into operatory areas for the College of Dentistry. The third floor was used as a chemistry laboratory for dental students plus the Department of Anatomy, Histology, and Embryology. The basement level was subdivided into mechanical technique laboratories for dental students.[9,14]

Lindsley Hall was also remodeled at this time. The amphitheatre was subdivided so that the portion which extended through the second floor was converted into College of Medicine administrative offices; the first floor portion remained as an amphitheatre. The remainder of the second floor was composed of a large lecture room and the Chemistry Department for medical students. On the third floor, part of the old anatomy dissecting area was converted into a library (Figure 28). The fourth floor comprised the School of Pharmacy.[9] These three buildings are depicted as they appeared in 1913 on Map #1.

Once ensconced in its new facilities in Rogers Hall, the College of Dentistry flourished and remained very stable throughout the 1911–1919 decade. Joseph Archibald Gardner, D.D.S. proved to be a quite able Dean and Professor of Crown and Bridge Dentistry from 1911–1923 (see Appen-

"Finally, the physician should bear in mind that he himself is not exempt from the common lot, but subject to the same laws of mortality and disease as others, and he will care for the sick with more diligence and tenderness, if he remembers that he himself is their fellow sufferer."

Thomas Sydenham, M.D.

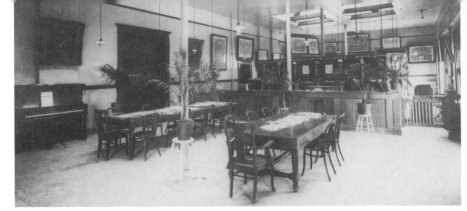

FIGURE 28. *University of Tennessee, Memphis Medical Units, Library in Lindsley Hall, 1911*

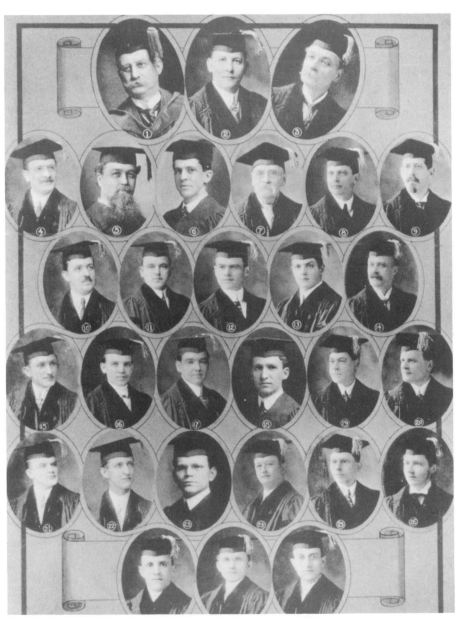

FIGURE 29. *University of Tennessee College of Dentistry Faculty, 1911–12*

dix C). He was supported by a very strong, distinguished faculty (Figure 29). Dr. Joseph Thompson Meadors, who had been Dean when the U.T. Dental College was located in Nashville, was Professor of the Principles of Operative Dentistry (Figure 24). The basic sciences were taught by a well-qualified, enthusiastic medical faculty.[11,13]

Arthur Rice Melendy, M.D., D.D.S., of Nashville (Figure 30), had the honor of being elected President of the American Dental Association for 1911–1912. Twice, he also served as Treasurer for the American Dental Association—from 1905–1911 and again from 1915 until his death on May 22, 1928.[7]

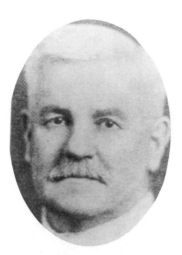

FIGURE 30. *Arthur Rice Melendy, M.D., D.D.S. (1859–1928) President of the American Dental Association, 1911–12*

The first dentist in Tennessee to limit his practice to oral surgery was John Jones Ogden, D.D.S. (Figure 31). He graduated from the U.T. College of Dentistry in 1916 and was appointed a Chief Demonstrator in Clinic from 1916–1917. During the war years of World War I, he served as a 1st Lieutenant in the U.S. Army Dental Corps. Dr. Ogden returned to Memphis and served intermittently on the University of Tennessee College of Dentistry faculty as a Professor of Oral Surgery for many years. From 1920 until his death in 1963 he was a Fellow of the American Society of Oral Surgeons and was very active in promoting that dental specialty. He is well-known as the designer of the parallel forceps used universally in anterior maxillary tooth extractions. Dr. Ogden was a Fellow of the American College of Dentists, a Vice President of the American Dental Association, and in 1932 he was elected President of the Tennessee State Dental Association.[10,11,12]

Perhaps the most famous dentist in Memphis during the 1911–1919 era was Justin Dewey Towner (Figure 32), who received his D.D.S. degree from Vanderbilt University in 1898. In 1909, he was the co-organizer and Dean of the short-lived University of Memphis College of Dentistry.[12] When this school merged with the University of Tennessee College of Dentistry in 1911, he became Professor of Oral Hygiene and Prophylaxis. Dr. Towner established the Department of Mouth Hygiene, Oral Prophylaxis, and Periodontia, which was considered the first of its kind in any dental school. He occupied this Chairmanship for 24 distinguished years as a well-respected Professor at the University of Tennessee.[10]

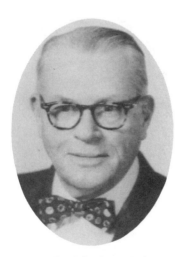

FIGURE 31. *John Jones Ogden, D.D.S. (1894–1963) First oral surgeon specialist in Tennessee*

His teaching activities, published scientific articles, service as President of six professional societies, numerous presentations, and the Towner periodontal instruments that he designed for surgical elimination of periodontal pockets—all contribute to a significant influence which transcends state and national accomplishments.[6] Among many honors, he was elected as President of these organizations: the American Academy of Periodontology, the International College of Dentists, the Pierre Fauchard Academy, the Tennessee State Dental Association, and Omicron Kappa Upsilon.[10,11,20] On May 5, 1952, he attended the Tennessee State Dental Meeting for the fifty-fourth time. On September 1, 1955, Dr. Justin Towner, Sr. was honored by his many friends and colleagues by the unveiling of his portrait at the University of Tennessee College of Dentistry.[20]

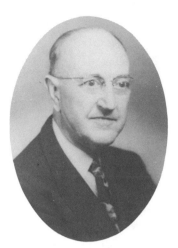

FIGURE 32. *Justin Dewey Towner, Sr., D.D.S. (1877–1966) First periodontist specialist in Tennessee*

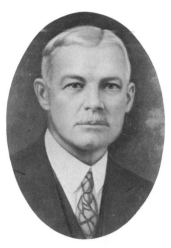

FIGURE 33. *Edward Coleman Ellett, M.D. (1869–1947) Dean, University of Tennessee College of Medicine, 1911–12*

When the Tennessee State Dental Association gathered in June of 1917 in Memphis for its fiftieth anniversary annual meeting, Dr. David Mahlon Cattell presided. Dr. Cattell had had a distinguished academic career that included the following diverse teaching accomplishments. He was Professor of Dental Anatomy, Operative Techniques, and Superintendent of Clinics at Vanderbilt University College of Dentistry from 1903 to 1909. Dr. Cattell was Registrar, Professor of Dental Anatomy, Operative Dentistry, and Dental Techniques, as well as Superintendent of the Faculty at the University of Memphis College of Dentistry from 1909 to 1911. He was Registrar, Professor of Dental Anatomy, Operative Dentistry, Dental Techniques, and Superintendent of Clinics at the University of Tennessee College of Dentistry from 1911 through 1917.[10,11]

Dr. Brown Ayres, as President of the University of Tennessee, remained the titular head of the University in both Knoxville and Memphis during the 1911–1919 period, as attested by his photograph in the center of all the various colleges' faculty composites (see Appendix A). There was no separate administrative head of the University of Tennessee in Memphis. The Deans of the U.T. Colleges of Medicine and Dentistry each retained local authority in Memphis.

While leadership in the College of Dentistry had remained consistent during this decade, Deans of the College of Medicine changed with much frequency. Dr. Heber W. Jones, who had been Dean of the College of Physicians and Surgeons, remained as Dean Emeritus of the College of Medicine and Professor of Clinical Medicine. Edward Coleman Ellett, M.D. (Figure 33) was the first Dean and served for only one year, 1911–1912 (see Appendix B), but remained a Professor of Ophthalmology until 1922. Dr. Ellett was perhaps Memphis' earliest celebrated ophthalmologist, who was known both nationally and internationally for expertise in this specialty, serving as chairman of the Section on Ophthalmology of the American Medical Association.[26] He practiced otolaryngology and ophthalmology from 1893 until 1917; following his service as a military physician in World War I, he confined his work to ophthalmology. Dr. Ellett was a major factor in the original organization of the American Board of Ophthalmology and Otolaryngology at a meeting in Washington, D.C. on May 8, 1916. He afterwards played a significant role in having this American Board conduct its first Diplomate Certification Examination in Memphis in Lindsley Hall during December, 1916.[1] Of the ten candidates, five were practicing in Memphis, and all five of these physicians passed the board examination.[26] Dr. Ellett served as President of the American Academy of Ophthalmology and Otolaryngology in 1926, and as President of the American Academy of Ophthalmology in 1932. He is well-remembered and recognized nationally for his advocacy of intracapsular cataract extraction and the use of the corneal-scleral suture, which he introduced into clinical practice in the United States after visiting Kalt's Clinic in Paris, France in 1910 to learn that technique.[1]

Officers of the Faculty

1 BROWN AYRES, Ph.D., L.L.D., D.C.L., *President of the University.*
2 JOSEPH A. GARDNER, D.D.S., *Dean of the Faculty.*
3 DAVID M. CATTELL, D.D.S., *Registrar of the College.*

FACULTY

JOSEPH ARCHIBALD GARDNER, D.D.S., *Dean of the College of Dentistry and Professor of Oral Surgery.*
23 JOSEPH THOMPSON MEADORS, D.D.S., *Professor of the Principles of Operative Dentistry.*
29 JUSTIN DEWEY TOWNER, D.D.S., *Professor of Oral Hygiene and Prophylaxis.*
DAVID MAHLON CATTELL, D.D.S., *Professor of Dental Anatomy, Operative Dentistry, Dental Technics, and Superintendent of Clinic: Registrar.*
6 STANLEY LOVEMAN RICH, D.D.S., *Professor of Prosthetic Dentistry.*
18 HARRY ADOLPH HOLDER, D.D.S., *Professor of Dental Histology.*
5 JAMES W. BRYAN, D.D.S., *Professor of Clinical Dental Surgery.*
4 MAXIMILIAN GOLTMAN, C.M., M.D., *Professor of General Surgery.*
22 WILLIAM ETHELRED LUNDY, D.D.S., *Professor of Orthodontia.*
20 CLARENCE JACKSON WASHINGTON, B.S., D.D.S., *Professor of Special Pathology and Therapeutics.*
14 CHARLES HERBERT TAYLOR, D.D.S., *Professor of Anesthesia.*
16 ELBERT WOODSON TAYLOR, D.D.S., *Associate Professor of Prosthesis.*
28 EUGENE ARMSTRONG JOHNSON, D.D.S., *Professor of Materia Medica and Therapeutics.*
9 LOUIS LEROY, B.S., M.D., *Professor of Pathology and Bacteriology.*
21 EDWIN DIAL WATKINS, B.S., M.D., *Associate Professor of General Surgery and Anesthesia.*
10 EDWARD C. MITCHELL, M.D., *Professor of Histology.*
27 ROBERT MANN, M.D., *Professor of Anatomy.*
11 ROBERT FAGIN, A.B., M.D., *Professor of Physiology.*
17 RAYMOND MANOGUE, B.A., B.L., *Professor of Dental Jurisprudence.*
HERBERT THOMAS BROOKS, A.B., M.D., *Professor of Histology.*
13 AUGUST JOHN PHILIP PACINI, B.S., Ch.E., M.D., *Professor of Chemistry.*
26 AUGUST HERMSMEIER WITTENBORG, B.S., M.D., *Associate Professor of Physiology.*
GEORGE GARTLY, M.D., *Associate Professor of Histology.*
24 JOSEPH EDWARD JOHNSON, M.D., *Associate Professor of Oral Surgery.*
15 WILLIAM PORTER JOHNSON, D.D.S., *Instructor of Crown and Bridge Work.*
19 WILLIAM GARDEN WALKER, D.D.S., *Instructor in Technical Laboratories and Clinical Demonstrator.*
8 W. T. SWINK, M.D., *Assistant Demonstrator.*
JOHN OWEN, M.D., *Instructor in Anatomical Laboratory.*
JOSEPH LEMUEL MEWBORN, D.D.S., *Lecturer on History of Dentistry in War Times.*
ARTHUR J. COTTRELL, D.D.S., *Lecturer on Metallurgy and Metal Casting.*
25 LAWRENCE JEHROME MCRAE, B.S., D.D.S., *Lecturer on Metallurgy.*
ENOCH A. MAY, D.D.S., *Lecturer on Dental Ceramics.*
7 LEROY M. MATTHEWS, D.D.S., *Lecturer on Celluloid.*
HENRY C. RUSHING, D.D.S., *Lecturer on Dental Ethics.*
12 ROBERT EGGLESTON BALDWIN, D.D.S., *Lecturer on Dental Economics.*

Officers and Faculty

1 BROWN AYRES, Ph.D., L.L.D., D.C.L., *President.*
2 EDWARD C. ELLETT, B.A., M.D., *Dean.*
3 EUGENE F. TURNER, *Registrar.*

FACULTY

4 HEBER JONES, M.D., *Dean Emeritus of the College of Medicine and Professor of Clinical Medicine.*

EDWARD COLEMAN ELLETT, B.A., M.D., *Dean of the College of Medicine and Professor of Ophthalmology.*

5 EUGENE MICHEL HOLDER, B.S., M.D., *Professor of Theory and Principles of Surgery.*

27 MAXIMILIAN GOLTMAN, C.M., M.D., *Professor of Clinical Surgery.*

13 GEORGE ROBERTSON LIVERMORE, M.D., *Professor of Genito-Urinary Diseases.*

19 ARTHUR GRANT JACOBS, M.D., *Professor of Pediatrics.*

14 JOHN M. MAURY, M.D., *Professor of Gynecology.*

37 RICHMOND MCKINNEY, A.M., M.D., *Professor of Diseases of the Nose, Throat, and Ear.*

15 GEORGE GILLESPIE BUFORD, M.D., *Professor of Diseases of the Nervous System.*

28 MARCUS HAASE, M.D., *Professor of the Skin and Syphilography.*

16 REUBEN SAUNDERS TOOMBS, M.D., *Professor of Clinical Medicine.*

18 LOUIS LEROY, B.S., M.D., *Professor of the Principles and Practice of Medicine.*

26 WILLIAM KRAUSS, Ph.G., M.D., *Professor of Tropical Medicine and Experimental Pharmacology.*

8 WALTER HIRAM PISTOLE, M.D., *Professor of Pharmacology and Therapeutics.*

17 PERCY WALTHALL TOOMBS, A.B., M.D., *Professor of Obstetrics.*

6 HERBERT THOMAS BROOKS, A.B., M.D., *Professor of Normal and Pathological Histology and Embryology.*

31 WILLIS C. CAMPBELL, M.D., *Professor of Orthopedic Surgery.*

21 EDWARD CLAY MITCHELL, M.D., *Professor of Bacteriology.*

12 EDWIN DIAL WATKINS, B.S., M.D., *Professor of Chemistry.*

25 ROBERT FAGIN, A.B., M.D., *Professor of Physiology.*

38 ROBERT MANN, M.D., *Acting Professor of Anatomy, Operative Surgery, and Demonstrator of Anatomy.*

9 AUGUST JOHN PHILIP PACINI, B.S., Ch.E., M.D., *Director and Demonstrator of Chemical and Pharmaceutical Laboratories.*

29 AARON DAVID HEINEMAN, M.Ph., M.D., *Professor of Theory and Practice of Pharmacy.*

LOUIS WARDLAW HASKELL, JR., A.B., M.D., *Associate Professor of Clinical Surgery.*

36 OTIS SUMTER WARR, L.I., M.D., *Associate Professor of Medicine and Chief of Clinic.*

EUGENE FREDERICK TURNER, *Registrar.*

```
┌─────────────────────────────────────────────────────────────┐
│                        ASSISTANTS                           │
│    WILLIAM EGBERT RAGSDALE, M.D., Assistant to Chair of     │
│       Pharmacology and Therapeutics.                        │
│ 35 WOODSON ANDERSON STEVENS, B.S., M.D., Assistant to Chair │
│       of Diseases of Nose, Throat, and Ear.                 │
│    W. LIKELEY SIMPSON, M.D., Assistant to Chair of          │
│       Ophthalmology.                                        │
│ 23 JOHN T. MORSE, Ph.G., M.D., Assistant Neurologist.       │
│ 11 WALTER THOMAS SWINK, M.D., Assistant to Chair of         │
│       Diseases of the Nervous System, and Assistant         │
│       Demonstrator of Anatomy.                              │
│ 33 WILLIAM THOMAS PRIDE, A.M., M.D., Assistant to Chair of  │
│       Obstetrics.                                           │
│  7 PERCY AUGUSTUS PERKINS, M.D., Assistant to Chair of      │
│       Surgery.                                              │
│    ISAAC GREENWOOD DUNCAN, B.S., M.D., Assistant to Chief   │
│       of Clinic.                                            │
│    JAMES DICK BRIDGER, M.D., Assistant to Chair of Diseases │
│       of Children.                                          │
│    CHARLES ROBERT MASON, M.D., Assistant to Chair of        │
│       Materia Medica and Therapeutics.                      │
│ 10 HARRY BROWN SEARCY, A.B., M.D., Assistant                │
│       Ophthalmologist.                                      │
│ 24 GEORGE GARTLY, M.D., Assistant to Chair of Pathology,    │
│       Assistant Demonstrator of Anatomy.                    │
│    JAMES PATRICK OWENS, M.D., Assistant to Chair of         │
│       Anatomy.                                              │
│    ROBERT BAILEY NELSON, M.D., Instructor in Prescription   │
│       Writing and Pharmacy.                                 │
│ 22 ROBERT LEONARD TAYLOR, B.S., M.D., Instructor in Botany  │
│       and Medical Latin.                                    │
│    ROBERT LATTA CROWE, Ph.C., Instructor in Dispensary.     │
│ 32 JOHN WILLIAM FARLEY, LL.B., LL.M., Lecturer on Medical   │
│       Jurisprudence.                                        │
│    A. HERMSMEIER WITTENBORG, A.B., M.D., Lecturer on        │
│       Biology.                                              │
│ 30 B. B. O'BANNON, D.D.S., Lecturer on Dental Surgery.      │
│ 20 R. B. BRETZ, A.B., M.D.                                  │
│ 34 HOWARD WALKER, B.S., M.D.                                │
└─────────────────────────────────────────────────────────────┘
```

From 1912 until 1917 Herbert Thomas Brooks, M.D. was Dean of the
U.T. College of Medicine. He was on leave for treatment in California from
1917–1919 due to illness and officially resigned in 1919. Lucius Junius
Desha, Ph.D., a Professor of General and Biological Chemistry, served as
Acting Dean until September, 1917. From October, 1917 until July 1, 1919
August Hermsmeier Wittenborg, M.D., who was Professor of Anatomy,
assumed the title as Acting Dean. Leverett Dale Bristol, M.D. was
appointed as Dean on July 1, 1919, but he did not actually assume the office
until August 1, 1919. He resigned after a brief tenure of only 12 days,
supposedly because of the hot, humid Memphis climate and a violent
disagreement with Dr. Marcus Haase, who virtually ran the Memphis City
Hospital in a dictatorial fashion. He later had a distinguished career in
Public Health. On August 13, 1919 Dr. Wittenborg again filled the breech,
serving as Acting Dean until May 1, 1920.[1,9,17]

The University of Tennessee College of Medicine had accumulated a
distinguished faculty by its mergers of 1911, as is illustrated by Figure 34.
Many of these gentlemen will be discussed later in this chapter under their
medical accomplishments.

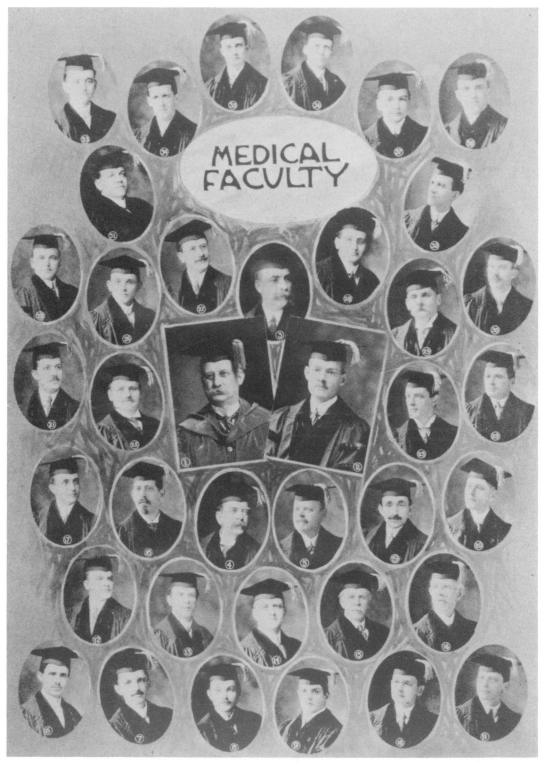

FIGURE 34. *University of Tennessee College of Medicine Faculty, 1911–12*

There were many serious problems for the University of Tennessee College of Medicine when it was moved from Nashville and amalgamated with other medical schools in Memphis. The first problem was its academic standing. It was given a Class "B" rating in 1913 after an inspection by the Flexner Committee, which gave a list of stipulations that would enable it to reach an "A" in rating by the A.M.A. Council on Medical Education.[9] Obtaining a Class "A" rating was an important point, because it would make the school more attractive to prospective students, and it would also ensure academic respectability. The second serious problem was financial need. The unvisionary Tennessee State Legislature would only appropriate paltry funds for the University, making even minimal improvements in the facilities, library, teaching aids, and faculty salaries difficult. Therefore, the University depended in no small measure mostly on either voluntary or part-time faculty.[2]

Dr. Hyman summarized the early academic problem as follows:

"Enrollment in the College of Medicine in the Fall of 1913 consisted of a freshman class of 65 students; enrollment had been stimulated by the announcement that it would be the last class admitted on the basis of 15 units of high school credits, which essentially was graduation from an approved high school. The sophomore class consisted of 82 students, the junior class of 80 students, and the senior class of 81 students. About three-fourths of these students had taken their previous training in the Memphis Hospital Medical College and the remaining one-fourth were derived from the combined University of Tennessee in Nashville, and the College of Physicians and Surgeons.[9]

As part of the program to qualify the College of Medicine for Class "A" rating, it had been agreed that beginning with the class admitted in September, 1914, one year of college training would be required. Anticipating that it would be difficult to secure an adequate enrollment unless some extraordinary plans were adopted, the University decided to offer one year of premedical training in Memphis, beginning in September, 1914. A course of training was organized, including the required premedical subjects: biology, chemistry, physics, and English. I agreed to teach the biology for an addition to my salary of $150 annually, giving me a total of $1,500 annually. An instructor for the chemistry course was employed. The English course was taught by one of the teachers at the Memphis University School, which was located immediately adjacent to the Rogers Hall property. A course in physics was taught by Dr. Sidney T. Moreland, an experienced and competent teacher in this subject. There was also a course in German offered by one of the teachers at the Memphis University School.[9]

The course in biology was given in the Histology-Embryology Laboratory, and the course in chemistry was offered in the laboratory on the second floor of Rogers Hall where the dental students were taught. It was necessary to establish a new laboratory for physics, and this feat was done by tearing out part of the basement of Rogers Hall. Thus, a reasonable well-equipped laboratory for physics was established there. The wisdom of establishing this one-year course of premedical training became obvious probably when classes were enrolled in September, 1914. The freshman medical class numbered only 14 students. The class in premedical training numbered 21 students, and looking forward to 1915, the enrollment of the freshman medical class was 16 students. Of these, ten had been premedical students

35

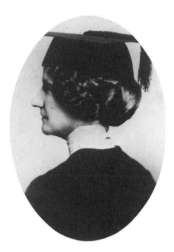

FIGURE 35. *Sara Conyers York, M.D. (1878–1970) First woman medical graduate of the University of Tennessee College of Medicine, 1913*

in Memphis in 1914–15. In the spring of 1915, the Trustees of the University felt that enough improvements had been accomplished in the College of Medicine to request that it be inspected again for reclassification. The A.M.A. Council on Medical Education team of inspectors came to Memphis in the late Spring. I had very little to do with this at the time, but recall going into the office of the Registrar-Bursar, Mr. Turner, and seeing the President of the University, Dr. Brown Ayres, perspiring freely as he tried to explain to one of the examining group how eight and five had come to add up to 15 Carnegie units on the application of one of those students who had been enrolled in the Fall of 1913. This, of course, had been done by the Registrar, Mr. Turner. The chief inspection that came my way was that of the course of biology which I was teaching, and a Professor from the Ohio State University went into quite great detail in attempting to determine whether the program which I was offering was adequate to merit approval. In spite of deficiencies and of the consequence of careful examination, the College of Medicine was placed in Class "A" rating as a consequence of the inspection in 1915. It was proving very difficult indeed to attract students into the College of Medicine."[9]

Among the 37 medical graduates of the University of Tennessee College of Medicine in 1913 was Sara Conyers York (Figure 35), the first woman to receive an M.D. degree from the University of Tennessee, Memphis.[1,12] After a difficult time of convincing the school authorities of her desire to become a physician, Sara Conyers York was admitted to medical school at age 32. She was a widow, had earned her living as a school teacher, and graduated first in her medical school class. She practiced in Crockett and Lauderdale Counties, Tennessee. In 1916 Minnie Enyeart McClellan became the first woman to receive a D.D.S. degree from the University of Tennessee College of Dentistry.[27] At graduation in 1914 Emma L. Hutchinson became the first woman to graduate with a Bachelor of Pharmacy degree from the School of Pharmacy, which at that time was a part of the College of Medicine.[27] Table 1 gives a breakdown of the number of graduates from the College of Medicine, the College of Dentistry, and the School of Pharmacy during the years 1912–1919.[27]

In the Fall of 1911 when the University of Tennessee College of Medicine began the Memphis phase of its history, one of the junior faculty members

Table 1

The University of Tennessee, Memphis—Graduates: 1912–1919

	College of Medicine	College of Dentistry	School of Pharmacy
1912	53	10	6
1913	37	13	5
1914	77	10	11
1915	70	11	4
1916	55	17	7
1917	58	9	8
1918	18	14	0
1919	20	22	5

was August Hermsmeier Wittenborg, an Assistant to the Chair of Pathology.[28] Dr. Wittenborg was destined to become one of the University's greatest teachers (Figure 36). He was born in Matorf, Germany on September 4, 1883 and obtained his A.B. degree from the Kaiser Wilhelm Gymnasium in Hanover. His original surname was Hermsmeier, but when he moved to Memphis in 1905, he was adopted by his uncle, Martin Wittenborg, a prominent jeweler.[17] He entered the College of Physicians and Surgeons in 1906 and received his M.D. degree in 1910 with highest honors.[5,15]

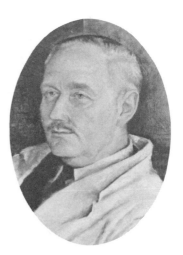

FIGURE 36. *August Hermsmeier Wittenborg, M.D. (1883–1941) Professor of Anatomy*

Following his graduation from medical school, Dr. Wittenborg returned to Europe for continuing study at several leading medical centers, including Berlin and Vienna. Returning to Memphis in 1911, he entered the private practice of urology for a short time and also became associated again with the College of Physicians and Surgeons as an Instructor in Physiology.[9] The high number of gonorrhea cases seen in urological practice at that time made his private practice less appealing, and he both enjoyed and preferred an academic life. Also, Dr. Wittenborg's hearing impairment may have been a factor in his decision to teach full-time and abandon his private practice. Soon, he became one of the U.T. College of Medicine's first full-time faculty members.[1] In the 1911–12 school session, he was listed as an Assistant to the Chair of Pathology. In 1912–13 he was a Lecturer for Biology, and for the 1913–14 session he rapidly became a full Professor of Anatomy, Histology, and Embryology. He assumed charge of all teaching, both lectures and laboratory in anatomy. Robert Mann, M.D. had been the previous Acting Professor of Anatomy and Operative Surgery since 1911–13.[5,28]

The microscopic anatomical courses, which had formerly been taught by Herbert Thomas Brooks, M.D., who was Professor of Pathology, were transferred to Dr. Wittenborg in anatomy.[5] Perhaps one of the most significant contributions that Dr. Wittenborg made to the University of Tennessee was his decision to hire Orren W. Hyman as an Assistant Professor of Histology and Embryology for the 1913 Fall session.[9,24]

It has already been mentioned that Professor Wittenborg served as Dean of the U.T. College of Medicine from early October, 1917 to August 1, 1919, again from August 13, 1919 to May 1, 1920, and again from May 2, 1921 to Autumn of 1921.[1] During these critical times in the history of the College of Medicine, his devotion and courage earned a major share of credit for the College's actual survival.[9]

Another important contribution which Dr. Wittenborg made to the University of Tennessee was his unrelenting stand against cheating. Today, the University of Tennessee, Memphis, has a uniform Honor Code for all of the Colleges. Each student, before matriculation, signs the following pledge:

"I have read carefully the Honor Code of the University of Tennessee, Memphis and fully understand its meaning and significance, and I agree to abide by this

Honor Code while a student in this institution and agree to accept all of its implications without reservation."

Such was not the case in the University's early days, as exemplified by the following reminiscence from Dr. Hyman's writing—

"In the spring of 1914 Dr. Wittenborg as leader, and Dr. Desha and I in support, decided to try to put a stop to cheating in the examinations given by the clinical faculty. We went to the Executive Committee with a suggestion—that each time a final examination was given in the Spring, that not only the teacher in charge of the course should be in charge of the examination, but that one of the pre-clinical full-time faculty should also be present as the assistant proctor or monitor. This was agreed to, and the examination to which I was assigned was one given on urology to junior students.[9]

The students were seated in the examination room when the Professor and I entered. When the Professor entered there was clapping all over the room. Incidentally, this was not uncommon, as it was the practice in those days for the students to applaud their Professor whenever he appeared to give a lecture. As I entered the room following the Professor, there were loud hisses in all parts of the room. The Professor then wrote his questions on the blackboard, sat down on the small platform adjacent to the blackboard, spread "The Commercial Appeal" ostentatiously before him, and began to read. I was left, of course, as the sole proctor for the examination. I walked around and eventually saw one student apparently looking at some material in his cupped hand. After watching this for a few minutes, I went to him and asked him to show me what was in his hand. He opened his hand without protest, and it contained an eraser. Both the student and his neighbors enjoyed a chuckle at my expense.[9]

During one of the incidences in which a student had been caught cheating in one of my quizzes, and it had been reported to the Executive Committee, I had been accompanied to the meeting of the Executive Committee by Professor Wittenborg and Professor Desha. After the presentation of the case, in which both Professor Wittenborg and I were the accusers, the Executive Committee seemed quite hesitant about finding the student guilty, or administering any discipline. I stated to the Committee that they would of course do what they chose, but if this man entered my classroom again, I would walk out simultaneously. The student was dismissed from the College. This incident recalls to me especially the unjustified confidence of the very immature."[9]

The name Wittenborg to the medical students of today conjures up memories of anatomy labs, the penetrating odor of formalin, and an old building on the Memphis campus. But from the early years through 1940, Wittenborg was synonymous with a pipe, a beckoning hand, and a popular professor carrying a large load of anatomy books. Both among his colleagues and his students, Dr. Wittenborg enjoyed a unique distinction. He was held in high esteem and affection, touching profoundly those with whom he came in contact. Invariably, students came to him with their personal problems. Around any campus, the academic faculty say you can always tell what a teacher means to his school when the graduates return for a visit. At the University of Tennessee College of Medicine, they always sought out Dr. Wittenborg.

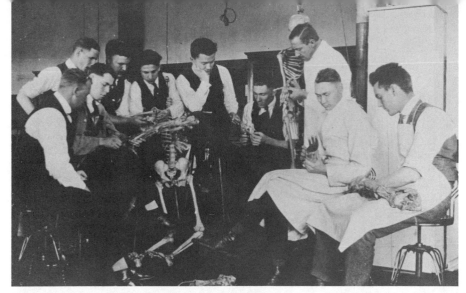

FIGURE 37. *Professor Wittenborg (third from the right) teaching his anatomy students*

The stories told about Dr. Wittenborg have become famous legends. Few medical students ever completed his classes in anatomy without acquiring a nickname. Many physicians are still known to their colleagues by the humorous names that he bestowed upon them. His anatomy students returned the favor by referring to Dr. Wittenborg as "Old Witt", a byplay not only on his name, but on his personality as well. One anecdote illustrates his sharp Teutonic wit. While Dr. Wittenborg delighted in giving nicknames to each of his students, he frowned on any of them trying to become too familiar or chummy with him, always maintaining his dignity. One day in the anatomy laboratory, a student desperately needed help in locating an artery just as Dr. Wittenborg passed by. Without thinking, he inquired, "Hey, Doc—can you help me?" Wittenborg whirled around and growled, "If you want to get familiar, why don't you just call me Gus!"[1] He did not adhere to that school of thought which believes that medical students can learn anatomy when merely left to their own devices with textbook and cadaver. He followed the dynamic method of quizzing his students, as Socrates did in the days of Greece, and his penetrating questions quickly came to the main points under discussion. There are many physicians who remember a high stool which Dr. Wittenborg kept by his desk in front of the class. It was his custom to call a student before his classmates, seat him on the stool, and by searching questions drive home the important points of anatomy to the entire class through the frequent use of homely similes, embryological references, and correlations between morphology and physiology (Figure 37). As stated in Wittenborg's eulogy by Drs. Hyman, Crowe, Nash, and Corbin: "He believed that it was inexcusable for the anatomy teacher not to give the student the benefit of his anatomical experience, and thus to help him to acquire more easily a working knowledge of this important and difficult subject."[9] Figure 38 shows Dr. Wittenborg with his medical anatomy class, standing in front of Rogers Hall in 1919.

Progressive heart disease compelled his leave of absence from University

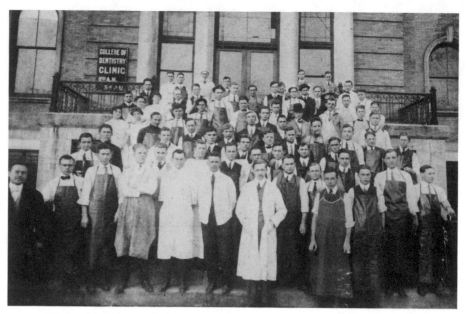

FIGURE 38. *Dr. Wittenborg with the medical anatomy class, standing before Rogers Hall in 1919*

duties during the academic year immediately preceding his death, which occurred during a visit with his son, Martin H. Wittenborg, M.D., in Ann Arbor, Michigan on August 21, 1941.[1,9] Formal dedicatory services naming the Anatomy Building "Wittenborg Building" were held in Memphis during the June commencement of 1951.[17] The following inscription on a bronze plaque inside the Wittenborg Building succinctly summarizes his greatest achievement:

"By his life and his teaching, he inspired in his students loyalty, integrity, and courage."

The accomplishments of Orren W. Hyman, Ph.D., who probably exerted greater influence on the University of Tennessee, Memphis than any other individual in his 48 years of association with it, will be discussed in greater detail during the 1920's decade. However, his recollections about the early development years of the U.T. Medical Units are of historical importance and significance. Dr. Hyman was born in Tarboro, North Carolina in 1890. Receiving his B.A. degree in 1910 and his M.A. degree in 1911 from the University of North Carolina in Chapel Hill, he was educated as a zoologist, graduating with Phi Beta Kappa honors.[3,22]

Dr. Hyman's first academic position was Assistant Professor of Biology at the University of Mississippi in Oxford; he also taught a histology laboratory course to premedical students. For these labors his salary was $1,000 annually. Drs. Herbert T. Brooks, Otis S. Warr, and August H. Wittenborg had visited the University of Mississippi in the late spring of 1913 with the purpose of offering the Professorship of Physiology and Pharmacology to Dr. William E. Nicely. While Dean Brooks and Professor Warr consulted with Dr. Nicely, Dr. Wittenborg visited in Hyman's laboratory and there detected a keen, competent academician. While Dr. Nicely declined the University of Tennessee's offer, Orren Hyman and Professor Wittenborg finally hammered out a mutual agreement of $1,350 for Hyman to become an Assistant Professor. His duties at the U.T. College of Medicine were to consist of teaching the medical students histology and embryology, and assisting other professors in quizzing the medical students on gross anatomy.[9]

He hurled himself into these tasks with his customary enthusiastic vigor. The previous laboratory material in histology was pitifully inadequate, so he prepared entirely new study sets for all of his students. His efforts at staying one jump ahead of his students in gross anatomy are best described in his own words:

"As I had never dissected the human body, my work as quiz master for medical students had a poor prospect. I was to quiz the students on the upper and lower extremities, leaving the quiz work on the abdomen, head, and neck to more experienced personnel. As a consequence, I decided that I should dissect these parts of the cadaver ahead of the students, so as not to rely entirely upon my knowledge of the textbook. In order to do this, I would go to the anatomical laboratory on the fourth floor of Rogers Hall in the evenings after dinner. The building, of course, was dark, and the fourth floor was lit only by light streaming through the windows from the street lights, giving quite an eerie appearance to the dissecting room with some 60 or 70 bodies in various states of dissection. A body had been assigned to my use, and each table had suspended above it a single incandescent light on the end of a cord. When I would enter the dissecting room, thumps could be heard all over the room as the rats jumped down from the cadavers and landed on the floor of the dissecting room. Under these conditions I would turn on the light and dissect away until about 11 or 12 o'clock, getting well ahead of the students that I would be quizzing for the next day or two."[9]

Beginning with the Fall term of 1917, it had been decided that the University of Tennessee College of Medicine would require two years of premedical training for admission. Therefore, because it would be impractical, it was also decided to discontinue the premedical course in Memphis after the school term 1916–17. Dr. Hyman had applied for Officer's Training School for the United States Army during the spring of 1917, but because of his small size, it was decreed that he was too light for military service. He returned to Memphis in the fall of 1917 in September to serve as Registrar-Bursar and also as an Associate Professor of Histology and Embryology. He was awarded a scholarship in the Department of Biology at Princeton University, and he resigned from the University of Tennessee as of August 31, 1919 to pursue his graduate training leading to the degree of Doctor of Philosophy.[9]

Charles Morgan Hammond (1879–1964) received his M.D. degree from the Memphis Hospital Medical College in 1902 and practiced medicine in Memphis, as well as in Mississippi and Arkansas. In 1903 he constructed the first artificial respirator in the world, which was the prototype and forerunner of the "iron lung". In 1909 his research efforts resulted in the first motor-driven respirator. Dr. Hammond applied for a patent on January 12,

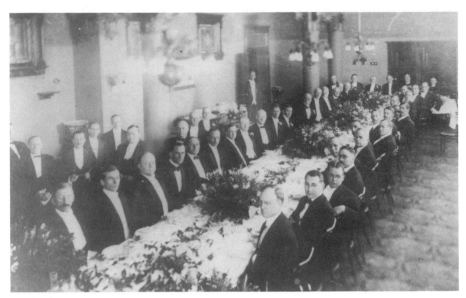

FIGURE 39. *Banquet at the Hotel Peabody in 1914 honoring Dr. Richard Brooke Maury (1834–1919) on the occasion of his 80th birthday (courtesy of William P. Maury, Jr., M.D.)*

1911, and his patent was issued from Washington on February 24, 1914. Earlier in 1912 this "mechanical lung" had passed its first clinical test at the Memphis City Hospital. In 1914 his device was the first artificial respirator to save a human life. By 1919, Dr. Hammond had built a cabinet-type respirator, but due to a lack of financial backing, he was never able to transfer his invention into mass production. When he failed to renew his patent after it expired, his claim to be the first inventor of the respirator was obscured, but it was later vindicated.[1,12]

The Maury family in Memphis have been readily identified with obstetrics and gynecology for many years. Dr. Richard Brooke Maury (1834–1919) in partnership with Dr. Robert Wood Mitchell had opened in Memphis the first Infirmary for the Diseases of Women in 1885.[12] Dr. Maury had obtained an M.D. degree from both the University of Virginia and the University of New York. He studied gynecology at the Women's Hospital in New York and had further training in Great Britain. He rendered distinguished service as a surgeon for the 28th Mississippi Cavalry Regiment, C.S.A., during the War Between the States. In 1886 Dr. Richard B. Maury was elected a Fellow of the British Gynecological Society, and in 1906 he became President of the American Gynecological Society.[1,12,16] He is seen in the Memphis Hospital Medical College faculty photograph of 1898 (Figure 10). In 1887, he performed the first abdominal section in a case of extrauterine "tubal" pregnancy in the United States.[1] Figure 39 depicts a banquet given in 1914 at the Hotel Peabody by the Memphis and Shelby County Medical Society to honor Dr. Richard Brooke Maury with a silver cup on the occasion of his 80th birthday. He is seated at the head of the table with Bishop Thomas Frank Gailor.

John Metcalf Maury (Figure 40), the son of Dr. Richard Brooke Maury, received his M.D. degree from the University of Pennsylvania in 1890. He interned at the St. Agnes Hospital and took further training in gynecology at the Joseph Price Hospital, both located in Philadelphia. He returned to Memphis and held surgical appointments at St. Joseph Hospital, Memphis City Hospital, and the Lucy Brinkley Hospital. Dr. John Maury was a Professor of Didactic Gynecology at the College of Physicians and Surgeons in Memphis from 1906–1909, and he was Professor of Didactic and Clinical Gynecology at the same institution from 1909–1911. With that medical school's merger with the University of Tennessee College of Medicine in 1911, he became a Professor of Gynecology at U.T. from 1911–1933 (Figure 34). Dr. Maury was an excellent teacher and a highly regarded gynecologist nationally.[1,12,28] His nephew, William P. Maury, Jr., M.D., who graduated from the University of Tennessee College of Medicine in 1937, continued his family's tradition of excellence in gynecological practice in Memphis.

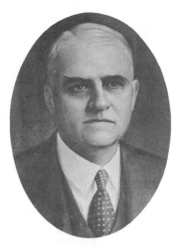

FIGURE 40. *John Metcalf Maury, M.D. (1868–1933) Professor of Gynecology*

Dr. William Krauss was born in 1861 in Germany, came to the United States as a young man, and earned a Ph.G. at the University of Maryland in 1883. Afterwards, he received his M.D. degree in 1889 from the Memphis Hospital Medical College and returned for graduate work in pathology in Germany at the Universities of Kiel and Wurzburg. His interest focused on the technical and laboratory aspects of medicine. Dr. Krauss introduced the use of the oil immersion microscopic lens in Memphis for high-power diagnostic work, and he persistently encouraged his fellow physicians to utilize the clinical pathologic tests for diagnostic purposes, that today we regard as standard procedure. He was heavily involved in important advances in public health endeavors statewide in Tennessee and was a national figure among public health authorities. Dr. Krauss was a Professor of Pathology and a Lecturer on Tropical Medicine at the College of Physicians and Surgeons in Memphis from 1906–1909; then he became a Professor of Pathology and Tropical Medicine at the newly merged University of Tennessee College of Medicine in 1911 (Figure 41). Dr. Krauss was also a recognized authority on malaria, having published in 1897 the first of several important papers on the pathological aspects of malarial hematuria. This Renaissance individual also became a pioneer radiation therapist in Memphis, and like many of these early radiologists, he suffered radiation burns on his left hand that eventually cost him his life.[1,12,16,28]

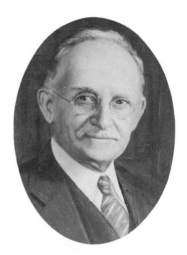

FIGURE 41. *William Krauss, M.D. (1861–1935) Professor of Pathology and Tropical Medicine*

As a native Memphian, Richmond McKinney (1874–1942) attended the Memphis Hospital Medical College and graduated in 1894. He specialized in otolaryngology and held the Professorship in Laryngology, Otology, and Rhinology at the University of Tennessee College of Medicine from 1911 until his retirement in 1938. Dr. McKinney was a charter member and President of the American Bronchoscopic Society. He was noted as a swift, deft surgeon. His nephew, James Wesley McKinney, M.D., continued the family medical tradition as an ophthalmologist in Memphis.[16]

One of the early, great teachers of medicine at the University of Tennessee College of Medicine was James Bassett McElroy (1866–1943). He was born in Mississippi, received his M.D. degree from the College of

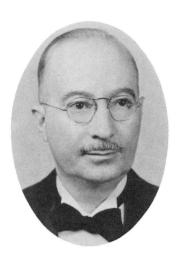

FIGURE 42. *Raphael Eustace Semmes, M.D. (1886–1982) Professor of Neurosurgery*

Physicians and Surgeons in 1893 in Baltimore, and in 1914 became Professor of Medicine at the University of Tennessee, Memphis. Earlier, from 1904–1914 he had also been a member of the faculty for the old Memphis Hospital Medical College. His nickname among the medical students was "Big Jim". Dr. McElroy was an international authority on malaria and nephrotic diseases.[1,16,27]

A native Memphian and a member of the University of Tennessee College of Medicine faculty since 1912, Raphael Eustace Semmes, M.D. was internationally acclaimed for his innovative contributions in the field of neurosurgery (Figure 42). Dr. Semmes received his M.D. degree from the Johns Hopkins University in Baltimore in 1910, where he first studied under the Father of Neurosurgery, Dr. Harvey Cushing. Afterwards, he followed Cushing to Harvard University for further training. He returned to Memphis with a deep sense of mission to propagate and develop this new field, and he became the first neurosurgeon in Memphis. He served as an outstanding faculty member for 43 years, and was Professor and Chairman of the U.T. Department of Neurosurgery.[1,12,27]

Dr. Semmes was a grandnephew of Rear Admiral Raphael Semmes, who was the Captain of the famous Confederate raider, C.S.N. Alabama. He was also a cousin of Dr. Alexander Jenkins Semmes of New Orleans, who was a brilliant physician, a scholarly medical writer, and later a Roman Catholic priest. As a Captain in the Army Medical Corps during World War I, Dr. Eustace Semmes was assigned to Base Hospital 87 in Toul, France, where he had a unique opportunity to surgically treat numerous battle casualties with head and spinal cord injuries. This war-time surgical experience not only saved soldiers' lives, but it rapidly advanced neurosurgical knowledge and operative techniques which would benefit the larger civilian population in the future.[4,12]

Dr. Semmes is especially recognized for his work on the intravertebral disc: in 1939—his famous paper on "Subtotal Hemilaminectomy and Extradural Removal of Ruptured Intravertebral Discs", and in 1943—his classic paper, published in collaboration with Dr. Francis Murphey, on "Ruptured Cervical Intravertebral Discs".[1]

With Dr. Francis Murphey he founded the famous Semmes-Murphey Clinic for Neurosurgery in Memphis in 1938; more information will be detailed on that subject later. Dr. Eustace Semmes was on the Founders' Group for the American Board of Surgery and the American Board of Neurological Surgery in 1937. On October 1, 1931 he was one of the four founding members of the Harvey Cushing Society, which met in Memphis in 1938. In 1939 Dr. Semmes was elected President of the Harvey Cushing Society.[1] He has been quoted as stating: "My greatest contribution has been the use of local anesthesia in the field of neurosurgery".[1,12]

Willis Cohoon Campbell, M.D. (Figure 43), the founder of the world renowned Campbell Clinic, was undoubtedly the most famous orthopedic surgeon in Memphis. He was born in 1880 in Jackson, Mississippi and obtained his M.D. degree from the University of Virginia in 1904. After two years of further medical training, he began a successful pediatric practice in Memphis. Later, he decided to study orthopedic surgery in London, Vienna, Boston, and New York. He returned to Memphis in 1909, organized the first orthopedic service at the University of Tennessee College of Medicine in 1911, and served as its Chairman until his death in 1941.[12,16,27]

In addition to serving as president of several various medical societies, Dr. Campbell was also President of the Clinical Orthopedic Society (1928), the American Orthopedic Association (1931), and the Southeastern Surgical Congress (1933).[16] He played a leading role in the organization of the American Board of Orthopedic Surgery and was elected as its President from 1937–1940. He was the first Secretary and the second President of the American Academy of Orthopedic Surgeons (1933) which was an organization that he both conceived and fostered; it now consists of over 12,000 members.[1,16]

As a pioneer specialist in orthopedic surgery, Dr. Campbell was famous nationally and internationally for his innovative work on the repair of injured knee ligaments, an important contribution to sports medicine. The use of sulfanilamide to prevent infections was also one of his major innovations. His pioneer work on the surgical reconstruction of stiff joints and on bone grafting to promote healing of non-united fractures brought patients from all over the nation and the world to the Campbell Clinic.[1,16] The three major books that Dr. Campbell published which are universally regarded as classics are: *Orthopaedics of Childhood* (1927), *A Textbook of Orthopaedic Surgery* (1930), and *Operative Orthopaedics* (1939). Many updated editions of *Operative Orthopaedics* continue to be published internationally in five languages by the staff at the Campbell Clinic under the editorship of Hoyt Crenshaw, M.D. (Appendix J).[1]

Dr. Thomas Palmer Nash's college roommate at the University of North Carolina, Dr. Orren W. Hyman, had been at the University of Tennessee College of Medicine for two years when in 1915 he recommended Dr. Nash for a faculty position in the Chemistry Department. At that time, T. P. Nash was the Assistant Editor of the Charlotte, North Carolina "News"; previously, he had been a high school mathematics teacher.[21] Dr. Nash joined the Chemistry Department staff in 1915 under Dr. Desha and was assigned to the instruction of premedical students in organic chemistry and dental students in a mixture of inorganic, organic, and physiological chemistry.

In 1919, following military service in World War I, Nash returned to the University of Tennessee and left a few months afterwards for graduate study at the Cornell University Medical School, where he obtained his Ph.D. degree in Biochemistry in 1922. That same year he again returned to the University of Tennessee in Memphis to serve as Professor and Chief of the Chemistry Department. He was one of the first faculty members to become actively involved in basic science research.[1,21] Further information on Dr. Nash's many teaching and research accomplishments will be detailed in Chapter Three.

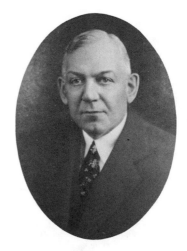

FIGURE 43. *Willis Cohoon Campbell, M.D. (1880–1947) Professor of Orthopedic Surgery (courtesy of Health Sciences Museum Foundation)*

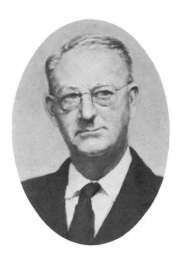

FIGURE 44. *Robert Latta Crowe, PH.C. (1887–1953) Professor and Dean of the School of Pharmacy (1936–53)*

Arthur Grant Jacobs, M.D. was the first Professor of Pediatrics at the University of Tennessee College of Medicine and served as Chairman of the Pediatrics Department from 1911–1921 and again from 1939–1940. He obtained two M.D. degrees—one from the University of Virginia in 1896 and one from the Medical College of Ohio in 1897. He pursued graduate studies at the University of Berlin, the University of Vienna, and the Memphis City Hospital. From 1905–1911, Dr. Jacobs was Professor of Pediatrics at the College of Physicians and Surgeons in Memphis, and in 1912 he was appointed the Head Pediatrician at the Baptist Memorial Hospital.[29]

While William Krauss, M.D. was the nominal Chief Administrative Officer for the School of Pharmacy from 1911–1928 (Appendix D), the real motivating force in pharmacy at the University of Tennessee was Robert Latta Crowe, PH.C. (Figure 44). Dr. Crowe was born in 1887 near Newbern, Tennessee and graduated from Ohio State University as a pharmaceutical chemist in 1910.[18] That September, he enrolled in the College of Physicians and Surgeons in Memphis with a twofold purpose: to study medicine and to play football. Because of his previous pharmaceutical qualifications, he was placed in charge of the school's dispensary and also taught both pharmacy and pharmacology, while completing his medical studies. He decided that teaching and pharmacy should be his life's vocation, so he never formally received his M.D. degree, although he was licensed by examination to practice medicine in Tennessee.[1,18,19]

When the University of Tennessee School of Pharmacy was moved in 1911 to become a Division of the newly merged University of Tennessee College of Medicine in Memphis, Dr. Crowe commenced teaching full-time in pharmacy. He helped to nurture and guide the School of Pharmacy from its beginning here in Memphis until his death in 1953. In 1959 it would become the College of Pharmacy (Appendix D). Figure 45 depicts President Ayres and the faculty of the University of Tennessee School of Pharmacy in 1911–12.[18] Dr. Crowe was appointed as Chief of the Pharmacy Division in 1926 and was made Dean of the School of Pharmacy in 1936. His name has always been synonymous with the profession of pharmacy in Tennessee. He organized the Memphis Retail Drug Association and labored incessantly to improve the teaching program at the University of Tennessee and to elevate the professional standards of pharmacy.[1,18,19]

Dr. Hyman's memoirs stated:

"During the year 1916–17 it became increasingly obvious that the United States was about to enter the first World War. Indeed, in the Spring of 1917, this decision was completed. A ferment in the faculty was noticeable throughout the year, and an increasing number of the members of the faculty were asking for leave in order to join the Armed Forces. Two important changes occurred during this year. Mr. E. F. Turner, who had served as Registrar-Bursar, resigned in the Summer of 1916 and went to Oklahoma City in the employment of the school system. Mr. Sidney Moreland, Professor of Physics in the premedical course, was made Registrar-Bursar. His daughter, Elizabeth Moreland, had served as Librarian for the past two years. A

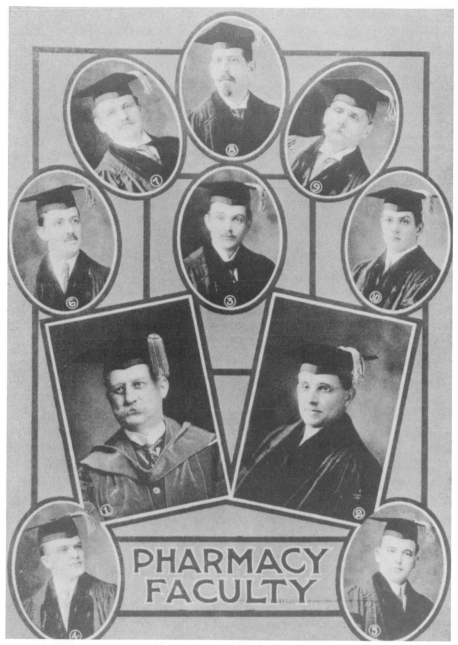

FIGURE 45. *University of Tennessee School of Pharmacy Faculty, 1911–12*

Mr. Martin Davis served as Assistant to the Registrar-Bursar. I would not mention his name except that during the course of the year, he began to have the records of the Memphis Hospital Medical College fed into the furnace. All of the scholastic records were burned before this was discovered, and the University was left with the financial records only of that institution."[9]

Living up to the nickname for Tennessee—"The Volunteer State"—

earned in the Mexican War, the University of Tennessee, Memphis' health professionals rapidly volunteered for military service when the United States did enter World War I in April of 1917. Appendix I lists the University of Tennessee, Memphis alumni or faculty members who sacrificed their lives in the service of their country. We lost three physicians who were affiliated with the University. Grover Carter, M.D. was a Captain in the 121st Brigade of the Royal Field Artillery in the British Army. He received his M.D. degree from the University of Tennessee in 1917 and was killed in action in France on October 16, 1918. The second loss was Norwin Batte Norris, M.D., who served as a Lieutenant (j.g.), (MC) U.S. Navy. He received his M.D. degree from the University of Tennessee in 1917 and was killed in action in October of 1918 while serving aboard the U.S.S. Ticonderoga. The third loss was Robert Boyden Underwood, M.D., who was a Captain, (MC) U.S. Army. Dr. Underwood received his M.D. degree from the University of Nebraska in 1904, was a member of the University of Tennessee Medical Faculty from 1914–1917, and died from pneumonia in Rouen, France while serving as an Army physician.

The medical, nursing, and hospital care during World War I was far advanced from the primitive medical care settings of the War Between the States. Efficient, clean field hospitals that were established near the front lines assured more rapid triage and treatment of wounded soldiers. Traumatic injuries from high velocity shells, shrapnel, and bombs, plus burn and poison gas injuries, required new methods of treatment. With 60 million men involved in a vast global conflict that eventually resulted in approximately 8 million deaths and over 19 million wounded individuals, new methods of treatment in orthopedic surgery, neurosurgery, general surgery, plastic surgery, skin grafting, burn care, and mental stress ("shell shock") made rapid advances. Medicine mobilized to meet these new challenges, and it made great strides in applying the science of infectious diseases to military sanitation. A massive vaccination program practically eliminated such previous wartime scourges as smallpox, tetanus, typhoid, and diphtheria.[12]

Numerous Tennessee physicians, surgeons, dentists, nurses, and pharmacists served in base and field hospitals in France. Dr. Battle Malone organized the Memphis General Hospital Red Cross Unit which was staffed by many University of Tennessee, Memphis personnel as Hospital Unit P, including 12 medical officers, 20 nurses, and 40 enlisted corpsmen. Figure 46 depicts some of the Tennessee physicians serving in France. Chief Nurse of Unit P was Myrtle Archer, who later trained in a French hospital in Compiegne to be an expert in a new, superior method for treating patients who were badly burned by poison gas.[12] Unit P left Memphis on November 17, 1917 and became the first Southern Medical Unit to serve in France under General Pershing. Even though nurses were technically prohibited from going to the front lines, Dr. Malone had a courageous group of young Tennessee nurses who worked heroically at the field dressing stations. Among these loyal ladies were: Myrtle Archer, Myrtle Bishop, Margaret

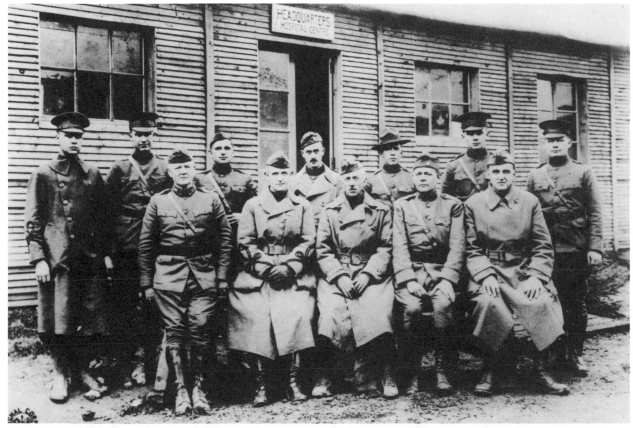

FIGURE 46. *Some of the Tennessee physicians serving in France during World War I (courtesy of Health Sciences Museum Foundation)*

Cummings, Jean Hope, and Edna Roach Campbell.[12]

Another famous medical unit that was composed of local health care personnel was Base Hospital 57, under the command of Major Frank D. Smythe and Major Edward Clay Mitchell, who would later become Chairman of the U.T. Department of Pediatrics from 1921–1939.[12,29] Edward C. Ellett, as an internationally acclaimed eye surgeon from the University of Tennessee College of Medicine, served as a Lieutenant Colonel in command of Base Hospital 115. This particular hospital specialized in treating head and neck wound injuries. Many other local physicians who garnered vast wartime experience and later returned to be involved with the University of Tennessee College of Medicine included: Joseph Edward Johnson, James Spencer Speed, Alphonse Meyer, Raphael Eustace Semmes, and Lucius McGehee.[12,27]

Dr. Joseph Edward Johnson (Figure 47) began practice in 1903 as a general surgeon in Memphis, but by 1908 he began to specialize in plastic surgery. His extensive practical experience that he acquired as a wartime plastic surgeon in France certainly enhanced his career as a surgical giant in that exacting surgical subspecialty. As his fame grew after World War I, Dr.

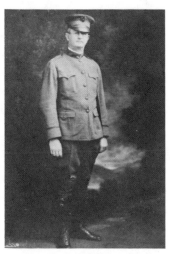

FIGURE 47. *Joseph Edward Johnson, M.D. (1872–1931)*

49

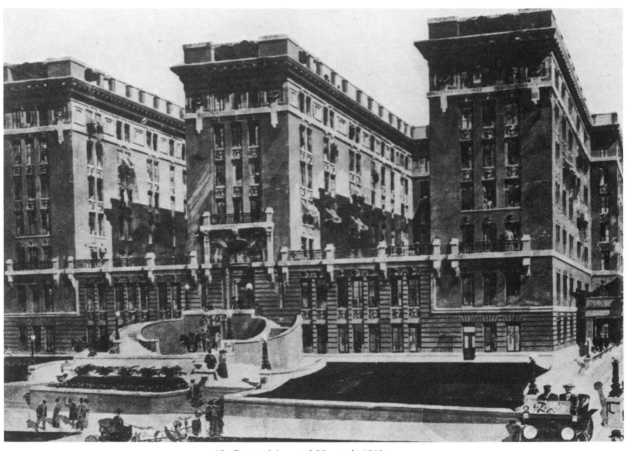

FIGURE 48. *Baptist Memorial Hospital, 1918*

Johnson attracted patients from throughout the United States and other nations, including movie stars from Hollywood.[12]

The Baptist Memorial Hospital, which was originally called the Tri-State Baptist Hospital, opened in July of 1912 just a short distance east of Lindsley Hall on land that was donated by the previous College of Physicians and Surgeons. By 1918 the first of many subsequent additions to this Memphis hospital increased its bed capacity to 250, making it one of the South's larger hospitals.[12] Its architectural design featured an elaborate Italian facade (Figure 48). When Sarah Conyers York graduated in 1913 from the University of Tennessee College of Medicine, she began her internship at age 35 at Baptist Memorial Hospital. Because she was the first female intern that the hospital had ever had in its program, there was confusion on the administrator's part in regard to where she would live, since only men lived in the interns' and residents' quarters. He solved this dilemma by having her stay in a patient's room as her assigned room rather than the men's dormitory. Dr. York also served as a clinical assistant in the U.T. Anatomy Department and appears in full dress for the occasion in Figure 49.

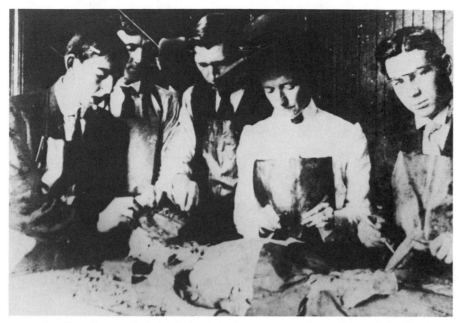

FIGURE 49. *Sara Conyers York, M.D., assisting in an anatomy demonstration (courtesy of Health Sciences Museum Foundation)*

As the teen's decade drew to a close with the end of World War I in 1918, several other significant events were occurring. Following her training in public health nursing in Chicago, Mrs. Lena A. Warner organized in 1911 a local program for public health nursing in Memphis. In 1916 she was appointed Director of Rural Health and Sanitation for the University of Tennessee Agricultural Extension Service and remained in that position until her retirement in 1946. She was also very influential in the recruitment of Tennessee nurses to serve in World War I.[25] On January 28, 1919 Dr. Brown Ayres, President of the University of Tennessee, died. He was succeeded by Dr. Harcourt A. Morgan, who assumed the reins of leadership for the University.[24] Dr. Willis Campbell became Chief of Staff for three special Memphis institutions: the Crippled Children's Hospital and School (1918), the Campbell Clinic and Hospital (1919), and the Hospital for Crippled Adults (1923).[12] Figure 50 depicts the graduating class of 1919 for the University of Tennessee College of Dentistry.

This chapter will end with the recollections of a student graduate of the U.T. Medical Class of 1917. Gettis Troy Sheffield (Figure 51) was born in 1893, grew up on a farm about 16 miles from Tupelo, Mississippi, and attended Mississippi College for two years. From there he returned to Itawamba County to teach in a country school from 1912–13, earning $50 a month.[23]

In 1913, with the money that he had earned from teaching and the proceeds that he had received from selling a horse and buggy, Sheffield pulled together enough money to go to Memphis and enter the University of Tennessee Medical School. Once there, he found that his lack of a college degree did not impede his studies.

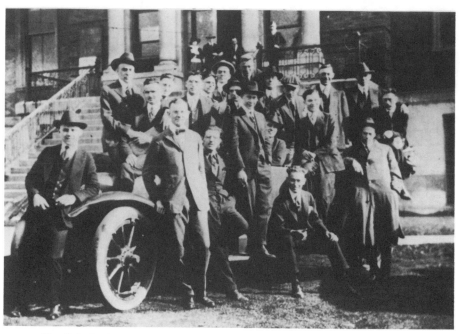

FIGURE 50. *1919 Graduating Class, University of Tennessee College of Dentistry*

"There were a lot of persons with B.S.'s and B.A.'s, and I led the class straight for a year and a half," Sheffield said. "So it goes to show you, you don't have to have a college degree to study medicine."[23]

Once in school, Sheffield lived in a boarding house, where he ate two meals a day. He bought a Remington No. 10 typewriter and typed his notes, which he then sold to his classmates.

"I remember the first paper that I turned in," he said. "Dr. Hyman said 'N.G.' (no good) 'Practice shading.' I needed practice on my drawing, you see." Dr. Orren W. Hyman was at that time an Assistant Professor of Histology and Embryology.[23]

Sheffield recalled that his classmates referred to Dr. Hyman as "Red" behind his back because of the color of his hair. In later years, Dr. Hyman was known by the nickname "Pinkie" because of his ruddy complexion. G. T. Sheffield continued to be a model student throughout his career at the University of Tennessee. He recalled that Dr. August H. Wittenborg, the Professor and Chairman of Anatomy, frequently called upon him in class.

"You see, I had a pretty good power of concentration," Sheffield explained. "And after a while they'd ask questions to certain ones, and Dr. Wittenborg would say, 'Tell 'em Sheffield.'"[23]

In 1915, Sheffield married Berda Stidham, who had been a classmate of his in Itawamba County, and in 1916 his first son, Edward, was born.

"I borrowed money from Peter to pay Paul," he said. "Finally, I borrowed some money from the bank in Tupelo and some from my Grandfather Sims. I sold notes. In my last year, I worked at the W. L. Douglas Shoe Store on South Main Street from one o'clock in the afternoon until ten o'clock p.m. for $1.50, and then I had an old Elgin seven-jewel watch that I pawned many, many times to get a little money to eat on."[23]

Eager to serve in World War I, Dr. Sheffield enlisted in the Army and was assigned during the war as a 1st Lieutenant in the 64th Coast Artillery Corps as a physician (Figure 52). In France, he was stationed in Andard, near Angers, at a camp where influenza was the biggest killer. He recalled that one French battalion near his own unit lost 75 men to the flu. His own battalion lost only 25 men because the viral strain was weaker by the time it hit them.

"We couldn't do a darn thing except let them stay in bed," Sheffield said.[23]

Upon his return to the United States, Dr. Sheffield practiced medicine for two years in Itawamba County. From there, he accepted a position at a state mental and tuberculosis institution in Jackson, Mississippi where he worked for five years, until he was appointed examiner at the Veterans Administration Regional Office in Jackson. He was transferred to several VA Hospitals across the United States, and his final five years with the VA were spent in Biloxi, Mississippi.

The changes in medicine and in his particular field of psychiatry have been most dramatic since 1917 to the present date, according to an interview with Dr. Sheffield in 1985.

"We didn't have a bloomin' thing to treat people with," he said. "The only thing we had was aspirin, codeine, morphine, laudanum, and things like that. Medicine has been written over a dozen times since I graduated."[23]

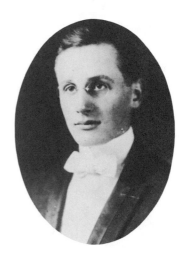

FIGURE 51. *Gettis Troy Sheffield, M.D., (1893–   ) as a 1917 University of Tennessee College of Medicine graduate*

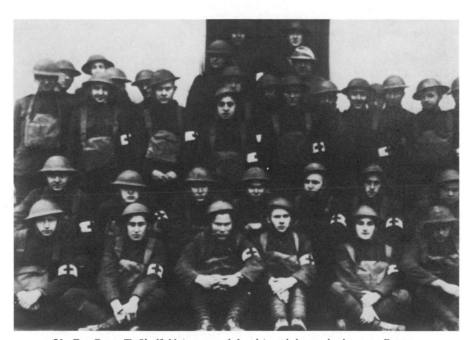

FIGURE 52. *Dr. Gettis T. Sheffield (top row, left side) with his medical unit in France*

REFERENCES

1. Bruesch, Simon R.: Personal Communication, 1985.

2. Bruesch, Simon R.: Chapters on "City of Memphis Hospitals" and "Medical Education" in *History of Medicine in Memphis*, editors—Stewart, Marcus J. and Black, William T., Jr., (McCowat-Mercer Press, Inc.: Jackson, TN.), 1971.

3. *Commercial Appeal:* November 11, 1968 ("Dr. O.W. Hyman").

4. *Commercial Appeal:* March 2, 1982 ("Dr. R.E. Semmes").

5. Conner, Cindy: "August H. Wittenborg", *Tennessee Medical Alumnus* 17:2–4, 1984.

6. *Dental Survey*—editorial—vol. 29:348–349, March, 1953 ("Dr. Justin Towner").

7. Hamer, Philip M.: *The Centennial History of the Tennessee State Medical Association 1830–1930*, (Tennessee Medical Association: Nashville, TN.), 1930.

8. Hyman, Orren W.: "U.T. Health Branch Is Medical Center of National Importance" in *The Commercial Appeal*, Sunday Magazine Section, June 18, 1933.

9. Hyman, Orren W.: *Early Development of the Medical Units, University of Tennessee*, (Privately Typed Manuscript Bound by Miss Kate A. Stanley, Registrar, University of Tennessee Medical Units: Memphis, TN.), 1970.

10. Jones, Madison: *History of the Tennessee State Dental Association*, (Tennessee Dental Association: Memphis, TN.), 1958.

11. Justis, Sr., E. Jeff: Personal Communication, 1985.

12. LaPointe, Patricia M.: *From Saddlebags to Science*, (The Health Sciences Museum Foundation: Memphis, TN.), 1984.

13. Montgomery, J.R., Folmsbee, S.J., and Greene, L.S.: *To Foster Knowledge: A History of the University of Tennessee 1794–1970*, (The University of Tennessee Press: Knoxville, TN.), 1984.

14. Morse, Charles R.: "History of the University of Tennessee", *University of Tennessee Magazine*, vol. 50:352–357, 1920.

15. *Science*, vol. 94:407–408, 1941 ("Dr. August H. Wittenborg").

16. Stewart, Marcus J. and Black, William T., Jr.: *History of Medicine in Memphis*, (McCowat-Mercer Press, Inc.: Jackson, TN.), 1971.

17. *University Center-Grams:* June, 1951 ("Dr. August H. Wittenborg").

18. *University Center-Grams:* August, 1951 ("Dr. R.L. Crowe").

19. *University Center-Grams:* August, 1953 ("Dr. R.L. Crowe").

20. *University Center-Grams:* October, 1955 ("Dr. Justin Towner, Sr.").

21. *University Center-Grams:* June, 1960 ("Dr. T.P. Nash").

22. *University Center-Grams:* June, 1961 ("Dr. O.W. Hyman").

23. *U.T.C.H.S. Record:* March 15, 1985 ("Dr. Gettis T. Sheffield").

24. Wittenborg, August H.: "The University of Tennessee Health Services Departments at Memphis", (Private Papers), 1933.

25. Wooten, Nina E. and Williams, Golden: *A History of the Tennessee State Nurses Association*, (Tennessee Nurses Association: Nashville, TN.), 1955.

26. Medical Accomplishments Report—U.T. Memphis Department of Ophthalmology.

27. University of Tennessee, Memphis—Records: 1911–1919.

28. University of Tennessee College of Medicine Bulletins 1911–1914.

29. Medical Accomplishments Report—U.T. Memphis Department of Pediatrics.

CHAPTER THREE

1920–1929

$\mathcal{T}$HE Roaring Twenties began with a bang at the University of Tennessee Medical Units in Memphis with a controversy over the appointment of Dr. McIver Woody as Dean of the College of Medicine. Dr. August H. Wittenborg had again served commendably as Acting Dean in late 1919 and 1920. After a search for the most appropriate individual, McIver Woody, M.D. was selected as the new Dean for the U.T. College of Medicine in 1920.

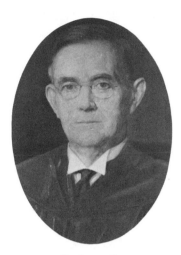

FIGURE 53: *James Bassett McElroy, M.D. (1866–1943) Acting Dean, College of Medicine, 1921–1923*

The Search Committee was pleased with their selection since Dr. Woody, as a native of Kentucky, was considered a Southerner, was a graduate of Harvard Medical College, and had gained practical teaching experience at that distinguished institution.[11,30] Dr. Woody actively assumed the Deanship in Memphis in July of 1920. Dr. Hyman related in his memoirs that the new Dean "was a man who possessed great energy, but very little tact."[11] This lack of persuasive abilities and insensitivity for the feelings of his colleague professors proceeded to alienate numerous faculty members during the Fall and Winter Terms. By the Spring of 1921, general academic dissatisfaction with Dean Woody had reached such a high pitch, that it was thought to be prudent to call a general meeting of the faculty. Local members of the University of Tennessee Board of Trustees (Mr. C. P. J. Mooney and Mr. Bolton Smith) and the new President of the University, Dr. Harcourt A. Morgan, were also invited to attend the meeting in Memphis. After a bruising round of bitter talk and accusations, with the President and Trustees attempting to defend Dr. Woody, the meeting adjourned on an unresolved and unamicable basis.[4,9,11]

After such an unpleasant confrontation, Dr. Woody elected to resign as Dean, effective July 21, 1921.[11] To replace him, the President and Trustees appointed James Bassett McElroy, M.D., who was at that time Professor of Medicine (Figure 53), as Chairman of the Faculty and Acting Dean. Dr. McElroy was a very scholarly Professor of Medicine, introduced European medicine to Memphis, and was an expert on nephrology and malaria.[7] Dr. McElroy, who was a favorite of the students, assumed his duties for the 1921–22 school year. At approximately this same time period, Dr. Wittenborg contacted Dr. Hyman, who was completing his Ph.D. degree studies at Princeton University, and he urged Orren Hyman to return to the University of Tennessee to assume a dual capacity: Registrar-Bursar and Assistant Professor of Histology and Embryology.[11,37]

Even though Dr. Hyman had made an informal agreement with the University of North Carolina to commence work in Chapel Hill as an

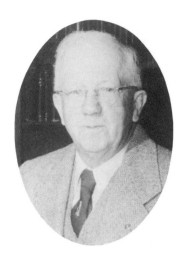

Associate Professor of Biology in the Fall of 1921, Dr. Wittenborg's persuasive powers prevailed. The University of North Carolina released Dr. Hyman from his obligation, and he accepted the offer to become a full Professor of Histology and Embryology and the Registrar-Bursar at the University of Tennessee, Memphis for the Fall Term of 1921.[11,37]

Next occurred perhaps the most fortuitous and brilliant maneuver that President Morgan ever made. He requested that Dr. Hyman stop off in Knoxville and visit with him on his journey from North Carolina to Memphis. In their discussion he made it clear that while Dr. Hyman was to be titled as the Registrar-Bursar, in reality he wanted him to take command of the situation at the Medical Units in Memphis, straighten it out administratively, and turn a deteriorating predicament around. This agreement is best described in Dr. Hyman's own words:

"The President told me that while I was to be titled Registrar-Bursar, they were expecting me to take charge of the situation in Memphis and make things take a turn for the better. This, of course, flattered me, and I made the mistake of assuming the responsibility without having any authority granted to exercise the control which President Morgan had expected and which I had agreed to exercise. I found this matter quite difficult in many respects, but it was years later before I had an active rebellion against my attempted use of authority and had to have President Morgan confirm my authority. By this time, however, my title had been changed so as to give some show of authority. I later decided that this difficulty, in which I found myself for several years subsequently to July, 1921, had been in my interest and in the interest of the Medical Units. Since I had no authority other than that of the Office of Registrar-Bursar, it was necessary for me to accomplish any of the changes which I thought were desirable by the persuasion of the faculty rather than by the exercise of authority."[11]

After 1921 on an actual day to day basis, Dr. Hyman controlled the University of Tennessee Medical Units in Memphis, even though titular authority had always rested with the University President in Knoxville. It is difficult to express adequately the tremendous influence that Dr. Hyman exerted in so many facets of University life in his 48 years of association with the University of Tennessee, Memphis. He handled the reins of administrative leadership with deft hands for many positive, productive years and played perhaps the most vital, decisive role in the evolution of this University from a small, struggling institution to one of the leading medical centers in the United States. As faculty, alumni, and students—we all owe a tremendous debt to Orren Williams Hyman.

Dr. Hyman received his Bachelor of Arts degree in 1910 and a Master of Arts degree in 1911 from the University of North Carolina where he was educated as a zoologist. He earned Phi Beta Kappa, but his honors were not all scholarly, for he also earned his letter in varsity tennis.

As has already been described in detail in Chapter Two, he came to the University of Tennessee after one year as an Instructor at the University of Mississippi. Later, he took time off from his duties at the University of Tennessee to obtain his Doctor of Philosophy degree from Princeton University in 1921. He returned to the University of Tennessee, Memphis as Assistant Professor of Histology and Embryology, and he was also named as the Registrar-Bursar, which started his career as an administrator.[23,35] In 1923, Dr. Hyman was appointed as Dean of the College of Medicine and remained in that position until 1957 (Appendix B). In the intervening years his title was to change considerably. From 1921–1925 he was listed as either the Registrar-Bursar or the Business Manager of the Medical Units, Memphis. From 1926–1942 he was listed in the various U.T. catalogs as the Administrative Officer of the Colleges in Memphis. Even though he was appointed as Dean of the College of Medicine in 1923, he continued to serve also in the strong leadership position in actuality as the Chief Executive Officer of the Medical Units. From 1943–1948 he was listed as Dean of Administration of the University of Tennessee Health Units in Memphis. From 1949–1961 he served as the Vice President in charge of the U.T. Medical Units. These administrative titles are listed in Appendix A.

His reputation as a medical educator won him an appointment by President Truman in 1951 to the 24 member National Science Foundation Board of Directors. He also received many other honors, including the Newspaper Guild's "Memphis Man of the Year" in 1953. Southwestern University conferred upon him the degree of Doctor of Laws in 1938. Also, Dr. Hyman held honorary membership in Alpha Omicron Alpha honorary medical fraternity and the Omicron Kappa Upsilon honorary dental fraternity. He served as President of the Memphis Rotary Club in 1940.[6,10,23,29,35]

Dr. Hyman was widely known as an avid hunter of quail, doves, ducks, and pheasants. Although he was certainly not renowned as a deadly shot, many humorous stories arose concerning his hunting exploits. As the University of Tennessee President, Andrew Holt, depicted him at Dr. Hyman's retirement dinner—"no duck has ever dodged a more deadly hunter".[35] Once when he was goose hunting with Dr. Crowe, Dr. Hyman was given the job of digging out the pit on a Mississippi River sandbar. He plunged into this task with his usual enthusiasm, digging out a very deep pit with even a ledge to lie down on in it, while Dr. Crowe was out by the water, setting decoys, and fetching more supplies from their car which was over a mile away. A little later Dr. Crowe heard Dr. Hyman screaming for help— being of such short stature, Hyman had dug a pit so deep that it was impossible for him to climb out, and Dr. Crowe had to hand down a shovel and literally pull him out of the pit.[4,29]

During the quail season, it was often Dr. Hyman's habit to come in early to work in his office, slip out for a bit of shooting, and then return to the University to work late into the evening. One medical student from Texas was seething because of what he considered to be an injustice in his grade— and he stormed into Dr. Hyman's office to settle the matter with that "son of a bitch". The student sat there fuming most of the afternoon waiting for the Dean. Being a bit later than usual and in a great hurry, Dr. Hyman returned, rushed into the building still in his hunting coat, and entered his office with his shotgun in hand. The terrified medical student took one look,

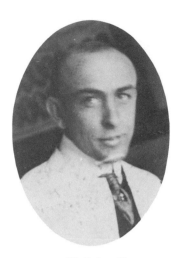

FIGURE 55: *Robert Sherman Vinsant, D.D.S. (1890–1967) Dean, U.T. College of Dentistry, 1924–1932*

screamed, and ran out of the office, and he never thought of complaining again.[4]

In 1955, the Hyman Administration Building was completed and named in his honor (Appendix K). Dr. Orren W. Hyman (Figure 54) retired in 1961 and was given a distinguished farewell dinner by his many University colleagues and friends. He remained as Vice President Emeritus for seven years with a research lab prepared for his use in the Wittenborg Building. On November 10, 1968 he died in Memphis, but he will long be remembered for the integrity and complete dedication which he brought to every task in making the University of Tennessee, Memphis the medical center that it is today.[6]

Dr. Joseph Archibald Gardner continued to serve as Dean of the University of Tennessee College of Dentistry until 1924 (Appendix C). In that year Robert Sherman Vinsant, D.D.S. was appointed as the Dental Dean and remained in that position until 1932. Previously, he had graduated from the University of Tennessee with honors and had served on the College of Dentistry faculty. Dr. Vinsant was a Fellow of the American College of Dentists.[16] Dean Vinsant is shown in Figure 55 with a student and patient in the U.T. Dental Clinic during the 1920's. From 1928–1933 Andrew Richard Bliss, Jr., Phm.D., M.D. served as the Dean for the School of Pharmacy (Appendix D), and in 1927 Ella George Hinton, R.N. was appointed Acting Director of the U.T. School of Nursing (Appendix E). The nursing topic will be discussed later in this chapter in greater detail. In 1928, the School of Biological Sciences would be organized under the Deanship of Dr. Thomas Palmer Nash, Jr. (Appendix G).

From the original three University of Tennessee Medical Center buildings, namely: Lindsley Hall, Eve Hall, and Rogers Hall—an ambitious building program surged forward in the 1920's that would lead to the completion of the Wittenborg Anatomy Building in 1926, the Goodman House Dormitory which was built in 1926 and acquired by the University of Tennessee in 1948, the Mooney Library in 1928, and the Crowe Pharmacy Building in 1928 (Appendix K). Earlier, the small Institute of Pathology Building was built in 1921 behind the City of Memphis Hospital, was vacated in 1951, and then occupied by the Institute of Clinical Investigations, and was finally demolished in 1980.

Under the inspired leadership of Mr. C. P. J. Mooney (editor of the *Commercial Appeal* and a University of Tennessee Trustee), Mr. Thomas A. Allen (Vice Mayor of Memphis and also a University of Tennessee Trustee), and Dean Orren W. Hyman, Administrative Director of the U.T. Health Division, the Tennessee Legislature appropriated $316,000 for the purchase of additional University land from East Street to Dunlap Street and from Union Avenue to Monroe Avenue; $300,000 worth of bonds were authorized, and the new Anatomy Building was built in 1926 (Figure 56). It was named in 1951 in honor of August H. Wittenborg, M.D. In 1927, bonds were again authorized and issued for the benefit of the University to build the Pharmacy Building in 1928 (Figure 57), which was later named in honor

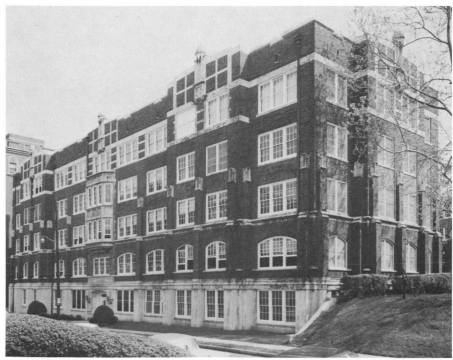

FIGURE 56: *Wittenborg Anatomy Building (built in 1926)*

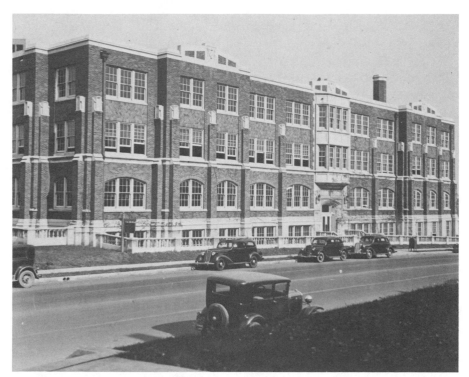

FIGURE 57: *Crowe Pharmacy Building (built in 1928)*

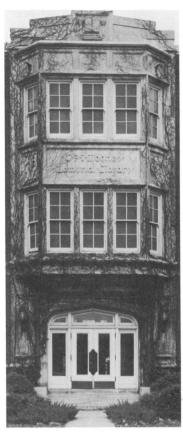

FIGURE 58: *C. P. J. Mooney Library (built in 1928)*

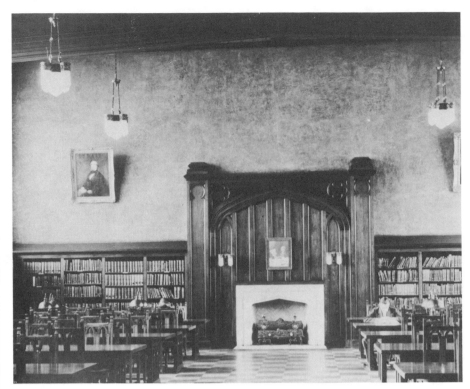

FIGURE 60: *Interior of the C. P. J. Mooney Library*

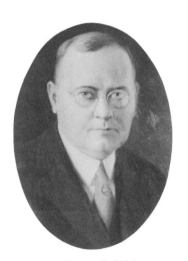

FIGURE 59: *C. P. J. Mooney University of Tennessee Trustee, 1918–1926*

of Robert L. Crowe, PH.C., and to construct the C. P. J. Mooney Library and Administration Building (Figure 58 depicts the library entrance). It was named at its opening in 1928 in honor of Mr. C. P. J. Mooney, who was a University of Tennessee Trustee from 1918–1926. A painting of Mr. Mooney (Figure 59) hung in the old library for many years until it was moved in 1985 to the new library facility.[10] Figure 60 illustrates the interior of the Mooney Library which hopefully will be utilized as a future Faculty Common Room.

The University of Tennessee Medical Center was originally conceived by architectural consultants (Jones & Furbringer) to resemble the traditional enclosed quadrangle with lawn and walkways of a British university, such as St. John's College at Oxford University or Trinity College at Cambridge University. Figure 61 illustrates this concept. After the Wittenborg, Crowe, and Mooney Buildings were completed in the late 1920's, the Dental Faculty Building was added as the new College of Dentistry Building in 1949, the Hyman Administration Building in 1955, and the Chemistry-Physiology Building in 1955 (named for Dr. Thomas Palmer Nash). These latter two buildings were connected to the Crowe Building by a series of cloisters, as was originally planned and depicted in Figure 61. However, an archway replaced the planned building enclosure of the quadrangle opposite the Mooney Library, and a paved parking lot occupied the land originally intended as an enclosed lawn between the Hyman Building and the College

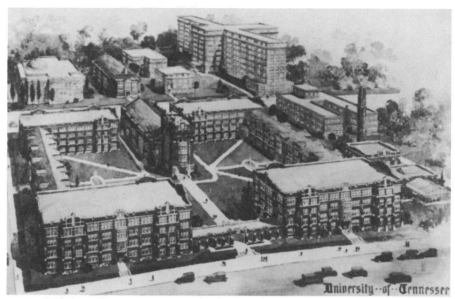

FIGURE 61: *Original Architectural Concept of the U.T. Medical Center Campus, 1920's (by Jones and Furbringer)*

of Dentistry. The center building, planned to connect the Wittenborg Anatomy Building and the College of Dentistry Building and extend toward the Union Avenue entrance, was never constructed. It was the intent in the 1920's that the main University would therefore face Union Avenue.[10,11] Figure 62 depicts the appearance of a Histology-Embryology Laboratory at the University of Tennessee in the early 1920's.

The new Anatomy Building was ready for occupancy by the Fall Term of 1926. The Department of Gross Anatomy was transferred from old Rogers Hall and was housed on the fourth and basement floors of the new building. The Histology Department was given the east half of the third floor, and the Department of Chemistry occupied the west half of the third floor and all of the second floor space. All of the prior activities of the Chemistry Department were transferred from Lindsley Hall and Rogers Hall to this new building. The Department of Physiology and Pharmacology was moved from its old space in Eve Hall and Rogers Hall to the first floor and half of the basement floor of the new Anatomy Building.[6,10]

There are several other important items regarding the subject of medical buildings in Memphis during the 1920's. The Methodist Hospital had its opening ceremonies for the first Methodist Hospital Building on All Saints' Day, November 1, 1921; it was built on the site of the former W. B. Mallory home on Lamar Avenue. This hospital was only in operation for six months when the Veteran's Bureau purchased it. The Methodist Hospital functioned in patient care from 1918–1921 in the Lucy Brinkley Hospital at the corner of Dunlap and Union and again in 1921–1924 in the same location.[4] The second Methodist Hospital was completed in September of 1924 at 1265 Union Avenue and has aided throughout the years as a clinical facility

61

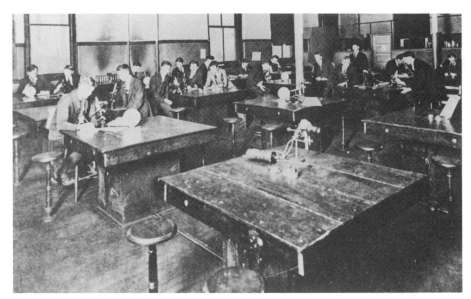

FIGURE 62: *Histology-Embryology Laboratory at University of Tennessee, Memphis in the early 1920's*

for training in collaboration with the University of Tennessee, Memphis.[16] Baptist Memorial Hospital opened in 1928 its Physicians and Surgeons Building, as the first such doctors' office building erected in the United States.[17] Figure 63 illustrates the appearance of surgeons and surgical nurses on a surgical team at the Memphis General Hospital in 1921.

During the history of the University of Tennessee, Memphis Library, there have only been three Library Directors: Miss Emily McCurdy (1917–1959), Miss M. Irene Jones (1959–1970), and Mr. Jess A. Martin (1971–to date).[18] All of these dedicated Librarians have rendered outstanding service in the academic literary area, which is so vital to any scientific community. Dr. Hyman gives a succinct description, regarding the hiring of Miss McCurdy, who served faithfully for 42 years:

"Miss Emily McCurdy had been graduated by the School of Pharmacy in 1916. She had been an excellent student and after a limited experience in the operation of a drug store, decided she would like to be in an academic position. Miss McCurdy was severely crippled and walked with the aid of crutches. She had, of course, an alert mind. She had been appointed Librarian in 1918 without any prior library training. It's only fair to add that there had been no one serving as Librarian prior to that time who had any better training. By 1921, however, the faculty wished to have a vigorous administration of the Library and an intelligent handling of library problems other than the securing and keeping of a few books in the Library. In the Spring of 1922, Miss McCurdy applied for and was granted leave-of-absence for the year 1922–23 so that she could take formal training in Library Administration. She went to the University of Illinois and spent the year in this activity, returning to the University with good information and good training concerning the management of a library. This was a very important addition to the scholarly program of the College of Medicine. There were an increasing number of men, both in the clinical

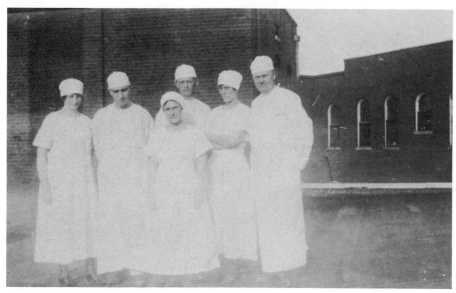

FIGURE 63: *Surgical team at the Memphis General Hospital, 1921 (courtesy of Health Sciences Museum Foundation)*

fields and the preclinical fields, who demanded a good current Library for their studies and for the preparation of their presentations to students."[11]

Enrollment in the University of Tennessee College of Medicine comprised a total of only 56 students during the school year of 1920–21. It was a time of crisis for the University, as the College of Medicine was in dire financial straits and about to be closed due to this lack of students.[11,37] Dr. Hyman, as Dean of the College of Medicine whose annual salary was only $1,500, and Dr. Wittenborg, who was Chairman of the Department of Anatomy, were giving part of their meager salaries simply to keep the College of Medicine operating.[25] The student number increased to 108 for the 1921–22 year, and by the Fall Term of 1922 enrollment had climbed to 173 students in the College of Medicine.[11] Much of the credit for the increase in the enrollment was due to the sudden popularity of the University of Tennessee, Memphis football team. In 1920 a group of enthusiastic medical, dental, and pharmacy students, without any football coach or financial aid, organized themselves into a team and played a six game football schedule. The first year record was three victories, two losses, and a tie.[27]

In 1921, the team was formally organized as the "University of Tennessee Doctors", and in 1922 it was able to hire as a coach, "Uncle" Bill Brennan, who was former umpire-in-chief of the Southern Association.[25,27] As Dr. Hyman was quoted: "The Doctors' football team put the University of Tennessee Medical Units on the map".[27] In numerous, awesome performances this team proceeded to achieve undefeated seasons in 1921, 1922, and 1923 with a winning streak of 33 consecutive games.[27] They scored 500 points to their opposition's 44 points. Tables 2 and 3 outline the 1922 and

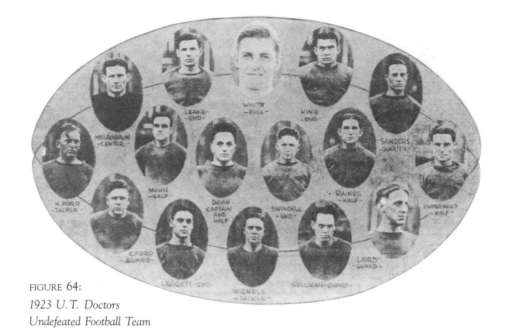

FIGURE 64:
*1923 U.T. Doctors
Undefeated Football Team*

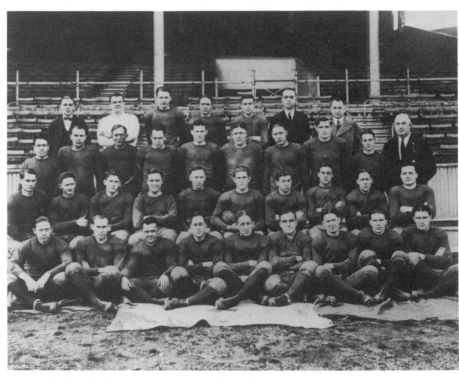

FIGURE 65: *1924 U.T. Doctors Undefeated Football Team*

1923 seasons.[25] Figures 64 and 65 depict the 1923 and 1924 U.T. Doctors Football Teams, respectively. They were nicknamed the "U.T. Docs".

These men were full-time students, who were confronted each day with a tremendously demanding scientific schedule. They had to keep up their grades, complete all of their laboratory work, and meet their clinical requirements—not just play football. This situation was a far cry from the usual physical education major athletes who dominate the 1985 college campus scene. Dusk came down early in Memphis on athletic fields without lights, and these men rarely appeared before 4:30, sometimes 5 o'clock, and sometimes only the Friday practice was the one that was a lengthy practice. This team practiced at old Hodges Field, which was located where the modern Veterans Hospital is now situated, and they played on the baseball diamond of Russwood Park, which was located across Madison Avenue from the Baptist Hospital. Crowds were feeble in strength, and ticket sales, even for this popular and winning team, had to struggle in order to keep up with minimal expenses. It was difficult to schedule teams who were willing to play the U.T. Docs. The reason for this dilemma was because in the opponents' minds, there was little to win in prestige and a great deal to lose; and of course the more the Doctors won, the more tedious it became to obtain games.[25,27,36]

The array of talent for this football team was quite diverse. One of its

Table 2
1922 Football Season

U.T. Doctors	45	Southwestern Presbyterian	0
U.T. Doctors	7	Union University	7
U.T. Doctors	14	Centenary	0
U.T. Doctors	28	Missouri School of Osteopathy	0
U.T. Doctors	19	University of Chattanooga	0
U.T. Doctors	22	University of Mississippi	0
U.T. Doctors	54	Rolla School of Mines	6
U.T. Doctors	14	Wabash College	7

Table 3
1923 Football Season

U.T. Doctors	12	West Tennessee Normal	0
U.T. Doctors	14	Union University	6
U.T. Doctors	55	Southwestern Presbyterian	0
U.T. Doctors	7	Carson Newman College	0
U.T. Doctors	6	University of Tulsa	6
U.T. Doctors	0	Loyola University	0
U.T. Doctors	14	Cumberland University	0
U.T. Doctors	6	Wabash	0

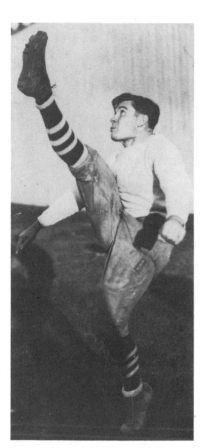

FIGURE 66: *Phil E. White, M.D. U.T. Doctors and former All-American fullback, 1923*

outstanding members was Phil E. White, who had been an All-American fullback from the University of Oklahoma and who later played professional football with the New York Giants. White went on to obtain his M.D. degree and became a practicing physician later; he is pictured in Figure 66, kicking one of his famous punts. The annual punting average for Phil White was seldom ever under 50 yards.[25] The Gotten twins both played for the successful U.T. Doctors Football Team. Henry Gotten, M.D. chose internal medicine after he graduated, while his twin brother, Nicholas Gotten, M.D., pursued a career in neurosurgery and served as a Professor of Neurology at the University of Tennessee. He was later President of the Southern Neurological Society. Another set of brothers, who were both outstanding players for the U.T. Doctors, was Julian "Big" Sullivan, M.D. and D.A. "Little" Sullivan, D.D.S., both of whom practiced their professions in Cleveland, Tennessee.[16,25] Figure 67 shows Hobart "Hobie" Ford, in a three-point stance, wearing the typical football gear of the 1920's. He received his D.D.S. degree in 1926. His son, Hobart Ford, Jr., also graduated from the U.T. College of Dentistry in 1943. Robert Thomas "Tarzan" Holt, D.D.S. played end; earlier in college he had been an All-Southeastern end at the University of Tennessee in Knoxville. He later had a distinguished career in the Veterans Administration.[29]

Figure 68 graphically illustrates the tough style of football played in 1923, as Sammy Sanders is shown running the ball through a hole in the line opened up by John Leake, Phil White, and Dutch Leggett. The team and its situation are best described by Dr. Sam Sanders in 1977:

"The nucleus of the 1921 team was a former halfback and captain of Washington and Lee (Dr. Sam Raines), four regulars from Maryville College, and outstanding fullback and triple-threat man from the University of Oklahoma (Dr. Phil White), an end from Virginia, and All-Southwestern halfback from Texas A & M (Dr. Sammy Sanders), an outstanding tackle from Tulane and points South, a high school halfback from New Orleans, and local high school prospects were enrolled. This group of 19, though small in number, were quite impressive when seen working out on Hodges Field. Most of the regulars played 60 minutes of every game. Our center, Cecil McLaughlin, played 60 minutes of every game for four years at Maryville College and 60 minutes of every game for the U.T. Doctors. The average weight of the team was about 175 pounds. Sammy Sanders was the lightest man on the team at 122 pounds. Paine and Ford were the heaviest at slightly over 200 pounds. Practice time was limited since all players were required to attend classes regularly, complete all classwork, and make up any work missed on away games. Coaching consisted of primarily developing teamwork. No one could have done a better job than our coach, "Uncle" Bill Brennan. Uncle Bill was one of the few coaches that could have molded the great array of football talent into the powerful working unit that it was."[25]

Financial stability for the University of Tennessee Doctors Team was always a problem. Generous contributions by Louis Levy, M.D., a prominent ear, nose, and throat surgeon; Jim Bodley, M.D., a distinguished Memphis general surgeon; and Charles Campbell, D.D.S., a well-known Memphis dentist, proved to be most helpful. Internally, Dr. Robert S.

Vinsant, Dean of the College of Dentistry, and Dr. Robert L. Crowe, a Professor in the Pharmacy School, gave both personal encouragement and financial support for the football team. At one time, Dr. Crowe even arranged to have a small band play for the team. One of the greatest benefits that this team rendered to the University was the definite increase in the number of students who were attracted to health professional careers because of the popularity that this team achieved. From a student body of 120, attendance increased to approximately 400 students within those three years in which the undefeated football team greatly influenced the decisions of numerous young men toward careers in the health professions. The U.T. Doctors contributed much more than simply winning football games and attracting prospective students to the University of Tennessee. All of these athletes became distinguished health care practitioners in their respective specialties. Table 4 depicts the future status of some of the players on those awesome U.T. Doctors Football Teams of the 1920's.[25,28,36]

The U.T. Doctors were undoubtedly a great football team. This fact was underscored during the 1922 season when they defeated Centenary 14 to 0. That same Centenary team had previously played and defeated Harvard University, which was considered to be the number one football team in the nation during 1922. On December 4, 1926 the U.T. Doctors played their final game against an All-Star team to help defray the cost of the deficit incurred over the previous two seasons. They won that final game 3 to 0. This game brought to a conclusion that tremendous six year era when the U.T. Doctors had accomplished so very much; it appeared that there was nothing left to conquer. They brought much honor and recognition to the University of Tennessee, and their record and accomplishments are still remembered, recognized, and unsurpassed in this present day. On October 11, 1979, Marcus J. Stewart, M.D. gave the principal speech at the dedication dinner which commemorated the naming of the present University of Tennessee athletic field facilities as the U.T. Doctors Field. A plaque was placed at the entrance to commemorate this tremendous team, their achievements, and their place in the University of Tennessee, Memphis history.

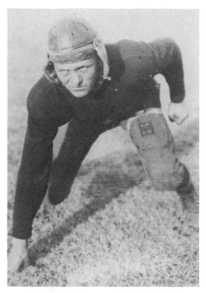

FIGURE 67: *Hobart ("Hobie") Ford, D.D.S. U.T. Doctors in 1920's football gear*

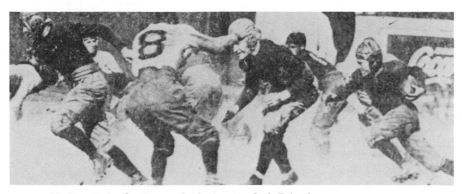

FIGURE 68: *Sammy Sanders, quarterback, running the ball for the U.T. Doctors, 1923*

Table 4
Where Some U.T. Doctors Players Are Now

Still Practicing:

"Ordie" King, D.D.S., Water Valley, MS

Sam Raines, M.D., Urologist, Memphis, Past Chairman of the Department of Urology at U.T.

"Sammy" Sanders, M.D., Ear, Nose & Throat, Memphis, Past Chairman of the Department of Ear, Nose & Throat at U.T. for 17 years

J. B. Futrell, M.D., General Practice, Rector, AR

Retired:

Bill Cockroft, D.D.S., now President and Chairman of the Board of United Inns

"Dutch" Leggett, D.D.S., New Orleans

Nick Gotten, M.D., Neurologist, Memphis. Past Chairman of the Department of Neurology at U.T.

Malcolm Prewitt, D.D.S., Memphis

D. A. Sullivan, D.D.S., Cleveland, TN

R. R. Swindell, M.D., Urologist, Amarillo, TX

Henry Gotten, M.D., Internal Medicine, Memphis

Charlie Campbell, former manager of the U.T. Docs, Memphis

One of the greatest players of the famous U.T. Doctors Football Teams was Sam Houston Sanders, Jr., M.D. For three years he had played halfback at Texas A & M University. On January 1, 1922 the Aggies had defeated Centre College 22–14 to win the first Cotton Bowl in Dallas and the national championship, since Centre had beaten number one-rated Harvard University one week previously. The Aggies' All-Southwestern halfback, Sam Sanders, had led them. Due to the influence of his earlier vow to become a physician when his sister died, and the support and encouragement of his coach, Dana X. Bible, Sanders set out to obtain a medical education with only $13 in his pocket.[3] It was the University of Tennessee's good fortune that he ended up as a student in Memphis. It was very difficult going to medical school and playing quarterback on the U.T. Doctors Football Team. With a couple of low grades and a deficiency in physics hanging over his head as he prepared for the second year of medical school, Sam had drawn the disfavor of the legendary Orren W. "Pinkie" Hyman. However, he had earned the support of Dr. August H. Wittenborg who encouraged Sanders to make up all of his academic deficiencies in one summer. He completed this arduous task, and the following fall he was back in school and ready to play football again. After an internship in New York, Dr. Sanders joined the staff of the U.T. College of Medicine as an assistant in the Department of Eye, Ear, Nose, and Throat in 1928. He advanced in academic rank until he was named Associate Professor in 1949. In April of 1954 it was Dr. Hyman who appointed him as Professor and Chairman of the Department of Eye, Ear, Nose, and Throat at the University of Tennessee in recognition of his leadership and academic prowess. He served as Chairman of that Department of Otolaryngology from 1954 to 1970 and continued teaching several years after that. Dr. Sanders has spent the majority of his life in Memphis and still continues a private practice at the age of 85. In recognition of his many services and generosity to the University as a student, a faculty member, and an alumnus, the University set aside a private dining room in the new Student-Alumni Center with appropriate memorabilia of the U.T. Doctors Football Team era and named it to honor Dr. Sanders. Dr. Sanders served as President and Director of the International Society of E.E.N.T.; he also was President of the Tennessee Academy of Ophthalmology and Otolaryngology. He was Secretary of the Tennessee Academy of Ophthalmology and Otolaryngology for 18 years. From 1950–1953 Dr. Sanders was Secretary of the A.M.A. Section on Laryngology, Rhinology, and Otology. In 1957 he served as Chairman of that Section. He is a Fellow of the American Academy of Ophthalmology and Otolaryngology, as well as numerous scientific societies including the American College of Allergists. Figure 69 depicts Dr. Sam Houston Sanders today with the accolade nouns that describe the many definitions of this outstanding alumnus.

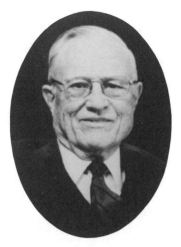

FIGURE 69: *Sam Houston Sanders, Jr., M.D. (1900–) Professor and Chairman, U.T. Department of Otolaryngology, 1954–1970*

Dr. Sanders relates a humorous story about the second game of the 1922 season which was against Union University in Jackson, Tennessee. It was a hard fought battle which ended in a 7–7 tie on a mud-clodded field—it was the only tie of the 1922 season.

"A funny story came out of that game. Sammy Sanders was injured and acting as water boy. Bo McMillin, the former quarterback of the famous Praying Colonels of Centre College was coaching Centenary of Shreveport, Louisiana and had sent a scout to the Union game to scout the Doctors—especially their quarterback, Sanders. Bo had good reason to remember Sanders. For it was on January 1, 1922 that Sanders and his Texas A & M Aggies defeated Centre, then national champions, by a score of 22–14 in a post-season tussle. Well, the scout couldn't locate Sanders, so he asked the Doctors' water boy (none other than Sanders) about their quarterback. He didn't recognize the water boy as Sanders until the following week when Centenary and the Doctors met in Shreveport, Louisiana for the classic contest, in which the Doctors defeated Centenary 14–0."[25]

Attending medical school was natural for Samuel Lucas Raines, M.D. who stated that he was "raised up with the profession".[2] His father, Newton Ford Raines, M.D. (1858–1925), was the son of Dr. William Nathaniel Raines, who arrived in the Whitehaven, Tennessee area in 1832 to "read medicine" under Dr. Alfred Eldridge. Newton F. Raines received his M.D. degree from Baltimore's College of Physicians and Surgeons in 1879 and practiced medicine at Raines, Tennessee in Shelby County. He also served in the Tennessee State Legislature in the 1890's and became Superintendent of the Shelby County Board of Health.[2,27]

69

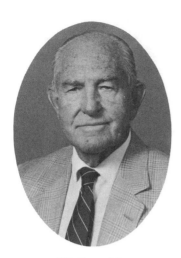

FIGURE 70: *Samuel Lucas Raines, M.D. (1900–   ) Professor and Chairman, U.T. Department of Urology, 1954–1964*

Sam Raines played baseball and football at both the Memphis University School and Washington and Lee University. The summer after he completed his studies at Washington and Lee University in 1921, he played semiprofessional baseball in Holly Springs, Mississippi. To quote Raines: "Baseball and football gave me identity and determination to do a few things."[2]

Dr. Raines, similar to many U.T. students, had good cause to remember Dr. Wittenborg, as he recounted in the following excerpt:

"Dr. Wittenborg came up to me in the dissecting room in Anatomy in my Freshman year and with that little twitching motion that he usually took to the left when he was telling a student something, he told me that Anatomy was about 40% of my first year classes and that I could not pass Anatomy and play football. He used the title 'HERR Raines' in addressing me, and then stood back to see my apparent reaction. I simply told him that I played four years of football and baseball at Washington and Lee and that I had finished barely below that Phi Beta Kappa level (which I did not qualify for) and that I expected to be able to play football and carry my courses here at the University of Tennessee. I further told him that if any time I seem to be dropping behind, all he had to do was to tell me, and I would stop football. We went ahead with our football schedule and went away on a trip, I believe, and won a couple of games rather substantially, and he came up to me and picked around at my cadaver one day and cleared his throat a time or two and then said, 'HERR Raines, I believe it will do', and then with that little tick that he frequently used when turning his head to the left, he strolled off down the aisle."[39]

It should be pointed out that Sam Raines received the Faculty Medal for having the highest academic average in the 1926 graduating medical class, in addition to playing halfback for the undefeated U.T. Doctors.

In another humorous student-day account, Dr. Raines stated:

"Dr. Hyman did a great deal for me in Histology, and I believe it was in his write-up that it was recorded that he felt kind of spooky when he went into the Anatomy dissecting room at night. I would like to point out that after I went on those football trips, I would go straight to the anatomy room on Sunday with the rats and everything else going on and dissect on my cadaver. One evening while I was there for some reason unknown to me, possibly I had pushed the cadaver when I didn't realize it, but the darn thing fell over on top of me. You can imagine how soon I cleared out of there! I hunted a lot with Dr. Hyman and got to know him and his family well and had a tremendous respect for him as well as many of our faculty members like Dr. Nash and so many others."[39]

After receiving his M.D. degree and completing his internship at the Memphis General Hospital, Dr. Raines spent two years at the Cleveland Clinic, where he decided to specialize in urology rather than pursuing a career in general surgery. After additional training in New York, young Dr. Raines returned to Memphis to begin what would be a distinguished career that has spanned more than 50 years. Except for the brief period during World War II when he served as a military physician, Dr. Raines has practiced in Memphis.[2]

While maintaining a private practice, Dr. Raines was appointed as

Chairman of the Department of Urology in the University of Tennessee College of Medicine from 1954–1964. He has been a member of the staff of the Methodist Hospital since 1940, and served as Chief-of-Staff from 1948–49 and again from 1964–69.[2,22]

Dr. Raines' outstanding medical career became nationally known in 1963 when he served as President of the American Urological Association (Figure 70). He had previously served as Secretary of the same organization and had received its Guiteras Award for outstanding contributions to the field of Urology.[27] At age 85, Dr. Raines still sees patients occasionally, although he retired from full-time active practice several years ago and turned over all the major surgery to his son, Richard B. Raines, who also received his M.D. degree in 1962 from the U.T. College of Medicine.

During the 1920's U.T. Memphis began to acquire more faculty who were to leave a lasting mark and exert a tremendous positive influence over their students, bringing both educational accomplishments, clinical excellence, and rudimentary scientific research to the University.

Dr. Harry Christian Schmeisser first joined the faculty of the University of Tennessee, Memphis on September 1, 1921, as Professor of Pathology and Bacteriology and Pathologist and Bacteriologist-in-Chief to the John Gaston Hospital. He continued in these duties for 33 years, relinquishing his administrative position on March 1, 1944 to Douglas H. Sprunt, M.D. Dr. Schmeisser was born September 20, 1885 in Baltimore, Maryland. He received his A.B. degree in 1908, his M.D. degree in 1912, and his Ph.D. in 1914 from the Johns Hopkins University in Baltimore. He also studied at the Universities of Marburg and Freiburg in Germany. During World War I between 1917–1919, he served as a Major in the United States Army Medical Corps with the American Expeditionary Force in France. His prior academic appointments were at the Johns Hopkins Medical School and the Emory University School of Medicine in Atlanta. In 1923, the Division of Pathology began offering one of the first courses in medical technology through the efforts of Dr. Schmeisser. Prior to that time, medical technologists were trained by each medical scientist. In the field of basic science investigation, Dr. Schmeisser is best known for transmitting fowl leukemia cells by experimental inoculation to other healthy fowls, thereby reproducing in the fowl all of the pathological changes seen in human leukemia. He was an excellent teacher, who was well remembered by all of his previous students. In Dr. W. A. D. Anderson's classic textbook, *Pathology*, there are numerous, excellent pathologic photographic illustrations with the caption, "Courtesy of Dr. H.C. Schmeisser".[31] Dr. Schmeisser is depicted in Figure 71. It is interesting to note that Dr. W. A. D. Anderson, who became such a nationally and internationally known pathologist through his famous textbook, served as an Instructor in the U.T. Department of Pathology from 1937–1940.[7]

In 1927 Dr. Anna Dean Dulaney came to the University of Tennessee, Memphis as an Instructor in Bacteriology. She devoted 33 years to the teaching of medical, dental, and pharmacy students and was a well-known

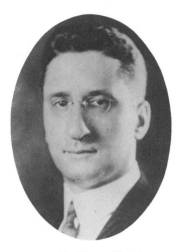

FIGURE 71: *Harry Christian Schmeisser, M.D., Ph.D. (1885–1964), Professor and Chairman, U.T. Department of Pathology, 1921–1944*

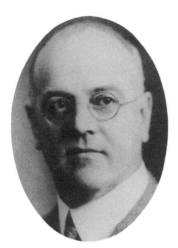

FIGURE 72: *Robert Boyd Bogle, M.D., D.D.S. (1875–1941) President, American Dental Association, 1928–1930*

figure to the numerous graduates of our University. She had obtained both her M.A. and her Ph.D. degrees from the University of Missouri. In 1943 Dr. Dulaney was one of the University of Tennessee's representatives at a special course in tropical diseases at Tulane University. This course was sponsored by the Markle Foundation, and 30 of the nation's top medical schools participated. At that time she was engaged in studies on malaria, with special interests in serological tests for the detection of latent malaria. In 1948 and in 1949 she spent six months at the Sloan-Kettering Institute for Cancer Research in New York City. While there, she organized a serological laboratory and conducted studies on mouse leukemia, a disease which in many respects resembles human leukemia. In 1950 she was appointed as a special consultant to the United States Public Health Service and took part in many conferences on cancer studies. During her distinguished academic career, she published more than 70 scientific papers, most of which were concerned with the serological or immunological aspects of disease. Dr. Dulaney was also a Fellow of the American Association of the Advancement of Science.[34]

George L. Powers, D.D.S., of Memphis, who was a leading figure in dental education and statutory regulation, was elected as President of the Tennessee State Dental Association in 1922. During his year in office he had a survey made of all the dental practice laws which had been enacted in Tennessee, and he did the entire dental profession a great service in editing and codifying these practice laws. In 1928 he achieved national prominence as one of the five dentists who organized the National Board of Dental Examiners as a standing committee of the American Dental Association.[16] Dr. Powers had received his D.D.S. degree from Vanderbilt University, but he practiced dentistry in Memphis and was a Lecturer on the faculty of the University of Tennessee College of Dentistry. He remained as a member of the National Association of Dental Examiners for 18 years, representing the Board of Tennessee. Dr. Powers was also a Fellow of the American College of Dentists.[12] In 1920 Dr. Richard Doggett Dean invented the first prosthetics surveyor known to dentistry. Like a topographical survey, it mapped the contours of the mouth and jaws to align dentures for a proper fit.[17] The U.T. College of Dentistry Chemico-pathological Laboratory was organized by Dr. Dean in 1924 and was the first of its kind in an American dental school. Robert Boyd Bogle received an M.D. degree from Vanderbilt University and a D.D.S. degree from Northwestern University. He practiced general dentistry for 23 years, then entered the exclusive practice of exodontia and radiography, a field in which he excelled. He was extremely concerned with dental education throughout the State of Tennessee and was President of the Tennessee State Dental Association in 1904. He was a Fellow of the American College of Dentists, as well as many other professional dental and medical societies. From 1928–1930 he served as President of the American Dental Association (Figure 72).[12,13]

Beginning with the 1924–1925 school term, the U.T. College of Dentistry required one year of college predental work for admission. President

Morgan approved the purchase of all new chairs for the U.T. Dental Infirmary. In 1925, the Education Council of the American Dental Association granted the University of Tennessee College of Dentistry a class "A" rating. The Dental Hygienist Program commenced in the 1926–1927 term with three students.[11,12,13]

To many of the students who received their education at the University of Tennessee, Memphis, Microbiology and Medical Bacteriology are synonymous with "Dr. Mike". Israel David Michelson, M.D. was born on July 8, 1897 in Baltimore, Maryland. He came to the University of Tennessee in 1923 from the Johns Hopkins University, where he received both the A.B. and M.D. degrees and was trained in Pathology under the tutelage of Dr. W. G. McCallum, successor to William Henry Welch, M.D., in the Chair of Pathology at the Johns Hopkins University School of Medicine. His internship was previously taken at the Mount Sinai Hospital in Baltimore. Although trained as a Pathologist and being a Diplomate of the American Board of Pathology, Dr. Michelson is best remembered as an inspiring teacher of Microbiology and Immunology to scores of medical, dental, graduate, pharmacy, and medical technology students. He is shown in Figure 73, working at his microscope. In response to the need of the University of Tennessee for a program of teaching in Medical Bacteriology, Dr. Michelson organized the effort and continued to teach the subject throughout his career. He served with distinction as a member of the University of Tennessee medical faculty for 44 years, advancing through the academic ranks from Instructor to Professor of Pathology and Microbiology. He was named Professor Emeritus upon his retirement from the University faculty in 1967. His excellence as a teacher was equaled only by his proficiency as a researcher. Many U.T. graduate students will remember Dr. Michelson as a Graduate Faculty Committee Member who always gave freely of his imaginative and innovative ideas for research problems in biomedical science. His principal research interests and scientific publications were on the subject of microbial genetics and anaerobic and fungal infections. He was a Fellow of the American Association for the Advancement of Science and a Diplomate of the American Board of Pathology. In addition he was Co-founder of the Memphis Society of Pathologists, and also, he was the Co-founder of the Memphis Medical Journal Club. On November 21, 1971 he was honored at a presentation ceremony in the Student-Alumni Center for the establishment of the Israel David Michelson Visiting Professorship in Pathology and a Commemorative Plaque with his head and name in marble, which was subsequently placed in the entrance foyer of the University of Tennessee Institute of Pathology.[40]

As a student, I recall "Dr. Mike", or "Black Mike" as he was often called, quite well. He was an excellent, but exacting Professor who was a stickler on working the full length of the long, arduous laboratory sessions, e.g. inoculating agar plates, checking cultures, etc., *ad infinitum*. It was spring quarter, and our class team (Dental-September, 1955) was doing quite well in the U.T. Intramural Softball League. We pleaded with him for a little more

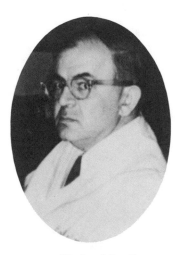

FIGURE 73: *Israel David Michelson, M.D. (1897–1977) Professor of Pathology and Microbiology, 1923–1967*

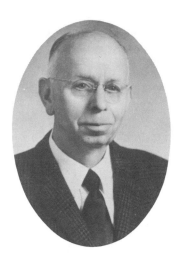

FIGURE 74: *Lemuel Whitley Diggs, M.D. (1900–)*
Emeritus Professor, Department of Medicine-Hematology, U.T. College of Medicine

time off, and after we had won several straight games, he begrudgingly let us out a bit early, then became our enthusiastic patron and let us slip off even earlier. His generosity paid off because the team did win the championship as "Black Mike's Boys".

In the spring of 1926, Dr. Hyman determined to establish a Division of Pediatrics, separating instruction in this specialty from that of General Medicine, with which it had been merged up to that particular time. Dr. Edward Clay Mitchell was appointed Chief of the Division of Pediatrics in 1926. Prior to his medical training, Dr. Mitchell had attended the West Point Military Academy. During World War I he was appointed Colonel, Medical Corps, U.S. Army and became Commanding Officer of a Base Hospital in France. It is interesting to note that of the first four individuals who served as Chairman of the U.T. Memphis Department of Pediatrics, two served in different wars, World War I and World War II, as Colonels, and both commanded overseas hospitals. Later in 1936, Dr. Mitchell succeeded in establishing an independent Department of Pediatrics, which was no longer merely a part of the Department of Medicine, as had been the custom in many medical schools for decades. He served as the Department and Division Chairman from 1926–1939. In 1928 Dr. Edward C. Mitchell established the first Children's Hospital in the City of Memphis. It was named the John Gaston Children's Hospital and was part of the John Gaston Hospital complex.[11,21]

In 1929 the City of Memphis extended only about one mile beyond East Parkway and had reached approximately 249,500 individuals in population.[14] It was in that year that Lemuel Whitley Diggs, M.D. (Figure 74) joined the faculty of the U.T. College of Medicine. He had obtained his B.A. and M.A. degrees from Randolph-Macon College in Virginia and his M.D. degree in 1926 from Johns Hopkins University School of Medicine.[4,7]

Dr. Diggs made outstanding medical contributions in five major fields of interest. He was an excellent teacher of Clinical Pathology, and many of his former medical students will recall his colorful, descriptive expressions, such as: "The phagocytic histiocyte surrounded by nucleated red cells reminds one of a sow suckling her piglets"; when describing a hypoplastic, fibrous bone marrow—"the fibroblast and megakaryocyte lived together like a rattlesnake and a gopher in the same hole"; "if you can't draw it, you don't see it"; and his famous admonition to medical students "when you get your stethoscope and ophthalmoscope, don't throw away your microscope".[7,14] The best testimony for his teaching prowess was found in the outstanding performance of his students during their staff years and later their medical practice. His second major achievement was the training of medical technologists. He was deeply involved in this pioneer program at U.T. Memphis and carried a major load of that responsibility from the time he first arrived. As a member of the Council of Hematology of the American Society of Clinical Pathologists, he was a prime mover in the setting of standards for medical technology and the certification of clinical pathology laboratories. The Governor of Tennessee appointed him Chairman of the Educational

Advisory Committee for the Tennessee Medical Laboratory Act.[14]

One of Dr. Lem Diggs' greatest medical pioneering efforts, however, was in the blood bank field. During the 1930's, Memphis held the sad distinction of having one of the highest mortality rates for obstetrical patients in the United States; the major cause of these deaths was loss of blood. Dr. Diggs established a blood bank at the John Gaston Hospital in 1938—the first one in the South, and the fourth one in the United States (hospitals in Chicago, Philadelphia, and Los Angeles had been the first three).[14] It had been demonstrated in the Spanish Civil War that refrigerated blood could be stored and given safely, with proper typing. Dr. J. Lucius McGehee, U.T. Professor of Surgery, helped to overcome the objections raised by older physicians in Memphis.[14]

The fourth area of medical accomplishment by Dr. Diggs was one of his main loves and life long interests, sickle cell anemia—which was to make him recognized internationally as an authority on this subject. In his early work he placed emphasis on autopsy data of sickle cell cases and clinical laboratory diagnosis. One of his major contributions was to assemble scientific publications reporting any aspects of sickle cell disease; this library research continued over more than 30 years and resulted in a collection of over 3,000 reprints as a reference source for other investigators throughout the U.T. Medical Units. The wives of the Bluff City Medical and Pharmaceutical Society donated both work time and money to provide funds to bind the sickle cell anemia literature. The 64 volumes comprise the world's best collection of publications on this topic. It has also been placed on microfilm at the National Institutes of Health.[7] Dr. Diggs developed numerous visual teaching aids over the years, consisting of several thousand lantern slides, scientific exhibits, film strips, and other teaching aids, each of which illustrate the various aspects of sickle cell anemia.[15]

His fifth major contribution was the publication of the several editions of *The Morphology of Human Blood Cells* in collaboration with Dorothy Sturm and Ann Bell (Appendix J). The magnificently well-illustrated plates by Dorothy Sturm, a Memphis artist, were issued earlier by Abbott Laboratories in Chicago and were circulated internationally among medical students and practicing physicians.[4,7] Dr. Lem Diggs was appointed as a Goodman Professor of Medicine in 1968 and Professor Emeritus in Medicine-Hematology in 1969.

One of the more dynamic, energetic clinical figures in the history of U.T. Memphis was John Lucius McGehee, Jr., M.D. (Figure 75). He was born in Como, Mississippi, received a B.A. from Millsaps College in 1898, and obtained his M.D. degree in 1901 from the old Memphis Hospital Medical College. After an internship at St. Joseph Hospital in Memphis, he took further pathology and surgical training in Chicago. He joined the U.T. College of Medicine faculty on a part-time basis in 1913 and developed his private surgical practice. During World War I, he spent 17 months as a surgeon in the U.S. Army in France, where he further forged his career in surgery.[4]

"The soul of an institution that has any pretense to learning comes to reside in its library, no less than does the soul of a professional or of an individual."

Harvey Cushing, M.D.

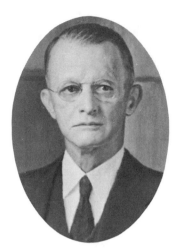

Dr. Lucius McGehee was both a skilled surgeon and an outstanding Professor at the University of Tennessee College of Medicine. He was widely known as the "Dean of Memphis' Surgeons".[4] The story of how Dr. McGehee became Professor and Chairman of the U.T. Department of Surgery is best told in Dr. Orren W. Hyman's own words:

"Dr. E. M. Holder had been Chief of the Division of Surgery for a number of years. It had been reported to me repeatedly that while he was one of the leading surgeons in the city and one of the most successful, he was also a very clever storyteller and that most of the time when he was supposed to be lecturing to the students on surgery, he was really engaged in telling stories and that these tended to be about the successful operations in his private practice. In the Spring of 1926, I asked for a conference with Dr. Holder and asked that he resign as Chief of the Division of Surgery. He did not protest greatly at this request, but when I suggested that he be made Professor Emeritus, he became quite incensed. I soon realized, of course, that the title 'Emeritus' implied senility and withdrawal from private practice, and promptly withdrew the suggestion. We wound up by publishing a statement that he had asked to be relieved of his administrative responsibilities, but would continue his activities as a member of the faculty. The resignation of Dr. Holder called for the nomination of someone to become Chief of the Division of Surgery. The three most likely men at that time were Dr. L. W. Haskell, Dr. J. L. McGehee, and Dr. R. E. Semmes. I asked these men to meet me at my office one evening, and they did so. When I told them of the resignation of Dr. Holder and the necessity of nominating someone to replace him, Dr. Semmes promptly withdrew his name from consideration, stating that he was confining his practice entirely to neurosurgery and that he felt a subspecialist should not become Chief of the Division of General Surgery."

"Dr. Haskell was a graduate of Johns Hopkins University and had had a number of years experience as a teacher in our College of Medicine. Dr. McGehee was a graduate of the Memphis Hospital Medical College, and he, too, had had a successful record as a surgeon in Memphis and as a teacher. It was impossible for me to make a selection between these two men, and they steadfastly refused either to agree upon the one, or one to withdraw. As a consequence, I proposed that I should spin a coin on the glass top desk where we were seated and make the decision on this basis. This was agreed to by all present, and the coin selected Dr. L. W. Haskell, who thereupon became Chief of the Division of Surgery and continued in that position until his death several years later, as a result of lung cancer."[11]

In 1932, Dr. Lucius McGehee became Chief of the Division of General Surgery for the U. T. College of Medicine, and he remained as Professor and Chairman of the Surgery Department until his retirement in 1948.

In 1929, Dr. Morton J. Tendler had diagnosed the first of several cases of sickle cell anemia in the Memphis City Hospital. On one of these patients the left lobe of the liver was mistaken for an enlarged spleen, and it was the consensus of the attending physicians that a splenectomy should be performed. This procedure was advised because surgical removal of the spleen was often effective in the treatment of a related disease, spherocytic anemia. Since this case would be the first time in history that a spleen was to be removed in sickle cell anemia treatment, the occasion was a momentous one, and both the senior staff members and the entire class of senior medical students were invited to the surgical amphitheatre in order to observe the operation. Dr. Lucius McGehee, as one of the senior Professors of Surgery, elected personally to perform this operation with most of his senior residents assisting. Dr. James B. "Big Jim" McElroy, Chief of Medicine, with his usual huge cigar in his mouth explained to the students, house staff, and visitors the rationale for this particular procedure and how it was theoretically supposed to benefit the patient. Dr. McGehee opened the abdomen and proceeded with the operation, but he was unable to find or to deliver the spleen. Perspiration broke out over his forehead, as he anxiously searched everywhere for the elusive spleen. He enlarged the original incision, resected a rib, and shifted his retractors to get even better visualization, but it was to no avail. He finally gave up in disgust and proclaimed to everyone that he would eat the spleen, if it weighed ten grams. Later, the unfortunate patient died and came to autopsy. Dr. McGehee had remained frustrated and was so eager to see why he had missed in finding the spleen that he literally climbed up on Dr. Schmeisser's Vermont marble autopsy table (which Dr. Schmeisser washed and wiped every day with a chamois skin). With both feet on top of the table, Dr. McGehee gazed down into his previous operative site, as the pathology resident diligently worked between his legs. As it turned out, the spleen was only a small nubbin, which was tightly adhered to the diaphragm and weighed only 7.5 grams. Thus, the spleen was saved for histopathologic examination, and Dr. McGehee was spared the indignity of having to eat it.[14,27]

Dr. Lucius McGehee was famous among U.T. medical students for his "Appendiceal Creed", which is stated in Table 5. He was both well-liked and well-respected by his students, residents, and medical colleagues, who described him as "a gentleman, scholar, and judge of good Scotch".[16] A caricature of Dr. McGehee at his retirement in 1948 states:

"Naow! If any of you medical students ever forget the 'Appendiceal Creed', don't come cryin' on *my* shoulder! You can skin your *own* skunks!"[16]

Table 5
"Appendiceal Creed"
by J. Lucius McGehee, M.D.

1) All deaths from appendicitis are unnecessary.

2) Patients dying do not die from appendicitis *per se* or from the operation, but die from the complications of appendicitis.

3) In every case of appendicitis, there is a time (the opportune time) during the course of the disease when the removal of the appendix would have resulted in recovery instead of death.

4) This opportune time precedes the development of complications, i.e. the cause of death!

John Lucius McGehee, IV, the grandson of this famous surgeon, received his M.D. degree from the University of Tennessee College of Medicine in 1980.[4]

During the 1926–1927 academic school year, Dr. August H. Wittenborg took a sabbatical leave from the University of Tennessee College of Medicine for one year to visit and study in Germany. While there, he purchased several valuable collections of important original German medical and scientific journal sets, which he generously donated to the University of Tennessee, Memphis Library. We are one of the few libraries in the United States to have such a fine collection of original German medical journals.[4]

Many of the medical accomplishments of Willis C. Campbell, M.D. were recorded in Chapter Two, when he first joined the University of Tennessee College of Medicine faculty. The famous Campbell Clinic and Hospital opened in January, 1919, but his spectacular chronicle continued on through the 20's and 30's until his death in 1941. He motivated the ladies of Calvary Episcopal Church to found the Crippled Children's Hospital at Lamar and LaPaloma in 1918. This facility was a tremendous haven of hope for crippled children. There were 55 beds, an accredited 12 grade school, a gymnasium, and a workshop where thousands of youngsters underwent treatment and training that put them back on their feet and into the working world.[41] In 1923, he organized the first Hospital for Crippled Adults, utilizing the empty Presbyterian Hospital Building on Alabama Street; St. Joseph Hospital offered the use of its operating rooms for these orthopedic patients. These patients were older children and young adults who needed orthopedic corrections before they could benefit from vocational guidance and re-enter the normal work force. Dr. Campbell and his staff devoted an immense amount of their time to this charitable work. In 1928, more funds were raised by Mr. B. B. Jones of Berryville, Virginia for a $200,000 hospital which was opened as 1928 ended. It was built next door to the Crippled Children's Hospital. A large part of the operating funds came from members of the Memphis Rotary Club and other Rotary Clubs from the Mid-South area; no patient was ever charged for being there, and no doctor ever received a fee for services. Dr. Campbell died in 1941, but he had provided in his will for the staff of the Campbell Clinic to continue orthopedic operations for the Hospital for Crippled Adults. More than 2,000 individuals benefited from its special services, but dwindling operating funds and the Federal action of establishing Medicare caused its closure in June of 1970.

Numerous stories surround the legend of Dr. Campbell. As has been stated, after he graduated from medical school, he did general practice and some anesthesia work for a brief time, then limited himself to pediatrics. Once, while he was on a house call, the mother of a sick child motioned for him to sit in one of her delicate antique chairs. It promptly collapsed beneath his 230 pounds, but he calmly got up from the floor, brushed his clothes off, and went to the bedside of the infant patient. Before Dr. Campbell could pick the child up or examine him, the mother stopped him screaming: "Don't touch that baby; you will crush him!"[41] This event ended his career as a pediatrician. He went to Vienna, Austria and trained in orthopedic surgery under the famous Dr. Lorenz.[29] Another humorous anecdote surrounding the time in which he worked as a pediatrician involved a mother who talked on and on and on about her baby's diarrhea. After many gory details, *ad infinitum ad nauseum*, she finally reiterated to him that the child's stools had now turned to "Kelly green". With his patience at an end, Dr. Campbell roared, "I don't give a damn if they're red, white, and blue!"[27,41]

In 1926 the Memphis Eye, Ear, Nose, and Throat Hospital, a three-floor brick building at 1060 Madison Avenue, was opened by several prominent local ophthalmologists and otolaryngologists. There were three operating rooms and 65 patient beds. This hospital was the only one of its kind in the South, and it had the only residency program in ophthalmology between St. Louis and New Orleans. It is remembered by thousands of people in the Memphis area because of the free clinics every afternoon that were given during the era of Edward Coleman Ellett, M.D., who was Memphis' most celebrated ophthalmologist. It was agreed with the Eye, Ear, Nose, and Throat Hospital that the University of Tennessee medical students would be sent to this new hospital for part of their training. This arrangement was attempted for approximately two years, but many difficulties developed in trying to correlate the records of the Eye, Ear, Nose, and Throat Hospital with those of the students' records and patients' records at the City of Memphis Hospital. There was also difficulty in securing good attendance at that hospital, both on the part of the Professors and on the part of the students. As a consequence of these difficulties, it was decided in the Fall of 1929 that students would resume their patient work in eye, ear, nose, and throat work at the City of Memphis Hospital. As a consequence of this decision by Dr. Hyman, several very active members of the medical faculty resigned, including Dr. Louis Levy and Dr. J. V. Stanford. Dr. Ellett served as Chief of the Eye, Ear, Nose, and Throat Hospital from its opening in August of 1926 until his death in 1947.[11,20,41]

In 1923 Miss Winifred Atkinson, a graduate of the Nightingale School of Nursing in London, England, was appointed Director of Nurses for the Memphis City Hospital. She immediately improved the curriculum and worked diligently to raise nursing standards. Miss Atkinson was quite instrumental in moving the Nursing School into the University of Tennessee. In 1926, a 50 year contract was arranged with the University of Tennessee, and the Nursing School became a Division of the U.T. College of Medicine. The University assumed responsibility for the academic classroom teaching of nursing students, and instruction was provided by faculty members of the School of Basic Sciences, the College of Medicine, and by two nurse faculty members. The program was administered by Miss Ella George Hinton, who remained the Acting Director, U.T. School of Nursing from 1927 through 1944. A baccalaureate degree was awarded to those individuals who completed two years of college academic work prior to

"The medical student is likely to be the one son of the family too weak to do any labor on the farm, too indolent to do any exercise, too stupid for the bar, and too immoral for the pulpit."

David Goit Gilman, Ph.D.

79

completing the three year nursing program.[24] The following ladies served as President of the Tennessee State Nurses' Association for the following years during the 1920's: Miss Myrtle Marion Archer (1920), Mrs. Daisy Gould (1920–1923), Mrs. Myrtle E. Blair (1924–25), Miss Abbie Roberts (1926–1927), and Mrs. Corrine B. Hunn (1928–1929).[38]

The University of Tennessee College of Pharmacy began as a Pharmacy Department within the U.T. College of Medicine when it was relocated in Memphis, Tennessee in 1911. Its first session was 1911–1912, and six students were in its first graduating class in the Spring of 1912. William Krauss, M.D. administered this Department of Pharmacy within the U.T. College of Medicine from 1911 through 1928. In 1928 it became a separate School of Pharmacy under the Deanship of Andrew Richard Bliss, Jr., Phm.D., M.D., who served until 1933 in this capacity. Earlier in 1924, the Department of Pharmacy applied for membership in the American Association of Colleges of Pharmacy; upon subsequent inspection it became a full member of this group. In 1959 the name of the School would change again to the name that it has today—The University of Tennessee College of Pharmacy.[1,8,19]

From 1911 until 1932 no academic work beyond the high school level was required to enter the pharmacy program. In 1932 the School of Pharmacy offered a program leading to the bachelor's degree. In 1944, and thereafter, pharmacy applicants were required to present evidence of the completion of one year of prescribed pre-pharmacy academic work in an approved college. This requirement was raised to two years when the American Association of Colleges of Pharmacy and the American Council on Pharmaceutical Education adopted a resolution that no student who began a pharmacy or pre-pharmacy curriculum in or after April of 1960 should be permitted to enroll in an academic program of less than five years.[1,8,19]

In 1911–1912, a two-year course leading to the degree of Graduate in Pharmacy (Ph.G.) was offered at the University of Tennessee. In 1913–1914, three courses were offered: a three-year course leading to the degree of Master of Pharmacy; a two-year course leading to the degree of Pharmaceutical Chemist (Ph.C.); and a two-year course leading to a Certificate of Proficiency in Pharmacy. In 1914–1915 a two-year course leading to the Ph.G. and a three-year course leading to the Ph.C. were the pharmacy options. Beginning in 1918, the Ph.G. course only was available, and this plan continued through 1923. In the fall of the school year 1923–1924, the course was extended to three years, but upon completion of the first two years, the student was eligible for the diploma of Graduate of Pharmacy; the degree of Pharmaceutical Chemist was conferred upon those students who completed the full three-year course. This plan was continued through 1924–1925, but beginning with the school session of 1925, pharmacy students were admitted to the three-year course only.[8,19]

In the early days of the School of Pharmacy, the academic sessions were seven months in length; however, these sessions later increased to nine months. The quarter system was adopted in July, 1947, with students in attendance the entire year. The present system consists of a three quarter academic year and a summer vacation. Beginning with the fall class of 1984, the College of Pharmacy began a four-year Doctor of Pharmacy degree program for all pharmacy students.[8,19]

There was a new college, almost unique in the United States, which was organized at the University of Tennessee, Memphis in 1928 as the School of Biological Sciences. The basic sciences, such as: anatomy, biochemistry, histology-embryology, pharmacology, physiology, pathology, etc., are the first subjects taught for the professional medical, dental, and pharmacy students. These departments were incorporated into this college with its own separate Dean in order to avoid duplication of the basic sciences in each of the professional schools; its second purpose was to provide a base for graduate training in medical sciences at the master's and doctoral level. It was not until 1961 that the Graduate School of Medical Sciences was established as an independent entity at the University of Tennessee, Memphis.[1]

In the Spring of 1928, the Department of Physiology and Pharmacology was divided into the Department of Physiology which remained in the Wittenborg Building and the Department of Pharmacology which moved into the new Crowe Building. In 1922, Dr. T. P. Nash had returned to the U.T. Medical Units after obtaining his Ph.D. degree from Cornell University Medical College. His degree was earned under the tutelage of Stanley R. Benedict, Ph.D., Professor of Biochemistry. In his doctoral studies, Dr. Nash devised a new sensitive method for determination of ammonia in blood and showed that the blood efferent to the kidney had a higher ammonia content than the blood afferent, thus establishing the role of the kidney in ammonia synthesis.[11,42] Dr. Nash taught both chemistry and biochemistry in Eve Hall. He played an important role in the design of the Wittenborg Anatomy Building, which in the late 1920's housed the Departments of Anatomy, Biochemistry, and Physiology; the Department of Biochemistry and the Department of Physiology later moved in 1954 to the Nash Biochemistry-Physiology Building, which Dr. Nash and other faculty members helped to design.

Together, Dr. Nash and Dr. Hyman organized the School of Biological Sciences, which was composed of the Basic Science Departments of the U.T. Medical Units. Dr. Nash served as Dean of this School from 1928 through 1960. He strongly promoted graduate training in the basic medical sciences, and in the late 1920's he established a position known as "Teaching Fellow". The purpose of this arrangement was to facilitate the enrollment of graduate students in the Basic Medical Sciences, since it enabled Dr. Nash to pay them a small salary to cover their living expenses while in school. Before his administrative duties became so heavy, Dr. Nash was very active in a personal research program on kidney function and on the mechanism of phlorhizin diabetes. He was a firm believer in the theory that basic research enhanced the quality and authority of any professor. He was an inspiring teacher; his lectures were illustrated by many demonstra-

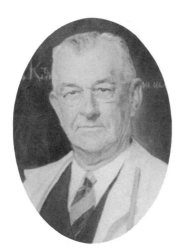

FIGURE 76: *Thomas Palmer Nash, Jr., Ph.D. (1890–1970) Dean, University of Tennessee School of Biological Sciences, 1928–1960*

tions, and his laboratory sessions were vigorously taught.[42] Dr. T. P. Nash is depicted in Figure 76. Many times when the University encountered difficulties in obtaining chairmen for the various basic science departments, such as biochemistry, pharmacology, and physiology, Dr. Nash served as Acting Chairman of these various departments. He was awarded the Southern Chemist Medal in 1958 in recognition of distinguished service to the profession of chemistry in the South. He was also a founder and the first Chairman of the Memphis Section of the American Chemical Society.[1,4,32,33,42] Dr. Nash also served as Associate Editor of the *Memphis Medical Journal.* He retired in June of 1960, having served 45 faithful years with the University of Tennessee. On May 24, 1960 his many friends and faculty colleagues gathered to honor him at a dinner at the Memphis Country Club.[32] His son, Thomas Palmer Nash, III, received his M.D. degree from the University of Tennessee in 1945.

In March of 1957, Dr. Hyman received a nostalgic letter from Dr. Edwin Orr Seiser, who at that time was a Captain in the U.S. Navy Dental Corps. Dr. Seiser had received his D.D.S. degree from the University of Tennessee in 1924. He reminisced as follows:

"But those fabulous days of the roaring 20's! What an amazing wealth of provocative memories come to mind when I review some of the activities of that harum-scarum mob; a mob of hoodlums that jolted staid old Memphis to its roots by staging the first nightshirt parade down Madison Avenue to Main Street, then down Main to the old Orpheum Theatre, where we broke down the doors after engaging the ushers and a squad of police in a free-for-all fight in the lobby. We took over the vaudeville acts and put on our own whooped version of a show that a Memphis audience had never seen before. The next time we did this, the City furnished us with a police motorcycle escort, many citizens joined us, and the doors of the Orpheum were thrown open to us. The slap-happy had been well advertised in advance, and that night the theatre was packed to the rafters. These wild forays became a regular feature of Memphis society after that. All of this, of course, was a build-up for the famous U.T. Docs undefeated 1922 Football Team."

"Even though the dentistry I practice today has little relation to that I learned in school, the fundamentals acquired there have afforded a foundation upon which has been created some compensating attainments."[26]

REFERENCES

1. Alden, Roland H.: "A History of the University of Tennessee Center for the Health Sciences", (A Taped Oral Interview by Dr. Howard E. Sandberg), 1979.

2. Mashburn, Janice: "Alumni Profiles—Samuel Lucas Raines, M.D.", *Tenn. Medical Alumnus*, Spring, 1981.

3. Braddock, Clayton: "Alumni Profiles—Samuel H. Sanders, Jr., M.D.", *Tenn. Medical Alumnus*, Summer, 1982.

4. Bruesch, Simon R.: Personal Communication, 1985.

5. *Commercial Appeal*: Feb. 12, 1960, ("U.T. Docs").

6. *Commercial Appeal*: Nov. 11, 1968, ("Dr. O. W. Hyman").

7. Diggs, Lemuel W.: Personal Communication, 1985.

8. Gann, Dorothy W. and Swafford, William B.: "A History of the University of Tennessee College of Pharmacy", *Tenn. Pharmacist 2:12–13, 1966.*

9. *Hamer, Philip M.: The Centennial History of the Tennessee State Medical Association 1830–1930*, (Tennessee Medical Association: Nashville, TN.), 1930.

10. Hyman, Orren W.: "U.T. Health Branch Is Center of National Importance" in *Commercial Appeal*, Sunday Magazine Section: June 18, 1933.

11. Hyman, Orren W.: *Early Development of the Medical Units, University of Tennessee*, (Privately Typed Manuscript Bound by Miss Kate A. Stanley, Registrar, University of Tennessee Medical Units: Memphis, TN.), 1970.

12. Jones, Madison: *History of the Tennessee State Dental Association*, (Tennessee Dental Association: Memphis, TN.), 1958.

13. Justis, Sr., E. Jeff: Personal Communication, 1985.

14. Kraus, Alfred P.: "A Reminiscent Journey with Lemuel Whitley Diggs, M.D.", *Tenn. Medical Alumnus*, Spring, 1968.

15. Kraus, Alfred P.: "Research and Service in Sickle Cell Disease at U.T. Memphis", *Tenn. Medical Alumnus*, Fall, 1972.

16. LaPointe, Patricia M.: *From Saddlebags to Science*, (The Health Sciences Museum Foundation: Memphis, TN.), 1984.

17. Lollar, Michael: "Medicine's Growing Pains" in *Commercial Appeal*, Mid-South Magazine Section: May 27, 1984.

18. Martin, Jess A.: Personal Communication, 1985.

19. Medical Accomplishments: U.T. College of Pharmacy.

20. Medical Accomplishments: U.T. Dept. of Ophthalmology.

21. Medical Accomplishments: U.T. Dept. of Pediatrics.

22. Medical Accomplishments: U.T. Dept. of Urology.

23. Montgomery, J. R., Folmsbee, S. J., and Greene, L. S.: *To Foster Knowledge: A History of the University of Tennessee 1794–1970*, (The University of Tennessee Press: Knoxville, TN.), 1984.

24. Murry, Ruth N.: Personal Communication, 1985.

25. Sanders, Sam H., Jr.: "The U.T. Docs Football Team: The Legend Lives On", *Tenn. Medical Alumnus*, Winter, 1977.

26. Seiser, E. O.: Personal Communication to Dr. Orren W. Hyman, 1957.

27. Stewart, Marcus J. and Black, William T., Jr.: *History of Medicine in Memphis*, (McCowat-Mercer Press, Inc.: Jackson, TN.), 1971.

28. Stewart, Marcus J.: "Facts on the Tennessee Doctors Football Team", Speech Given at the Dedication of the U.T. Docs Field in Memphis, TN.—Oct. 11, 1979.

29. Stewart, Marcus, J.: Personal Communication, 1985.

30. U.T. Registrar: 1920–1921.

31. University Center-Grams: April, 1954 ("Dr. H. C. Schmeisser").

32. University Center-Grams: June, 1960 ("Dr. T. P. Nash").

33. University Center-Grams: April, 1954 ("Dr. T. P. Nash").

34. University Center-Grams: Oct., 1960 ("Dr. Anna Dean Dulaney").

35. University Center-Grams: June, 1961 ("Dr. O. W. Hyman").

36. *U.T.C.H.S.* *"Record"*: Sept. 28, 1979 ("Tennessee's Forgotten Football Team").

37. Wittenborg, August H.: "The University of Tennessee Health Services Departments at Memphis", (Private Papers), 1933.

38. Wooten, Nina E. and Williams, Golden: *A History of the Tennessee State Nurses' Association*, (Tennessee Nurses Association: Nashville, TN.), 1955.

39. Raines, Samuel L.: Personal Communication, 1985.

40. The Israel David Michelson Visiting Professorship Presentation (November 21, 1971).

41. Coppock, Paul R.: *Memphis Memoirs* (Memphis State University Press: Memphis, TN.), 1980.

42. Wood, John L.: Personal Communication, 1985.

CHAPTER FOUR
1930–1939

*T*HE Black October Crash of 1929 devastated the American stock market on Wall Street; the result was financial disaster for the entire nation. Finally, after the great banking crisis of 1933, the stock market began to follow the gradual recovery of general business in the United States. The Net National Product (NNP) for 1919 was $95.2 billion; by 1933, the NNP for the United States had dropped to $48.6 billion. This halving of the monetary value of goods and services in the American economy caused financial and personal hardship, bank failures, riots, increase in the suicide rate, and political turmoil. We know this era in the 1930's as "The Great Depression".[16]

Naturally, the Depression years would exert deleterious effects on the University of Tennessee, Memphis, also. Dr. Hyman's memoirs do not address this particular financial problem directly in detail, and unfortunately, they end with the year 1939. He never was able to complete the 1940–1961 segment of his memoirs as Chief Administrator for U.T. Memphis.[5,6] The Tennessee Legislature of 1931 reduced the appropriation for the University of Tennessee drastically, in keeping with the inopportune times. Consequently, all faculty, staff, and teaching fellows' salaries were reduced by 10% in January of 1931, and again in July of 1931 by an additional 9%, for a total of 19% in cuts for that year.[5,6]

Table 6 reflects the student enrollment figures at the University of Tennessee, Memphis for all of the Colleges during the 1930's decade. The College of Medicine had increased from 306 students in 1927 to a high of 384 in the Fall Term of 1929 before the Depression. In 1930, this figure fell to 264, then fluctuated between 330 in 1931 to 306 in 1939— thus, surprisingly it remained fairly stable. The College of Dentistry had averaged 123 students per year from 1927 to 1929, then actually increased its enrollment in the early 1930's to 164 students in 1932. It then began to fall off, reached a low of 89 in 1936, and then climbed to 111 students at the end of the decade. The School of Pharmacy rose from 133 students in 1929 to a high of 164 in 1930; then it began a rapid decline—dropping to only 41 students in 1933. It gradually increased to an enrollment of 90 students in 1939. The School of Nursing actually did well during the Depression years, growing from 124 students per year to 217 students in 1939. The fledgling School of Biological Sciences averaged about six graduate students annually during the 1930's.[21,22]

As could be expected, the depressed 1930's did not witness a building surge as did the 1920's. However, in 1933 the University did acquire the Rex

"The lowest ebb is the turn of the tide."

Henry Wadsworth Longfellow

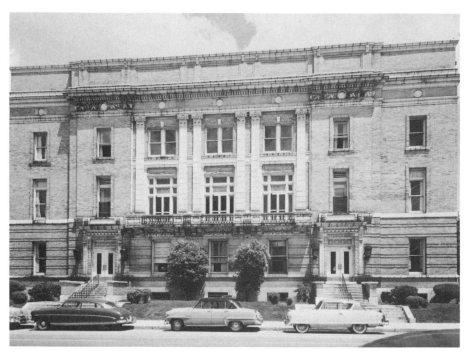

FIGURE 77. *Rex Club at Dunlap and Madison (University of Tennessee Student-Alumni Center from 1933–1969)*

Club, which had been built in 1906 as a private club. There was a standing indebtedness of $31,000 against this property which had not been used for a number of years. It had been on the market for a long time because of the indebtedness, the general depressed real estate market, and the need for substantial repairs. The University of Tennessee was able to purchase the property with the aid of the federal assistance program known as PWA (Public Works Assistance). The State Chairman for PWA in Tennessee was Mr. Thomas H. Allen, who was a University of Tennessee alumnus as well as a member of the U.T. Board of Trustees. With Mr. Allen's assistance, funds were secured through PWA to remodel the interior of the Rex Club and to place it in a usable state. It was renamed the University Center and utilized as a student/faculty center until 1969 (Figure 77).[6]

The old Memphis City Hospital, which had been built in 1898 on Madison Avenue, was demolished, and the John Gaston Hospital was built as the new City Hospital in 1936 (Figure 78). It provided clinical hospital training for numerous U.T. Memphis students for many years. A University dormitory for men was built on Monroe Avenue in 1939 and was utilized until 1974 when it was demolished (Appendix K).

Dr. Orren Williams Hyman, who had assumed the Deanship of the College of Medicine in 1923, continued to serve as Dean until 1957. His tenure of 34 years in this position will probably always remain as the longevity record. Dr. Lem Diggs stated: "Pinkie Hyman always kept a clean desk and gave straightforward answers".[3] Had it not been for the tenacity

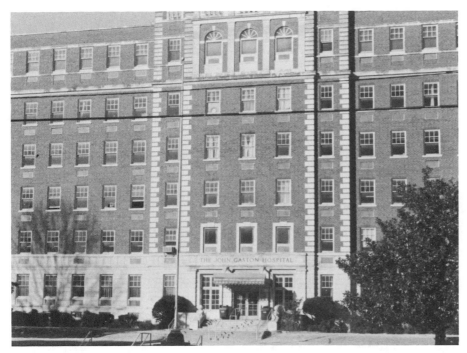

FIGURE 78. *John Gaston Hospital, built in 1936*

and adroitness that Dr. Hyman exhibited as a capable administrator and the generous donation of private funds by Dr. August H. Wittenborg to render financial stability, the University of Tennessee Medical Units would probably have folded in the depressed 1930's.[8,14,18] It is to their everlasting credit that they truly believed in a bright future for the University of Tennessee, Memphis.

Dr. Andrew R. Bliss remained as Dean of the School of Pharmacy until 1933. Dr. Hyman served in a titular capacity as the Acting Dean from 1933–1936, but in the actual management of the School of Pharmacy, Dr. Robert L. Crowe (Figure 44) prevailed. In 1936, Dr. Crowe was formally appointed as Dean of the U.T. School of Pharmacy.[4]

Miss Ella George Hinton continued as the Acting Director of the U.T. School of Nursing throughout the 1930's and managed the School successfully, as it rose in student enrollment from 124 (1930) to 217 (1939).[21]

From its beginning in 1911, the U.T. College of Dentistry suffered from lack of sufficient funds. When Dr. Hyman assumed control of the U.T. Medical Units in the early 1920's, he had an Administrative Committee of three persons. Dr. Gardner, as Dean of the College of Dentistry, felt outvoted by the medical members who, in his opinion, lacked interest in the dental program. There were few full-time dental faculty members, and morale was low within the College. The Dental Education Council of America inspected the U.T. College of Dentistry in 1923 and continued its "B" rating. Dean Gardner and most of the faculty resigned in 1923 except for

Dr. D. M. Cattell and Dr. Robert S. Vinsant. As was earlier stated in Chapter Three, Dr. Vinsant was selected as Dean, some of the Professors who quit were rehired, and the Administrative Committee pattern was dropped by Dr. Hyman; Dr. Vinsant subsequently reported only to Dr. Hyman. There were internal problems because of a town/gown squabble in which the local dentists objected to the College of Dentistry charging patients and claimed that the dental infirmary fees were too high.

In 1925, the U.T. College of Dentistry became the target of external criticism when Dr. James L. Manire, the 1914 President of the Tennessee State Dental Association and a local Memphis dentist, harshly censured the College during a meeting of the Memphis Dental Society. The crux of his criticism was directed at the operation of the U.T. Dental Infirmary and how much, if anything, it should be allowed to charge patients. This controversy with the Memphis Dental Society smoldered during the remainder of the 1920's, until it erupted again during the depressed 1930's. An all-out effort was made to close the U.T. Dental Infirmary, and local dentists demanded that only charity patients be treated. The State Board of Dental Examiners charged that the U.T. Dental Infirmary created unfair competition with local dentists and filed a legal suit. The University rejected these charges, fought them successfully during the first round in court, and an appeal by the State Board of Dental Examiners to the Tennessee Supreme Court in 1932 resulted in a dismissal of the suit. However, such controversy by the Memphis Dental Society did cause the ouster of Dean Vinsant in 1932.[7,8,13]

It was decided by Dr. Hyman that under the circumstances, it would be prudent to seek a new Dean from outside the local area—one who presumably would be indifferent to the animosities existing between the U.T. College of Dentistry and the practicing dentists of Memphis. Dr. Edgar D. Rose of Bowling Green, Kentucky, was chosen and served as Dean from 1932–1941. He received his D.D.S. degree from Vanderbilt University and taught both there in Nashville and at the University of Louisville. While he was Dean of the U.T. College of Dentistry, he also taught classes in Therapeutics and Periodontics. His technique in treating periodontal disease was widely used by practicing dentists.[8,19] Dr. Hyman described Dr. Rose's tenure thusly:

"After some negotiation, Dr. E. D. Rose, practicing at Bowling Green, Kentucky, was employed as Dean of the College of Dentistry. Dean Rose was a man of high personal ideals and an experienced dentist. He had had some experience in dental teaching on the level of postgraduate teaching in a variety of situations. However, he had very little understanding of the organization and operation of dental education in the College of Dentistry. He was assisted in the mechanics of operating the College by Dr. Richard Dean and other members of the faculty and so the College was held together and the instruction did not suffer too greatly. Dean Rose was a man of a great deal of courage and conviction. It soon developed that members of the local dental society wished him to take steps in the operation of the College of Dentistry which essentially would have returned control of the College to the dental society. Dean Rose realized that the College had to be operated under the direction of a Board of Trustees and without any other object than to prepare qualified dentists for the service of the people of Tennessee and the Mid-South. Looking forward a bit, this animosity between Rose and the profession in the City of Memphis became more and more embroiled and embittered, so that Dean Rose was given a very difficult time, and his health was materially affected."[6]

As Table 6 illustrates, Dr. Nash was able to maintain a steady program in the new School of Biological Sciences during the 1930's. An extremely important achievement occurred in September of 1932 when Edward Foster Williams, Jr. (Figure 79) was awarded the first Ph.D. degree to be granted within any portion of the University of Tennessee System. He accomplished his dissertation research under Dr. Thomas Palmer Nash, Jr. He served for two years as a Research Biochemist with the Killian Research Laboratories in New York City, New York from 1933–1935. Dr. Williams returned to the University of Tennessee, Memphis in 1935 as an Instructor and advanced steadily to the academic rank of Professor in the Department of Biochemistry in 1962. In 1968, he was named Goodman Professor of Biochemistry and held this position until his retirement in August of 1972. Dr. Williams was known as a particularly loyal member of the University of Tennessee faculty, and he taught many hundreds of students during his more than four decades of outstanding service.[13,15,21,22,23,24]

The accomplishment of awarding the first University of Tennessee Ph.D. was not achieved easily. The University of Tennessee faculty in Knoxville were highly skeptical and exhibited considerable reluctance to approve such a doctoral postgraduate program for U.T. Memphis. A Doctor of Philosophy degree represents the highest academic degree and accomplishment. Dr. Nash stated that the Chairman of the Graduate Committee for U.T. Knoxville was "tenacious" in his opposition. However, the U.T. Memphis

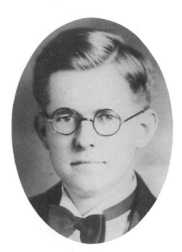

FIGURE 79. *Edward Foster Williams, Jr., Ph.D. (1906–1978) Awarded First Ph.D. in the University of Tennessee System in 1932. Goodman Professor of Biochemistry, 1968–1972*

Table 6
The University of Tennessee, Memphis—Enrollment 1930–1939

Fall Term	College of Medicine	College of Dentistry	School of Pharmacy	School of Nursing	School of Biological Sciences
1930	264	140	164	124	7
1931	330	157	121	127	6
1932	310	164	71	193	6
1933	313	122	41	200	5
1934	330	116	45	216	3
1935	327	95	49	202	4
1936	335	89	81	209	5
1937	308	115	97	193	1
1938	317	107	89	219	7
1939	306	111	90	217	9

medical faculty was competent, and with persistence by Drs. Hyman and Nash, the request from Memphis was finally approved. In the Fall Term of 1929, Edward Foster Williams, Jr. and Alan Hisey entered a doctoral program in Biochemistry at U.T. Memphis. Williams was awarded his Ph.D. degree in 1932, and Hisey received his Ph.D. degree in 1937.[9,13,21]

In 1930 a momentous decision was made when Dr. Hyman devised the Four-Quarter System, which consisted of offering every course four quarters of the calendar year. This system permitted medical and dental students the option of dropping out of school for a quarter or two to earn tuition money, then return to school without having to wait for the next school year to commence. If a student went straight through school, he could accomplish the normal four year curriculum in only three calendar years, since students went to school year-round without a summer break, if they so elected. The Four-Quarter System played a vital role in keeping enrollment fairly consistent in the College of Medicine and the College of Dentistry during the depressed 1930's, as Table 6 illustrates. In contrast, the School of Pharmacy, which was on a regular school year basis, witnessed a precipitous drop in its number of matriculating students.[5,6,23,24]

In 1936, the College of Dentistry followed suit with the College of Medicine in raising admission requirements to two years of college work, prior to professional school enrollment.[13] Dr. Richard Doggett Dean, who was a member of the U.T. College of Dentistry faculty and a U.T. dental graduate of 1922, obtained an M.D. degree from the U.T. College of Medicine in 1931. He played an important role in faculty influence in the 1930's and would become Dean of the College of Dentistry in 1943.[21] His wife, Marguerite Taylor Dean, also received her M.D. degree from the University of Tennessee in 1931 and was responsible for the Dental Hygienists' Program during the 1930's.[21]

The year 1931 was a banner year for the dental profession related to the University of Tennessee, Memphis. The national annual meeting of the American Dental Association was held at the Peabody Hotel in Memphis that Fall. Robert Boyd Bogle, M.D., D.D.S. (Figure 72) was the immediate Past-President of the A.D.A. in 1930. Dr. J. L. McDowell was President-Elect of the American Full Denture Society. Dr. Carl W. Hoffer was President-Elect of the American Academy of Periodontology, as well as President of the Tennessee State Dental Association in 1931. Dr. Oren A. Oliver was President of the American Society of Orthodontists.[7,8,9]

Dr. Hyman recounted an interesting story in 1931 regarding Dr. Haskell:

"In the Fall of 1931 I had a serious encounter with Professor Haskell, Chief of the Division of Surgery. During the previous summer, Dr. Gerald Penn, who had been recently graduated by the College of Medicine with high honors, had applied for appointment to the staff of the City of Memphis Hospital. I consulted Professor Campbell with reference to the appointment, and he agreed that I should go ahead and make it, but requested that I do so without his recommending it. Professor Campbell and Dr. Henry Hill, practicing orthopedists in Memphis, nourished great enmity toward each other for years, and in the Spring of 1931 this culminated in a fist fight at the Baptist Memorial Hospital. As a consequence, Dr. Campbell was debarred from the staff of the City of Memphis hospitals. It should be noted that Dr. Henry Hill had married a niece of Mr. Ed Crump, who at that time was at the height of his power in City control. When Dr. Haskell heard that Dr. Penn had been appointed to the hospital staff, (Dr. Penn had gone into practice with Dr. Henry Hill), Dr. Haskell became quite incensed and asked for an interview with me and Professor Campbell in my office one night. We met, and Dr. Haskell insisted that Dr. Penn's nomination should be withdrawn. I took the position that he was one of our own graduates and he had a fine record, and that I had sent forward the nomination with the knowledge and tacit approval of Dr. Campbell. Dr. Haskell, nevertheless, became quite excited, pounding my desk with his fist and announced that he would resign unless the appointment was recalled. I told Dr. Haskell that I sincerely trusted he would not resign since I considered him a highly effective and important member of our staff, but the nomination for appointment had been made in good faith and would stand. Thereupon, Dr. Haskell announced that I should have his letter of resignation the following day. As it happened, I was leaving for Knoxville on the night after this interview. When I returned to Memphis a day or two later, Dr. Haskell met me as I drove down Madison Avenue going home and stopped me, asking that his letter of resignation be torn up, that he had been mistaken in his behavior, and wished to remain on the University staff. Later in the morning when I came to my office, I found his letter and promptly destroyed it. Dr. Haskell served effectively for several years, and I was highly pleased that his resignation was not insisted on."[6]

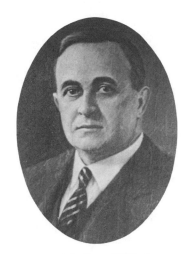

FIGURE 80. *Percy Walthall Toombs, M.D. (1880–1933) Professor and Chairman, U.T. Department of Obstetrics, 1911–1933*

Unfortunately, Dr. Haskell died in 1932; afterwards, Dr. J. Lucius McGehee was named as Professor and Chairman of the University of Tennessee Department of Surgery.[21]

George R. Livermore, M.D. was known as the "Father of Urology" in Memphis. He was Chairman of the U.T. Department of Urology during the 1920's and 1930's. Dr. Livermore is credited with introducing the cystoscope to physicians in the Mid-South area. Also, he served as President of the American Urological Association, 1932–1933, which held its annual meeting in Memphis at the Peabody Hotel in the Spring of 1931.[12]

Percy Walthall Toombs was born in 1880 in Greenville, Mississippi. He was the son of Reuben Saunders Toombs, M.D. (1844–1921), who helped to establish the College of Physicians and Surgeons in Memphis in 1906 and was a Professor of Clinical Medicine at the University of Tennessee College of Medicine when the schools merged in 1911.[1] Dr. Percy Toombs obtained his undergraduate training at Georgetown College in Kentucky and received his M.D. degree from Tulane University in 1905. After two years of medical practice in Greenville, Mississippi, he moved to Memphis where he was in private practice as well as Professor of Physiology at the College of Physicians and Surgeons from 1907–1911. He joined the University of Tennessee College of Medicine faculty in 1911 and served as Professor and Chairman of the Department of Obstetrics until his death in 1933 (Figure 80). Dr. Toombs was an outstanding obstetrician in Memphis, and was responsible for the development of the Maternity Pavilion at the Memphis General Hospital.[1,10,17]

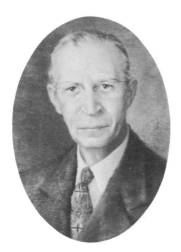

FIGURE 81. *Conley Hall Sanford, M.D. (1893–1953) Professor and Chairman, U.T. Department of Medicine, 1939–1953*

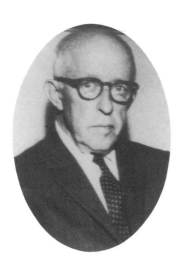

FIGURE 82. *Francis Murphey, M.D. (1906–   ) Professor and Chairman, U.T. Department of Neurosurgery, 1964–1972*

Conley Hall Sanford, M.D. succeeded Dr. James B. McElroy as Professor and Chairman of the U.T. Department of Medicine in 1939, upon the latter's death. He remained as Chairman and also Chief-of-Staff of the John Gaston Hospital until his untimely death at age 60 in 1953. In 1918, he obtained his M.D. degree from the University of Tennessee College of Medicine. Dr. Sanford interned at the Philadelphia General Hospital, continued postgraduate education in medicine, and joined the University of Tennessee faculty in 1920. In addition to his standard of excellence in academic teaching as well as in administrative duties, Dr. Conley Sanford was a well-known internist in private practice—typified as a quiet, dignified gentleman (Figure 81).[1,9,17,21]

The Semmes-Murphey Clinic was established in 1938 as the first neurosurgical clinic in Memphis and was located in the Baptist Hospital; later, it underwent subsequent moves within the City. It was as famous for neurosurgery as the Campbell Clinic was for orthopedic surgery.[9] Dr. Semmes' many medical accomplishments have been described previously in detail in Chapter Two. Dr. Francis Murphey was born in 1906 in Macon, Mississippi and obtained his M.D. degree in 1933 from Harvard University. Afterwards he took surgical training at the University of Chicago and completed his neurosurgical training under Dr. Eustace Semmes at the University of Tennessee in Memphis. He became a Professor of Neurosurgery in 1956, and from 1964–1972 he served as Professor and Chairman of the U.T. Department of Neurosurgery (Figure 82). Dr. Murphey combined superb surgical skills with an excellent aptitude for training residents. Also, he was known internationally for his contributions to the field of neurosurgery and his interest in neurosurgical research. He served as President of the Harvey Cushing Society (which is now called the American Association of Neurological Surgeons) in 1965, and in 1985 he was awarded the Harvey Cushing Medal for his original contributions (with Dr. Eustace Semmes) in the surgical management of ruptured cervical disks, and singularly for the removal of obstructive blood clots from internal carotid arteries. By keen diagnostic judgment and swift surgical action, he removed such an internal carotid clot from the neck of Edmund Orgill, then the Mayor of Memphis, and thus saved his life.[1,9]

Dr. Murphey held the offices of Secretary, Vice President, and President of the American Academy of Neurological Surgery. He is a Diplomate of the American Board of Neurosurgery and a member of the Society of Neurological Surgeons. In 1964, he served as Chairman of the American Board of Neurological Surgery.[1]

Figure 83 depicts a sketch of Dr. Eustace Semmes, Memphis' famous pioneer neurosurgeon, by Dorothy Sturm. Dr. Marcus Stewart recalled a humorous story that illustrated Dr. Semmes' wit—

"Dr. Semmes had a lady patient who was a chronic hypochondriac and was constantly telling him, in great detail, that she was always at death's door. One day after he had heard her same story of how she knew she was about to die for the umpteenth time, he growled: 'Pick a date and stick to it!'".[18]

Dr. Edward Coleman Ellett (Figure 33), Memphis' most outstanding ophthalmologist and the first Dean of the University of Tennessee College of Medicine, received honors in profusion. In 1926, he was President of the American Academy of Ophthalmology and Otolaryngology. Dr. Ellett served as President of the American Ophthalmology Association in 1932.[1] One of his most unusual marks of distinction was "Ellett Day", which occurred in 1935. Eye specialists of this area came to Memphis and operating rooms throughout the various hospitals in the City were filled with sight-saving procedures, which were done in his honor. Dr. Ellett performed some of the operations himself that day and explained his surgical procedures to visiting physicians. In 1939, he was awarded the prestigious Leslie Dana Medal—this Medal of the St. Louis Society for the Blind was engraved to hail "his outstanding achievements in the prevention of blindness". He was commended and nominated for membership by the Association for Research in Ophthalmology. In 1943, a half century after he began his medical practice, numerous physicians of Memphis paid formal tribute to him with an elaborate dinner. His career came to a sudden end on June 8, 1947, in Atlantic City, New Jersey, where he planned to take part in the American Medical Association's annual meeting. He was felled by a fatal coronary occlusion, which ended a brilliant medical career. His name lives on in Ellett Hall, a men's dormitory at Rhodes College in Memphis. His will left the residue of his estate equally to his two colleges, Rhodes College, Memphis and the University of the South, Sewanee.[2,11]

Daniel Harbert Anthony received his M.D. degree from the University of Tennessee in 1915 and served on the faculty as an Assistant in Ophthalmology from 1926–1930. He was responsible for developing the Anthony compressor, which is an instrument used in hemostasis in the enucleation operation of the eye.[11,21]

When the University of Tennessee acquired the Rex Club in 1933 and remodeled it as the University Center, the student bookstore and all of the other activities of the student welfare secretary were moved to the University Center. Mr. Robert E. Haney was employed in 1925 as the first student welfare secretary; he also served as the alumni secretary for the U.T. Medical Units in Memphis.[6]

Fortunately for the University and its numerous alumni, an assistant welfare secretary, Mr. F. June Montgomery, was hired in 1936. He graduated from the University of Tennessee in Knoxville in 1929, taught school and coached in middle Tennessee for three years, and then taught school for four years in Kingsport, Tennessee.[14] There were very few students with whom June Montgomery did not become acquainted during his 37 years of service at the University of Tennessee, Memphis. He is well-known and beloved by many persons for his keen interest in the lives of students and their families, over several generations. During the 1940's and 1950's when students particularly were struggling financially, June Montgomery offered financial aid, part-time jobs, encouragement, and advice. Mr. Montgomery (Figure 84) set the standard for personal interest and love of people that makes students

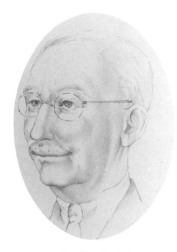

FIGURE 83. *Sketch of Dr. Raphael E. Semmes by Dorothy Sturm. (Courtesy of William P. Maury, Jr., M.D.)*

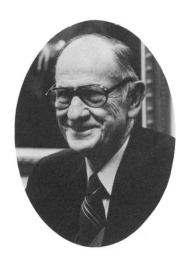

FIGURE 84. *F. June Montgomery (1907–   ) Director of U.T. Memphis Student Affairs, 1937–1969. Director of U.T. Memphis Alumni Affairs, 1941–1973*

feel at home when away from home and nourishes high regard for one's Alma Mater. In fond recognition of his continued interest and dedication and his many contributions both to student life and to alumni affairs, the University of Tennessee College of Medicine proudly established the F. June Montgomery Medical Student Loan Fund.

Dr. James S. Speed (1890–1970), one of Memphis' best-known orthopedic surgeons, will be discussed in greater detail in Chapter Five. In 1921, he joined Dr. Willis Campbell as an associate and also was appointed to the U.T. Memphis faculty.[21] However, in 1938 an important medical advancement occurred which directly involved him. Carl Hubbell, the nationally acclaimed and award winning pitcher for the New York Giants baseball team, was incapacitated by an injured elbow. Dr. Speed performed corrective orthopedic surgery on him (the surgical removal of six bony loose bodies from the elbow), obtained a successful outcome which permitted Hubbell to return to National League pitching, and extended his career for an additional five years. Dr. Speed had a keen interest in sports medicine. By a similar operation he extended the pitching career of Hal "Prince" Shumaker. He performed a repair operation on the torn cartilage in "Memphis Bill" Terry's knee, which allowed him to continue as a playing manager. He did a spinal fusion on Clyde "Slick" Castleman, another pitcher. Dr. Speed operated on another baseball great from Memphis—Lou Chiozza, a shortstop who had a badly broken leg between the knee and ankle. He was literally the New York Giants' team doctor.[18]

In the mid-1930's an important event, which affected the accreditation of the U.T. College of Medicine, occurred. It is best described in Dr. Hyman's own words:

"In the year 1935–36 the Medical College was inspected by the Council on Medical Education for the first time in many years. As a consequence of the inspection, the college was placed on probation largely because of the low expenditures per student and the lack of active research both in the preclinical departments and in the clinical departments. This, of course, was very disappointing to the President and to me and to the trustees. The information, however, was given only to the President, to Dean Nash, and to the members of the Medical Units Committee in Memphis. President Hoskins and I made a number of trips to Chicago and elsewhere in an effort to secure reconsideration of the ruling of the council. We were unsuccessful, however, and the Medical College remained on probation until many years later into the forties or fifties when another inspection restored it to full approval. So far as we could tell, the Council of the American Medical Association kept this ruling quite confidential, so that the operation of the college was scarcely affected by it, since neither the students nor the faculty were informed of the ruling."[6]

This chapter will end with two humorous stories concerning Dr. Wittenborg:

In his typical teaching fashion, Dr. Wittenborg had called upon a young medical student who was from a farm in East Tennessee to take his place upon the stool in front of the class. The student was asked twelve questions regarding the anatomy dissection at hand, and all of his answers were extremely poor. The thirteenth question asked by Dr. Wittenborg was: "Has your father sold the mule yet?" The puzzled student replied, "No, sir". To his answer, Dr. Wittenborg replied: "At the rate in which you are stumbling through anatomy in medical school, you had better write to him and tell him not to sell the mule!".[25]

Another humorous story regarding Dr. Wittenborg involved a very tall, thin, serious young man from Winchester, Tennessee, who always dressed formally in black and white and wore thick-rimmed glasses (he and all of the other male family members were morticians). Following his usual procedure of giving students nicknames, Old Witt called him "Physician", because he said that the student looked as if he were already a physician.

The young man decided to treat himself to a movie in downtown Memphis and did not study anatomy one night, thinking that the odds were in his favor of not being called upon. Therefore, he was not prepared to face the severe questioning that he was subjected to by Dr. Wittenborg the next day, as he unfortunately was the student called upon to take his turn on the stool in front of the class. After several answers of, "I'm sorry, I do not know", Dr. Wittenborg was infuriated. He then shook his head sadly several times and said to the student, "I have made a serious mistake. You are too dumb to be called 'Physician'—from now on we'll call you 'Surgeon'."[18]

REFERENCES

1. Bruesch, Simon R.: Personal Communication, 1985.
2. Coppock, Paul R.: *Memphis Memoirs* (Memphis State University Press: Memphis, TN.), 1980.
3. Diggs, Lemuel W.: Personal Communication, 1985.
4. Gann, Dorothy W. and Swafford, William B.: "A History of the University of Tennessee College of Pharmacy", *Tenn. Pharmacists* 2:12–13, 1966.
5. Hyman, Orren W.: "U.T. Health Branch is Center of National Importance" in *Commercial Appeal*, Sunday Magazine Section: June 18, 1933.
6. Hyman, Orren W.: *Early Development of the Medical Units, University of Tennessee*, (Privately Typed Manuscript Bound by Miss Kate A. Stanley, Registrar, University of Tennessee Medical Units: Memphis, TN.), 1970.
7. Jones, Madison: *History of the Tennessee State Dental Association*, (Tennessee Dental Association: Memphis, TN.), 1958.
8. Justis, Sr., E. Jeff: Personal Communication, 1985.
9. LaPointe, Patricia M.: *From Saddlebags to Science*, (The Health Sciences Museum Foundation: Memphis, TN.), 1984.
10. Medical Accomplishments: U.T. Department of Obstetrics and Gynecology.
11. Medical Accomplishments: U.T. Department of Ophthalmology.
12. Medical Accomplishments: U.T. Department of Urology.
13. Montgomery, J. R., Folmsbee, S. J., and Greene, L. S.: *To Foster Knowledge: A History of the University of Tennessee 1794–1970*, (The University of Tennessee Press: Knoxville, TN.), 1984.
14. Montgomery, F. June: Personal Communication, 1985.
15. Overman, Richard R.: Personal Communication, 1985.
16. Samuelson, Paul A.: *Economics* (McGraw-Hill Book Co.: New York, N.Y.) 1976.
17. Stewart, Marcus J. and Black, William T., Jr.: *History of Medicine in Memphis*, (McCowat-Mercer Press, Inc.: Jackson, TN.), 1971.
18. Stewart, Marcus J.: Personal Communication, 1985.

19. University Center-Grams: Dec., 1952 ("Dr. Edgar D. Rose").

20. University Center-Grams: Feb., 1956 ("Dr. F. Murphey").

21. University of Tennessee, Memphis—Bulletins (1927–1939).

22. UTCHS Graduate School of Medical Sciences: Report to the Southern Association of Colleges and Schools (1971–1981), 1982.

23. Wittenborg, August H.: "The University of Tennessee Health Services Departments at Memphis", (Private Papers), 1933.

24. Wood, John L.: Personal Communication, 1985.

25. Murry, Ruth Neil: Personal Communication, 1985.

CHAPTER FIVE
1940–1949

THE most significant event of the 1940's was, of course, World War II. The War itself and its aftermath were to influence the University of Tennessee, Memphis in a profound fashion.

Table 7 illustrates that the enrollment figures for the 1940 School Session were showing a recovery from the depressed 1930's, which reflected the general national pattern of economic recovery. During the war years, enrollment in all of the U.T. Colleges exhibited a steady increase, except for the School of Pharmacy which dropped to a low of 16 students in 1945. Even though the national manpower pool was being drained by the tremendous war effort, the accelerated demand for more physicians and dentists by the Armed Forces kept the student level in these Colleges high. Likewise, the need for nurses raised their enrollment to 238 students by 1945.

During 1947, 1948, and 1949 the number of returning veterans caused the matriculation figures to rise dramatically at the University of Tennessee. Following World War II, the U.T. School of Pharmacy's enrollment rose significantly from 28 students in 1946 to 209 students in 1949. Graduate students in the School of Biological Sciences increased from 8 students in 1946 to 26 students in 1949. The College of Medicine had 488 students enrolled in 1949, and the College of Dentistry surpassed the 300 mark at 307 students. The School of Nursing, in contrast, exhibited a decline in its number of students from 235 in 1946 to 106 in 1949.[34]

"Quality is no accident; it is always the result of intelligent effort. There must be the will to produce a superior thing."

Raskin

Table 7

The University of Tennessee, Memphis—Enrollment 1940–1949

Fall Term	College of Medicine	College of Dentistry	School of Pharmacy	School of Nursing	School of Biological Sciences
1940	306	109	90	157	9
1941	331	106	78	163	16
1942	342	113	69	148	13
1943	400	136	68	194	12
1944	414	115	36	220	2
1945	414	125	16	238	9
1946	387	124	28	235	8
1947	433	168	97	181	17
1948	422	233	149	138	23
1949	488	307	209	106	26

The number of faculty and staff members in the U.T. College of Medicine during the 1940's shows an interesting trend (Table 8). From 1940–1945, it remained fairly constant during these war years between 289 and 301 totals. After World War II and with the return of veteran physicians, it demonstrated a 47 percent increase by 1949 to a total of 441 members. A high percentage of the U.T. College of Medicine faculty were part-time or volunteers; few were full-time paid faculty.[6,34]

Some building expansion occurred (Appendix K) during the 1940's, beginning with the construction of the Bishop Thomas F. Gailor Memorial Hospital (Figure 85). It was built as a Psychiatric Hospital and Diagnostic Clinic, and it was named for Thomas Frank Gailor, D.D. (1856–1935), who was the third Bishop of the Episcopal Diocese of Tennessee, the first President of the National Council of the Episcopal Church in North America, and the Chancellor of the University of the South, Sewanee. Bishop Gailor was a tremendously admired humanitarian, who had long labored for the people of Tennessee, as evidenced by the dedication inscription on this building:

> *"First Citizen of Tennessee*
> *Whose love of his fellow men*
> *Made him the Bishop of*
> *All races and all creeds".*

When the West Tennessee Psychiatric Hospital was built in the 1960's, the U.T. Department of Psychiatry left Bishop Gailor Hospital to move to the new facility. Gailor Hospital was subsequently converted from an inpatient hospital to a series of various outpatient clinics.

The Polyclinic Dormitory was secured by the University in 1943 and was demolished in 1960. The old Memphis University School building was purchased by the University and converted to a dormitory in 1946, as the post-war enrollment increased (Table 7). It was demolished in 1965. A merger between the City of Memphis and Shelby County Health Departments into a joint Health Department was accomplished in 1942. This

---

Table 8
The University of Tennessee College of Medicine Faculty:
1940–1949*

1940–289	1945–301
1941–294	1946–326
1942–304	1947–358
1943–291	1948–383
1944–301	1949–441

These total faculty numbers include: Emeritus Professors, Professors, Associate Professors, Assistant Professors, Instructors, Lecturers, Assistants, Technical and Clerical Assistants, and other Officers/Fellows.

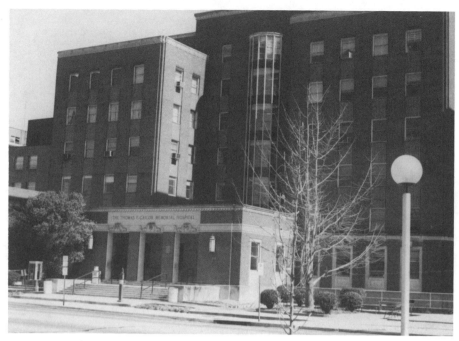

FIGURE 85. *Bishop Thomas Frank Gailor Memorial Hospital*

combined Health Department moved from the Court House to Lindsley Hall at 879 Madison Avenue in the University of Tennessee medical complex.[26]

Since the University of Tennessee's merger with the Memphis Hospital Medical College in 1913, the U.T. College of Dentistry had been housed in old Rogers Hall on Union Avenue for 36 years (Figure 86). A new dental building, designed by Walk C. Jones, was constructed and ready for occupancy in 1949 (Figure 87). It was located with its entrance at 847 Monroe Avenue and formed the northwest portion of the originally conceived collegiate quadrangle (Figure 61). The architecture of this new building was collegiate Gothic. It furnished excellent clinical, laboratory, and teaching facilities for 28 years, when the U.T. College of Dentistry again moved to its present, outstanding facilities in the Dunn Clinical Building at 875 Union Avenue.[10,14,23]

Dr. O. W. Hyman adroitly guided the U.T. Medical Units through the 1940's and continued in his dual role as Dean of the U.T. College of Medicine and Chief Administrative Officer. Dr. R. L. Crowe remained the Dean of the School of Pharmacy, and Dr. T. P. Nash continued as Dean of the School of Biological Sciences. However, important leadership changes occurred in the College of Dentistry and the School of Nursing.[34] For reasons of ill health, Dr. Edgar Dupree Rose resigned at the end of 1942 as Dean of the U.T. College of Dentistry. Dr. Hyman chose a respected member of the dental faculty, Dr. Richard Doggett Dean (Figure 88), to replace Dr. Rose.[11,34] Dr. Dean was born in Nesbitt, Mississippi in 1884,

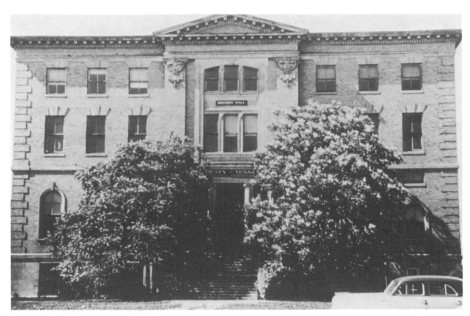

FIGURE 86. *Rogers Hall U.T. College of Dentistry (1913–1949)*

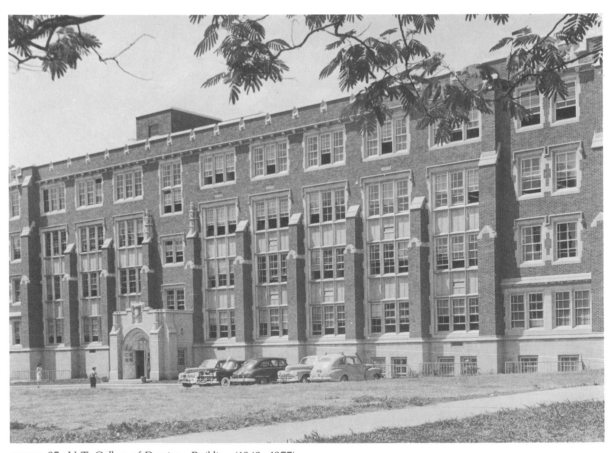

FIGURE 87. *U.T. College of Dentistry Building (1949–1977)*

obtained his B.S. degree from Mississippi State College in 1908, worked as an electrical engineer in Seattle, received his D.D.S. degree from the U.T. College of Dentistry in 1922, and later in 1928 obtained his M.D. degree from the U.T. College of Medicine. Dr. Dean was among the outstanding Deans that the College of Dentistry has had in its history, since he was born academically and scientifically inclined, as well as an inventive, competent clinician. He was a good administrator who led the transition of the College of Dentistry from its rather archaic, original setting in Rogers Hall into its modern, well-designed facilities on the main U.T. campus (Figure 86).

His wife, Marguerite Taylor Dean (Figure 89), was born in St. John's, Washington in 1893, attended the University of Washington, married Richard D. Dean, and followed her husband to Memphis when he was accepted as a student by the U.T. College of Dentistry. She received her M.D. degree from the University of Tennessee College of Medicine in 1928 and her B.S. from the University of Tennessee (Knoxville) in 1931. Dr. "M.T.", as she was affectionately known to the students, was Director of the U.T. Dental Hygiene Program from 1929–1943. She was a Professor of Oral Pathology in the 1940's. Both of the Dr. Deans made outstanding academic and research contributions to the University of Tennessee, Memphis in the areas of microbiology, serology, and oral pathology. Both of them were honor students in the U.T. College of Medicine. The Richard D. Dean and Marguerite T. Dean Odontological Society was founded at the University of Tennessee on December 6, 1948 as an honorary society for undergraduate students in the College of Dentistry. It was named by its founders to honor Dr. Richard D. Dean and his wife, Dr. Marguerite Taylor Dean. Its membership consists of outstanding junior and senior dental students who are selected by a combined Faculty-Student Election Committee. The purpose of this society is to propagate and perpetuate professional ideals and ethics; to exert its influence untiringly for the advancement of the dental profession in methods of teaching, practice, and jurisprudence; to elevate and sustain the professional character and education of dentistry; to promote among them mutual improvement and goodwill; and to disseminate knowledge of dentistry and dental discoveries.[2,23,34] Dr. Richard D. Dean died in 1950, and Dr. Marguerite T. Dean died in 1952 from a coronary occlusion.[14,32]

Omicron Kappa Upsilon is an Honor Society of dentists whose purpose is as stated in the preamble of the Society's first constitution: "To encourage and develop a spirit of those who shall distinguish themselves by a high grade of scholarship." The O.K.U. Society was organized in 1914 at Northwestern University Dental School in Chicago, Illinois; there are 46 chapters in the United States today. Psi Chapter was founded at the University of Tennessee College of Dentistry on May 15, 1929. Its charter members were: Drs. R. S. Vinsant, R. D. Dean, C. P. Harris, J. F. Brigge, W. E. Lundy, L. J. McRae, J. J. Ogden, J. D. Towner, and W. J. Templeton. The Alpha Omega Alpha Honor Medical Society was organized at the College of Medicine, University of Illinois, August 25, 1902. The Beta Chapter of A.O.A. was established at U.T. Memphis in 1941. The faculty charter

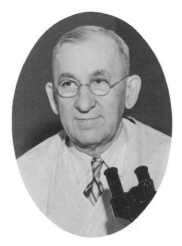

FIGURE 88. *Richard Doggett Dean, D.D.S., M.D. (1884–1950) Dean, U.T. College of Dentistry, 1943–1949*

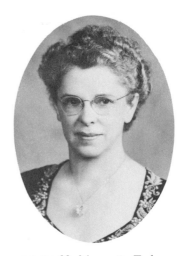

FIGURE 89. *Marguerite Taylor Dean, M.D. (1893–1952) Professor of Oral Pathology, U.T. College of Dentistry*

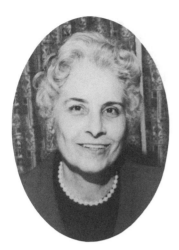

FIGURE 90. *Ruth Neil Murry, B.S.N., M.A. (1913–   ) Director, U.T. School of Nursing, 1945–1949 Dean, U.T. College of Nursing, 1949–1977*

members were: Drs. Lathan Augustus Crandall, Lemuel Whitley Diggs, Raphael Eustace Semmes, and James Spencer Speed. The student charter members were: Mr. Edwin Wheeler Couch, Mr. James Nicholas Etteldorf, Mr. Noble Owen Fowler, Jr., Mr. Jim Gilbert Hendrick, Mr. Milton Moses Liebeskind, Mr. Russell Horner Patterson, Jr., Mr. William Edward Sheffield, Mr. Ellison Fred White, Jr., Miss Mary Irene Griffith, and Miss Mary Evelyn Plummer.[2] The Society comprises three classes of membership: (1) undergraduate membership based entirely upon scholarship, personal honesty, and potential leadership; (2) alumni and faculty membership granted for distinctive achievements in the art and practice of scientific medicine; and (3) honorary membership awarded to eminent leaders in medicine and allied sciences. The motto of Alpha Omega Alpha is "To be worthy to serve the suffering". In its aim and purpose toward attaining highest ethical and professional standards, the Society is closely allied with the Council on Medical Education and Hospitals of the American Medical Association. Rho Chi, the National Honorary Pharmaceutical Society, was established at the University of Tennessee College of Pharmacy in 1948. The chapter at U.T. Memphis is Alpha Nu. The Society's objective is to promote the advancement of the pharmaceutical sciences through the recognition and encouragement of scholarship. All candidates selected for membership have completed the fifth quarter of the curriculum of the College of Pharmacy and must have shown the capacity for achievement in the basic arts and sciences, as well as the art and science of Pharmacy, as evidenced by strength of character, personality, and leadership.[2]

The Three-Year Diploma Program for the U.T. School of Nursing, which began in 1926, continued through the 1930's and the 1940's. Instructors' offices were located in the Marcus Haase Residence and on the wards of the John Gaston Hospital. Academic work was conducted both in the Marcus Haase Residence and in the Anatomy Building of the U.T. Medical Units. Classes continued, as in the 1930's, to be admitted four times per year. In the 1940's a Five-Year Program for students who had attended college prior to admission to the School of Nursing was instigated; a few students graduated from this program each year. Psychiatric nursing experience was added to the nursing curriculum after Bishop Gailor Hospital was opened in 1941.[21,34,35]

The lady who contributed the highest, most steadfast leadership and greatest influence on the University of Tennessee College of Nursing was Dean Ruth Neil Murry (Figure 90). She devoted 41 years of service to the University, 32 of which she was either Director (1945–1949) or Dean (1949–1977) of the U.T. College of Nursing. Through her dedicated commitment, exemplary ideals, and skillful foresight, the University of Tennessee College of Nursing produced graduates of the highest caliber across the United States. Throughout her illustrious career, she was always a strong believer and an outstanding leader in superior professional nursing education.[16,35]

Ruth N. Murry was born in Hattiesburg, Mississippi and attended college at the Pearl River Junior College and at Mississippi Southern College. Because of her interest in science, she attended the U.T. School of Nursing and graduated with a Diploma in Nursing in 1936. She took postgraduate training and qualified for a Certificate in Obstetrical Nursing from the New York Memorial Hospital, Cornell University Medical Center in 1937, and she obtained an M.A. degree from the University of Chicago in 1953. Miss Murry became the first Clinical Instructor in Obstetrical Nursing at the U.T. School of Nursing in 1938; she continued in that position through 1944. She became the Educational Director for the U.T. School of nursing in 1944, and the Director following year in 1945, became Director of the entire U.T. School of Nursing. When the School was formally recognized as the University of Tennessee College of Nursing in 1949, she became its first Dean and served with great distinction in that position until her retirement in 1977.[16,21,34] In January of 1978, she was named Dean Emeritus. After her retirement, Dean Murry established the first U.T. College of Nursing Faculty Development Fund in 1981.[16]

Dean Murry was President of the Tennessee State Nurses Association from 1948–1950. In 1949 she was named as Tennessee's outstanding Nurse Educator of the Year.[16,35] Her many other leadership and academic contributions to the University will be mentioned in the succeeding chapters. Her statuesque bearing, gentility of manner, alertness of mind, and professional demeanor—all of these laudatory characteristics typify Dean Ruth Neil Murry.

It is impossible to list in this history all of the young men and women alumni of the University of Tennessee, Memphis who have voluntarily stepped forward to serve their country's need when national security circumstances demanded it. Similar to the State of Virginia's monument to her sons lost at Gettysburg which states—

"When duty called, they answered; when honor called, they died."

—their sacrifice has not been forgotten.

It suffices to say that the University of Tennessee, Memphis has contributed more physicians, dentists, nurses, and pharmacists to the United States Navy than any other Health Sciences University in the Nation. It has also contributed numerous graduates to the other Armed Forces of the United States over the years. It is impossible to list all of the many honors, military awards, wounds, hardships, and man-hours of caring, competent service that U.T. Memphis alumni have devoted to their country. It was decided to list and describe the actions of those brave individuals who made the supreme sacrifice of their lives for their country (there have been 21 University of Tennessee, Memphis graduates from 1918–1967: see Appendix I) and those graduates who have reached flag rank in military service (Appendix H).

There were 13 U.T. Memphis alumni who died in World War II. Their actions are described in alphabetical order, according to surname:

"Literary men are . . . a perpetual priesthood."

Thomas Carlyle

103

Everett Benjamin Archer was a Major (MC) in the U.S. Army. He received his M.D. degree from the University of Tennessee in 1920 and died January 18, 1945 while serving as an Army physician in New Guinea during World War II.

Alton Coleman Bookout was a Lieutenant (MC) in the U.S. Navy. He received his M.D. degree from the University of Tennessee in 1938 and was killed in Manila Bay on December 7, 1941 when the destroyer on which he was serving was sunk by Japanese aircraft at the commencement of World War II.

Newton Alexander Cannon was a 1st Lieutenant (MC) in the U.S. Army. He received his M.D. degree from the University of Tennessee in 1941 and was killed in action on March 31, 1945 on Luzon, Philippines toward the end of World War II.

James Allison Fannin was a 1st Lieutenant in the U.S. Army Air Corps. He received his D.D.S. degree from the University of Tennessee in 1935 and was killed in an airplane crash in the Atlantic Ocean, while flying at night off Cape Charles, Virginia on January 14, 1942.

Earl O'Dell Henry was a Lieutenant Commander (DC) in the U.S. Navy. He received his D.D.S. degree from the University of Tennessee in 1935 and lost his life when the cruiser, U.S.S. Indianapolis, was sunk by a Japanese submarine on June 30, 1945 in the Pacific Ocean.

John Gilbert Hudgins was a Captain (DC) in the U.S. Army. He received his D.D.S. degree from the University of Tennessee in 1940 and died on January 22, 1945, following injuries which were received aboard a prison ship while being transported as a prisoner of war from the Philippines to Japan.

Claude Raymond Huffman was a Lieutenant (MC) in the U.S. Navy. He received his M.D. degree from the University of Tennessee in 1936 and died October 10, 1943 from chest wounds caused by shrapnel received aboard a destroyer under attack by the Japanese in the South Pacific.

Lee New Minor was a 1st Lieutenant in the U.S. Army Air Corps. He received his B.S. degree in Pharmacy from the University of Tennessee in 1940, volunteered for flight school in the U.S. Army Air Corps, and was killed on August 6, 1942 while serving with General Clare Chenault's "Flying Tigers".

David Edward Nolte was a Chief Pharmacist Mate in the U.S. Navy. He received his B.S. degree in Pharmacy from the University of Tennessee in 1927 and was killed in action on December 11, 1944 when his destroyer was hit by Japanese bombs and sank off the coast of Leyte, Philippines.

Lewis Cowan Ramsay was a Captain (MC) in the U.S. Army. He received his M.D. degree from the University of Tennessee in 1936 and was killed on November 4, 1944 in an airplane accident during World War II.

Robert Henry Robbins was a Captain (MC) in the U.S. Army. He received his M.D. degree from the University of Tennessee in 1937 and died June 5, 1943 from a fractured skull received in the North African theatre.

Wendell F. Swanson was a Major (MC) in the U.S. Army. He received his M.D. degree from the University of Tennessee in 1932, was taken prisoner after the fall of Bataan and Corregidor, and lost his life when the Japanese prison ship on which he was being taken to Japan was sunk December 13, 1944.

Jehu Creed Walker was a Major (MC) in the U.S. Army. He received his M.D. degree from the University of Tennessee in 1936 and was killed April 12, 1945 in an airplane crash in England, while serving as a flight surgeon with the 8th Air Force during late World War II.

The Bolton Bill of 1945, sponsored by Representative Frances Bolton of Ohio, provided for a Nurse Cadet Corps for the purpose of increasing enrollment in the School of Nursing and thereby increasing graduate nurses for the war effort. The U.T. School of Nursing qualified for student funds by completing the course of study six months prior to graduation, thereby permitting students to accept assignments in federal agencies. The majority of nursing students became cadets and served in a variety of areas. Following graduation, they were commissioned as either 2nd Lieutenants in the Army Nurse Corps or as Ensigns in the Navy Nurse Corps. During World War II, a large number of U.T. School of Nursing graduates volunteered for active duty and were represented in each branch of the service and each theatre of war. Two such graduates, Inez McDonald and Jean Kennedy, were captured by the Japanese after the fall of Bataan and were interned as prisoners of war in Santa Tomas until the end of World War II. Fortunately, both of these ladies survived and returned safely to the United States at the conclusion of the War.[16,21]

In January of 1943, approximately 115 officers and 140 enlisted men in the United States Army began training in a special School of Roentgenology, which was taught by personnel of the University of Tennessee and the John Gaston Hospital. This school was physically located in Eve Hall on the University of Tennessee campus. Those men assigned to the school took an intensive course in radiology lasting six weeks. During this time they lived in U.T. dormitories and ate their meals at the U.T. cafeteria in the old Student Center. This program functioned very successfully until the end of the war in 1945. The United States Public Health Service Laboratory of Tropical Medicine did important studies on malaria and attracted several eminent malariologists to the Memphis area. Dr. Melvin H. Kniseley performed much of his research on "sludged blood" on patients having malaria. He was on a leave of absence from the University of Chicago, and he also had an appointment in the University of Tennessee's Department of Anatomy. Dr. Kniseley developed the quartz-rod technique for direct observation of living blood vessels, using the conjunctiva in humans. His laboratory, which was housed on the top floor of the Crowe Building, concentrated on screening large numbers of molecules for anti-malarial activity, using malarious ducks. Throughout this time, the "quacking of ducks" resounded through the University of Tennessee quadrangle. Extensive studies were required to discover a substitute for quinine in the treatment of malaria during World War II when the Japanese controlled the world supply

"Perhaps no sin so easily besets us as a sense of self-satisfied superiority to others."

Sir William Osler

105

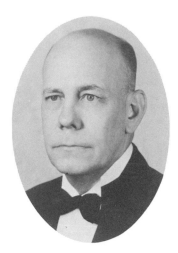

FIGURE 91. *Frank Thomas Mitchell, M.D. (1890–1966) Professor and Chairman, U.T. Department of Pediatrics, 1940–1960*

of cinchona. Arthur Pawley Richardson, M.D., who was Professor and Chairman of the U.T. Department of Pharmacology from 1941–1944; Lloyd Donald Seager, M.D.; Reginald Hewitt, Ph.D.; and James N. Etteldorf, M.D., who was on the University of Tennessee, Memphis faculty, worked diligently on the studies that resulted in the recommendation of the use of Atabrine, which remains the drug of choice for the treatment of malaria. William R. Amberson, Ph.D., who was Chairman of the U.T. Department of Physiology from 1931–1938, did important work in the study of blood substitutes which proved to be a helpful contribution to the war effort in the 1940's. This research work involved a plasmapheresis with complete replacement of blood in dogs with a suspension of blood cells in a protein-free electrolyte solution. An outgrowth of his observations also resulted in the use of plasmapheresis in the management of poisoning, toxemia, and autoimmune diseases.[3,5,6,18,19]

Many graduates of the University of Tennessee, Memphis have held important commands within the medical care sector of the United States Armed Forces. It is impossible to list all such individuals, so it was decided to list only those University of Tennessee, Memphis alumni who had reached flag rank within the Armed Forces (Appendix H). There have been 19 such individuals: U.S. Army—7; U.S. Air Force—2; U.S. Navy—9; and U.S. Public Health Service—1.[27]

Frank Thomas Mitchell, M.D. was born in Memphis in 1890. He received his M.D. degree from the U.T. College of Medicine in 1914 and next took his internship at the New York Nursery and Child's Hospital in New York City. He completed further work in pediatrics at the old Memphis City Hospital. His first appointment to the U.T. faculty in 1915 to the Outpatient Division was later changed to Pediatrics in 1917. His advancements in academic rank were steady, and in 1940 he was named as Professor and Chief of the Division of Pediatrics; he continued as Chief of the U.T. Department of Pediatrics until his retirement in 1960. Dr. Mitchell was one of the most respected and honored of the many physicians in Memphis. His many previous students will long remember "Dr. Tom" and what they termed "Mitchell's Maxims"—these were expressions that he used to emphasize points in his teaching. Many Memphis pediatricians contributed to a portrait of Dr. Mitchell which was presented to the University of Tennessee in 1953. This portrait hangs in the conference room foyer of the Le Bonheur Children's Medical Center, for which he served as the first Chief-of-Staff for a period dating July, 1951 through 1956. Dr. Tom Mitchell served as President of both the Memphis Pediatric Society and the Tennessee State Pediatric Society. He was a charter member of the American Academy of Pediatrics, and in 1953, he received the prestigious Gillford G. Grulee Award of the American Academy of Pediatrics for his outstanding service as Director of Exhibits at the annual meetings of the American Academy of Pediatrics from 1930–1939 and again from 1951–1960. In 1951 he established the annual report on "Child Health Service in Tennessee", while he was Chairman of the American Academy of Pediatrics for Tennessee. He retired as the Chairman of the U.T. Department of Pediatrics in 1960. Dr. Tom Mitchell was well-respected and admired by his many medical students and served as a class sponsor for many of the medical graduating classes; he is so depicted in Figure 91.[6,7,33]

Raymond Harrison Rigden, M.D. was an Associate Professor on the faculty staff of the University of Tennessee Department of Pathology from 1940–1944. While in Memphis, he published several important scientific articles concerning the relationship of capillary permeability to inflammation, on aneurysms of both the coronary arteries and of the vertebral arteries.[3,24]

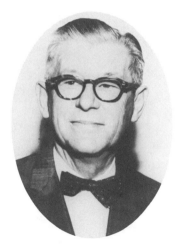

FIGURE 92. *Ralph Raymond Braund, M.D. (1903–1974) Medical Director, U.T. Cancer Clinic, 1945–1969*

Ralph Raymond Braund was born in 1903, received his M.D. degree from Tulane University in 1931, and interned at the U.S. Public Health Service Hospital in New Orleans. His surgical training was taken at the Memorial Hospital in New York, and he was certified by the American Board of Surgery in 1949. He was appointed as an Associate Professor in the U.T. Department of Surgery in 1945. In October of that year, a Cancer Clinic was opened in the John Gaston Hospital, sponsored by the American Cancer Society, the Memphis Medical Society, and the John Gaston Hospital staff. The principal motivating force behind this development was Dr. Ralph Braund, who was appointed Medical Director. He initiated a weekly tumor conference and held teaching clinics. With growth, by 1947 the Cancer Clinic had moved to new quarters at 787 Jefferson. It was incorporated in 1956 as the West Tennessee Cancer Clinic; the Cancer Clinic continued to grow, and in 1959 was able through a special gift to purchase the first cobalt radiation treatment unit in the Mid-South area. Through many generous gifts, especially from the Belz, Kriger, and Lowenstein families, a new building was opened in October of 1964 at Three North Dunlap. Dr. Braund also established the first Tumor Registry in the Mid-South during the 1950's. He served as President of the Society of Head and Neck Surgeons, President of the James Ewing Society, and President of the Tennessee Division of the American Cancer Society (he received their Outstanding Service Award in 1957). In 1960, he also received the Memphis Newspaper Guild's Outstanding Citizen Award. To commemorate the many outstanding contributions that Dr. Braund made toward both medicine and cancer research, the Belz family established the Ralph Raymond Braund Distinguished Visiting Professorship in 1986 (Figure 92).

Philip Merriweather Lewis, M.D., assisted by Dr. Ralph O. Rychener, in 1940 performed the first diathermy operation in the United States on an angioma of the retina. Dr. Lewis was President of the Memphis and Shelby County Medical Society in 1955 and President of the American Ophthalmological Society in 1966–1967.[3] Ralph O. Rychener, M.D. established the first Ophthalmology Residency Program at the John Gaston Hospital in 1945. Dr. Rychener served as President of the Memphis and Shelby County Medical Society and as President of the Tennessee State Medical Society. He was one of the original founders of the National

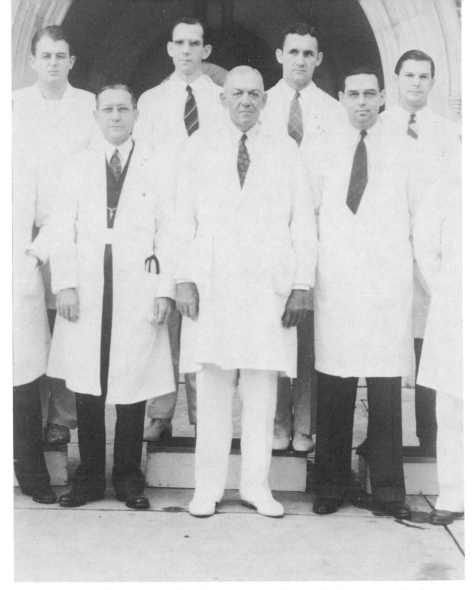

FIGURE 93. *Dr. Willis C. Campbell in 1941 with his residents/staff, left to right in the front row: Joe Frank Hamilton, M.D.; Willis C. Campbell, M.D.; Harold B. Boyd, M.D.; left to right in the back row: Dale E. Fox, M.D.; C. C. McReynolds, M.D.; Marcus J. Stewart, M.D.; and F. O. McGehee, M.D. (Courtesy of the Health Sciences Museum Foundation)*

Foundation for Eye Care and served as its first President until his death in 1962.[3,26] Dr. Edward Clay Mitchell, who had served as Chairman of the U.T. Department of Pediatrics from 1921–1939, also served as President of the American Academy of Pediatrics from 1941–42.[7]

Death dealt two severe, untimely losses to the University of Tennessee, Memphis in 1941 with the passing of two of its pioneer giants—August Hermsmeier Wittenborg, M.D. at age 58 and Willis Cohoon Campbell, M.D. at age 61. They will both be long remembered—for their many contributions—and in the fond memory of their students and residents. Dr. Willis Campbell is seen with some of his residents and staff of the Campbell Clinic in Figure 93.

Upon Dr. Campbell's death in 1941, James Spencer Speed, M.D. became Professor and Chairman of the U.T. Department of Orthopedics, and Chief-of-Staff of the Campbell Clinic.[1,12] Figure 94 depicts Dr. Speed around 1922, shortly after his association with Dr. Willis Campbell and the opening of the Campbell Clinic in January of 1921.[1] He was born in Rapid City, South Dakota in 1890, returned with his parents to Virginia, and graduated from the University of Virginia in 1912. His M.D. degree was received from Johns Hopkins University Medical School in 1916. He began his general surgery residency at Union Memorial Hospital in Baltimore, and he obtained valuable practical experience as a surgeon with the American Expeditionary Force in France during World War I.[1,4,25]

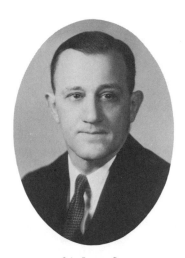

FIGURE 94. *James Spencer Speed, M.D. (1890–1970) Professor and Chairman, U.T. Department of Orthopedics, 1941–1962 (Courtesy of A. Hoyt Crenshaw, M.D.)*

Following the War, he completed another year of residency training at the Hospital for Women of Maryland in Baltimore and was ready to set up practice in a Southern city. Dr. Marcus Stewart described how Dr. Speed's affiliation with the Campbell Clinic developed, thusly:

"Armed with letters of recommendation to five or six prominent Memphis surgeons, including Dr. Campbell, Dr. Speed toured the facilities. Dr. Campbell was out of town, so he left a note with his card. Electing a solo practice in general surgery and gynecology, he rented half an office in Memphis and departed for Roanoke and a few weeks of vacation. But on arriving home, he found a telegram from Dr. Campbell requesting that he return to Memphis promptly for an interview. Dr. Campbell needed help; Dr. Speed was broke and needed a job. In only three days they reached an understanding. At this stage, Dr. Speed had little knowledge of orthopedic surgery, but he was interested, and Dr. Campbell assured him that with his training in general surgery, and his brief experience in traumatology in the war, he could learn the necessary orthopedic details within a year.

Another unusual circumstance was in their relationship. In those days, outstanding surgeons of professorial rank usually surrounded themselves with subordinates, who stayed three or four years and departed. But in this instance, at the end of a year, and according to their original agreement, Dr. Speed had become a partner. This was an entirely different psychological arrangement, permitting to each man the rapid development of an independent practice without consciousness of difference in rank, and without interference or jealousy. This rapport not only existed throughout their association, but established a tone which is true of the Campbell Clinic today."[1]

Dr. Speed became a nationally recognized orthopedic surgeon and a participant in many prestigious medical societies, among which were: the Clinical Orthopedic Society in 1923, the American Orthopedic Association in 1926, the American Academy of Orthopedic Surgeons in 1934, the American Board of Orthopedic Surgery in 1935 (he served for nine years), the Board of Trustees of the *Journal of Bone and Joint Surgery* in 1956, and the Advisory Board of the National Shriners Hospital in 1957. Dr. Speed also served as President of the Clinical Orthopedic Society in 1944. He was elected as an honorary member of the British Orthopaedic Association. In 1951 another great honor was bestowed upon him when he served as President of the American Orthopedic Association.[1,4,25,26]

Dr. Speed once said, "Surgical judgment is that very indefinable quality

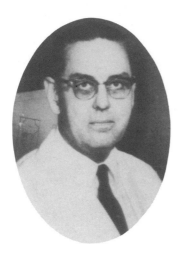

FIGURE 95. *Harold Buhalts Boyd, M.D. (1904–1981) Professor and Chairman, U.T. Department of Orthopedics, 1958–1971*

based upon experience; experience is based upon poor surgical judgment."[1]

When Dr. Speed retired from the University of Tennessee and as Chief-of-Staff at the Campbell Clinic in 1962, he was succeeded by Dr. Harold B. Boyd. Harold Buhalts Boyd was born in Chattanooga, Tennessee in 1904. After attending Emmanuel Missionary College in Michigan, he entered the College of Medical Evangelists (now named Loma Linda University) and received his M.D. degree in 1932. He took his surgical residency in Kern County Hospital, Bakersfield, California from 1932–1934. His orthopedic residency was taken at the Campbell Clinic from 1934–1936. Dr. Boyd remained on the Campbell Clinic Staff from 1938 until 1974; he was Chief-of-Staff from 1962 until 1971.

Dr. Harold Boyd was a member of the U.T. College of Medicine faculty in the Department of Orthopedics from 1940 until 1977. He was Professor and Chairman of the U.T. Department of Orthopedics from 1958 until 1971 (Figure 95). He was certified by the American Board of Orthopedic Surgery in 1938, and also served as a member of the Board from 1964 through 1968, when he was Vice President. Dr. Boyd was a nationally known orthopedic surgeon and held leadership positions in many professional societies. Within the American Academy of Orthopedic Surgeons, from 1947 to 1952 he served as Secretary, and in 1953, he was elected President. Dr. Boyd was also an honorary member of the British Orthopaedic Association, and he was President of the Tennessee Chapter of the American College of Surgeons in 1965. He served as a Trustee from 1966 to 1972 on the *Journal of Bone and Joint Surgery*. In 1973 Dr. Boyd was given an award as Tennessee Physician of the Year. Dr. Boyd was also widely known internationally as an orthopedic surgeon, and in 1953 Brazil awarded him the National Order of the Southern Cross.

He contributed more than 60 articles to the scientific literature and participated in six editions of *Campbell's Operative Orthopaedics.* His interest in research continued throughout his lifetime, and his original contributions in clinical areas consisted of: dual-onlay bone grafts for non-unions, an anatomical approach for exposure of the radial head and neck and proximal end of the ulna, amputation of the foot with tibiocalcaneal fusion, and disarticulation of the hip. His research interests also included such areas as compression plates for the fixation of forearm fractures, total hip replacements, and the electrical stimulation of the bone for non-union.[4,9,25] The best summation of Dr. Boyd's medical accomplishments and description of him as an individual is found in his memorial in the *Journal of Bone and Joint Surgery:*

"Dr. Boyd had the main ingredients that are necessary to be a good physician and surgeon: intelligence, integrity, compassion, humility, and dedication, sprinkled with a dash of humor. He also possessed the quality of greatness: the ability to evaluate a problem logically, separate the important from the less important issues, review the alternatives, and arrive at the most appropriate solution. This unique quality, coupled with his thoughtfulness and genuine interest in people, endeared him to his patients as well as his colleagues."[9]

Hugh Milby Alexander Smith, Jr. was born in Knoxville, Tennessee in 1909. He obtained his M.D. degree from the U.T. College of Medicine in 1933 and interned at the Cincinnati General Hospital from 1933–1934. He was a Fellow at the Willis C. Campbell Clinic from 1934–1936 and was certified by the American Board of Orthopedics in 1939. He served on the medical faculty of the University of Tennessee, Memphis and was the Associate Editor for the second edition of *Campbell's Operative Orthopaedics*, which was published in 1949.[25]

One of the many young Memphis physicians, returning from service in World War II, was Marcus J. Stewart, who was appointed as a Clinical Assistant in the U.T. Department of Orthopedics in 1947. Dr. Stewart told a humorous story relating to his appointment by Dr. O. W. Hyman:

"I had just returned from overseas Army service after World War II, re-affiliated with the Campbell Clinic, and made an appointment with Dr. Hyman to request a clinical appointment on the U.T. Medical Faculty to maintain my academic connection. Dr. Hyman agreed readily and as I was about to leave his office, he stated, 'Dr. Stewart, I hear that you like quail hunting.' I replied that I certainly did. Dr. Hyman then asked, 'Why haven't you ever invited me to go with you before?' I responded, 'Dean, when I was a medical student here, we didn't exchange that many words.' I told him that I would be delighted to take him quail hunting on our place and that we always hunted on horseback. He shook his head and said that he had never been on a horse but once and that was a mistake, but he would try. When the day of the hunt arrived, I told Pigeon, a workhand on our place, to put the Dean on the smallest, calmest, gentlest horse that he could find and to take real good care of him. Dean Hyman had a delightful day of quail hunting and bagged, as usual, only three birds. Later, he thanked me profusely and said that the horseback part of it had gone fine except that it was amazing that whenever he had to mount or dismount, it seemed that the horse was always standing next to a tree stump or in a gully. In his quiet knowing way, Pigeon had done a fine job of taking good care of Pinkie and seeing that he wasn't hurt."[25]

Marcus J. Stewart, M.D. (Figure 96) was born July 13, 1911 in Whiteville, Tennessee. He obtained his B.S. degree with honors from Milligan College, and after working for one year, he entered the University of Tennessee College of Medicine and received his M.D. degree in 1938. He became a member of Alpha Omega Alpha, the honor fraternity. Dr. Stewart interned in the John Gaston Hospital in Memphis and did his residency in orthopedic surgery at the Campbell Clinic; he also did graduate work in fractures at the University of London in England in 1942.[25,26]

Beginning in 1947 as a Clinical Assistant, Dr. Stewart progressed steadily through the academic ranks to Professor in the U.T. Department of Orthopedics and has served his University in many productive ways, and from 1970–1981 he was a Trustee of the Statewide University of Tennessee Systems. Dr. Stewart has been heavily involved in numerous professional societies. He has served on or chaired five different committees within the American Academy of Orthopedic Surgeons. He was a founding member of the American Orthopedic Foot and Ankle Society, and he was also a founding member and served as President of the American Orthopedic

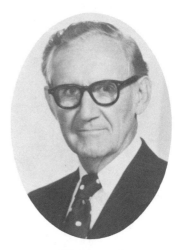

FIGURE 96. *Marcus J. Stewart, M.D. (1911–) Founder and First President, University of Tennessee Medical Alumni Association Trustee, University of Tennessee, 1970–1981*

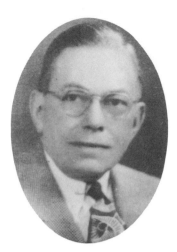

FIGURE 97. *Oren Austin Oliver, D.D.S. (1887–1965) President of the American Dental Association, 1941–1942*

Society for Sports Medicine from 1977–1978. In 1945, he became a Fellow of the American College of Surgeons. He was a founding member of the American Trauma Society in 1973, a founder and the first President of the Memphis Orthopedic Society in 1978, and President of the Tennessee State Orthopedic Society in 1955. After becoming a Diplomate of the American Board of Orthopedic Surgery in 1948, Dr. Stewart served as an examiner for 20 years.[18,25,26] He was President of the Clinical Orthopedics Society in 1958.[25]

Dr. Marcus Stewart was one of the founding members and was elected as the first and second President of the University of Tennessee Medical Alumni Association. In 1947, he was a founding member of the Willis C. Campbell Orthopaedic Club; he served as Secretary from 1947–1953, and in 1955 he served as President of this group. In addition, he served as President of the Willis C. Campbell Foundation from 1965 to 1980. From the time that he entered military service in the Army Medical Corps in 1941, Dr. Stewart has been actively involved with the U.S. Army Reserve. He is a retired Colonel in the U.S. Army Reserve and has served as a consultant to the Surgeon-General of the U.S. Army from 1947 to the present time. For his services during World War II in establishing rehabilitation programs in the U.S. Army, he was awarded the prestigious Legion of Merit award. During World War II he commanded several large Army Field Hospitals in England and Europe.[18] From 1959–1972 he served as a member of the President's Committee for Employment of the Physically Handicapped. He served as Chairman of the Governor's Committee for Employment of the Handicapped for the State of Tennessee under both Governor Clement and Governor Ellington.[25] Dr. Stewart was cited for his outstanding work on the Council on Sports Medicine of the United States Olympic Committee from 1978–1980 and again from 1980–1984. In addition to his medical accomplishments, Dr. Marcus Stewart served the Memphis community as one of the most respected Presidents of the Memphis Rotary Club from 1983–1984. Also, he was Chairman of the Board of Directors for Les Passees Rehabilitation Center from 1964–1965. In 1971 he became the third graduate to receive the Distinguished Alumnus Award from Milligan College. In 1976 he received the Outstanding Alumnus Award from the U.T. College of Medicine. In 1983 he gave the Commencement Address to Milligan College, 50 years after graduating from there in 1933.[25] His academic contributions to medicine include 22 contributions to scientific books and over 50 published scientific articles.[18,25,26]

The 1940's decade saw three University of Tennessee College of Dentistry graduates become President of the Tennessee State Dental Association: 1940—E. Jeff Justis, Sr., D.D.S.; 1944—C. N. Williams, D.D.S.; and 1949—Glenn A. Bibee, D.D.S.[10] Oren Austin Oliver, D.D.S., an orthodontist from Nashville, Tennessee (Figure 97), served as President of the American Dental Association from 1941–1942.[10,11] William Booth Cockroft received his D.D.S. degree from the University of Tennessee College of Dentistry in June of 1928. He played football on the famous U.T. Doctors

Football Team of the 1920's, and he still continues to serve as their unofficial Corresponding Secretary. After returning from service in World War II, he was elected President of the National Veteran's Dental League in 1948. He relinquished his dental practice in Memphis in 1961 to become a full-time businessman. He is the President and Chairman of the Board of United Enterprises, Inc. and its nine subsidiaries (e.g. United Inns). His son, Robert Lawrence Cockroft, followed his father's footsteps to the University of Tennessee, Memphis and received his M.D. degree in December of 1966.[11,23]

James Nicholas Etteldorf, M.D. (Figure 98) was born in 1909 in Lennox, South Dakota and graduated with his Ph.C. degree in 1931 and his B.S. degree in 1932 from South Dakota State University. He came to the University of Tennessee, Memphis in 1932, where he taught part-time (being paid $36 per month) and attended the School of Biological Sciences part-time. His initial goal was to pursue a Ph.D. in Pharmacology, but he decided in favor of the broader training of medicine and obtained his M.D. degree from the U.T. College of Medicine in 1942.[17,31,34] His internship and pediatric residency were taken at the John Gaston Hospital, plus one additional year at St. Louis Children's Hospital.[6]

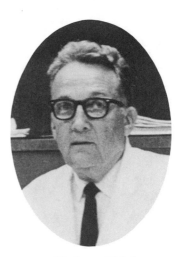

FIGURE 98. *James Nicholas Etteldorf, M.D. (1909–) Goodman Professor, U.T. Department of Pediatrics, 1955–1977*

Dr. Etteldorf credits the hard times of the 1930's with framing the foundations for his later achievements:

"If times are tough, it brings out the best in you," Etteldorf asserted. "If you have things too easy, it might jeopardize your ability to progress, provided there is an underlying dedication to achieve and serve. For me, hardship was a good experience. It taught me to seize all opportunities and make the best of them. Sometimes I wonder if people don't have it too easy. I am pretty much a self-made individual because I came through such a difficult time."[6,31]

The many medical accomplishments of Dr. Jim Etteldorf include: the first exchange transfusion to a child in Memphis and the first use of penicillin in treating meningitis in Memphis; he was the first physician in the Mid-South to procure and use ACTH for the treatment of leukemia and for the treatment of nephrosis; he was the first person to successfully treat tuberculosis meningitis in Memphis; he pioneered the technique of peritoneal dialysis for managing renal failure and salicylate poisoning in children. His earlier work in obtaining a substitute for quinine (Atabrine) for the treatment of malaria was mentioned previously. From 1948–1976, Dr. Etteldorf served as Director of Pediatric Research at the University of Tennessee, Memphis.

Dr. Etteldorf administered a postdoctoral training grant, which was awarded to him in the late 1950's and funded by the National Institutes of Health for a record 18 years. This program provided for the development of pediatric subspecialties in the U.T. Department of Pediatrics. Dr. Etteldorf was especially proud of this achievement:

"This grant was really the basis for us getting started in the subspecialty program." he said. "The grant was tied in very closely with the basic science departments, and

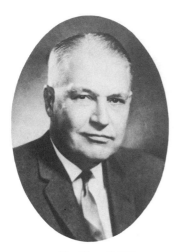

FIGURE 99. *Harwell Wilson, M.D. (1908–1977) Professor and Chairman, U.T. Department of Surgery, 1948–1974*

my earlier training and contacts in these departments meant a great deal. I was able to get the collaborations of the Divisions of Biochemistry, Physiology, and Pharmacology in establishing a basic training program for physicians who had finished their pediatric residencies and were enrolling in additional three-year programs to prepare for careers in academic medicine and subspecialty activities. This training required acquisition of clinical expertise and also led to the M.S. degree after completing a research project and thesis."[6,31]

Among the outstanding graduates of this postdoctoral training program in key positions across the United States is Robert L. Summitt, M.D., current Dean of the U.T. College of Medicine.

Except for medical school and his training in St. Louis, Dr. Etteldorf served on the faculty of the U.T. College of Medicine from 1934–1976. He was appointed as Chief-of-Staff for Le Bonheur Children's Hospital from 1961–1965, and his portrait hangs in the foyer of the Le Bonheur Auditorium. From 1955–1976 he was a Professor in the U.T. Department of Pediatrics and received the Goodman Professor Award in 1970. He was certified by the American Board of Pediatrics in 1947, was Secretary of the Board from 1955–1974, and he served as an examiner from 1959–1976. Dr. Etteldorf is a Fellow of the American Academy of Pediatrics, served on the Editorial Board (1955–1974) of the *Journal of Pediatrics*, was elected as a member of the Society of Pediatric Research and the American Pediatric Society, and in 1985 was honored as the first recipient of the Tennessee Chapter of the American Academy of Pediatrics as "Pediatrician of the Year".[6,7,31] He was also the first recipient of the U.T. Award for Outstanding Research and Residency Training in 1982.[6]

In the area of pediatric research, Dr. Etteldorf has published 101 articles in scientific journals and pediatric textbooks in the research areas of kidney diseases, fluid and electrolytes, diabetes, endocrinology, and the beneficial role of cyclophosphamide in the management of malignancies and the nephrotic syndrome in children, singularly or in combination with steroids.[28,31] One of the major pediatric events of each year is the Wild Game Dinner, hosted by "Dr. E.", as Jim Etteldorf is affectionately known, in conjunction with the Etteldorf Lectureship, which he established in 1959 in honor of his beloved wife.[6]

Dr. Harwell Wilson was born in Lincoln, Alabama on May 23, 1908. He received his medical education at Vanderbilt University, obtained his M.D. degree in 1934, and served both his internship and surgical residency at the University of Chicago Clinics. He joined the faculty of the U.T. Department of Surgery in 1939. During World War II, Dr. Wilson was on leave of absence from the University of Tennessee, Memphis. He served with distinction in the United States Army Medical Corps, received the Legion of Merit, and completed his service at the end of the war with the rank of Lieutenant Colonel.[29] After the War, he rejoined the faculty of the University of Tennessee, Memphis, and in September of 1948 he was appointed Professor and Chairman of the U.T. Department of Surgery (Figure 99). He held this position until he retired in June, 1974 at which time he was succeeded by Dr. James Pate. Subsequently, Dr. Wilson was promoted to Professor Emeritus. In academic achievements, Dr. Wilson was the author of over 100 articles published in the surgical literature and contributed to chapters in several surgical textbooks. He was a very active Fellow of the American College of Surgeons and was the National Treasurer for the American College of Surgeons for many years. He was a member of the American Surgical Association and the Southeastern Surgical Congress; in the latter organization he served as President in 1961. Dr. Wilson was also President of the Southern Surgical Association in 1970. In addition to these honors, he was a member of numerous medical and surgical professional associations.[29,34]

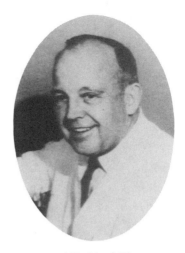

FIGURE 100. *Lloyd Clayton Templeton, D.D.S. (1901–1968) Professor and Chairman, U.T. Department of Oral Surgery, 1960–1965*

After an extended illness, Dr. Harwell Wilson died October 10, 1977. On August 1, 1980 friends of the late Harwell Wilson, M.D. commemorated his interest and good works in both medicine and surgery by establishing the annual Harwell Wilson Distinguished Visiting Professorship at the University of Tennessee, Memphis. This lecture is one of the group of similar such Distinguished Visiting Professorship Lectures which have been published annually by the University of Tennessee, Memphis since 1983. Dr. Wilson was deeply dedicated to his profession as Professor and Chairman of the Department of Surgery of the U.T. College of Medicine. As a distinguished surgeon on the Memphis scene, he was widely respected by his professional peers, and he was deeply admired by his students and residents.

Dr. Clarence Riley Houck was one of several brilliant basic science graduates of Princeton University who were appointed to the University of Tennessee, Memphis faculty (the other two were: Orren Williams Hyman, Ph.D. and Richard Roll Overman, Ph.D.). In 1947, C. R. Houck, Ph.D. joined the U.T. Department of Physiology as an Assistant Professor. Dr. Houck was most famous for his pioneer research work in peritoneal dialysis. He developed the original technique of dialysis to maintain the health of experimental dogs which had had both kidneys removed. Locally, this research stimulated Dr. Jim Etteldorf and others to conduct the first peritoneal dialysis studies in children. On a national scale, it laid the groundwork for the later research and development of a National Kidney Dialysis Program. From personal experience, I can vouch that Dr. Houck was an outstanding lecturer in physiology, making both his lectures and laboratory sessions interesting and stimulating to his students. It was a tragic loss for the University when this fine, young basic researcher died on December 10, 1955 at age 34.[3,6,13,34]

Dr. L. C. Templeton (Figure 100) was one of the most outstanding oral surgeons of Memphis. He was born November 14, 1901 in Winchester, Tennessee, completed the first two years of Dental College at Vanderbilt University, and graduated with his D.D.S. degree in June of 1928 from the University of Tennessee College of Dentistry.[11,23] From 1928–1938 he was a member of the full-time faculty at the University of Tennessee College of Dentistry, except for the summer of 1933 when he studied exodontia under Dr. George Winter, who was a Professor at the Washington University

115

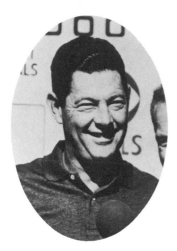

FIGURE 101. *Emmet Cary Middlecoff, D.D.S. (1921–   ) U.T. College of Dentistry graduate, 1944*

School of Dentistry in St. Louis, Missouri. He also spent a summer of training in oral surgery at the Mayo Clinic in Rochester, Minnesota in 1940.[15,20]

From 1943–1968 he limited his practice to oral surgery in Memphis. He remained a part-time faculty member at the U.T. College of Dentistry from 1939–1946. From December of 1960 until 1966, he served as Chairman of the Department of Oral Surgery at the University of Tennessee College of Dentistry. L. C. Templeton was an excellent teacher, and his quiet unassuming, but very effective manner was strongly felt by both students and faculty colleagues around him. As an educator, he was always intent on giving a part of himself to all of the participants, whether they be practicing dentists or dental students. Many of his students recall the touch of his strong, but delicate hands surrounding their own, as he taught them the proper techniques and skills with surgical instruments.[11,15,23]

In 1947, Dr. L. C. Templeton was inducted as a Fellow of the American College of Dentists and a Fellow of the American Society of Oral Surgeons. The following year he became a Diplomate of the American Board of Oral Surgeons. He was an active participant in many professional societies, and served as President of the Memphis Dental Society in 1947, President of the Southeastern Society of Oral Surgeons 1958–1959, and President of the Tennessee State Dental Association 1959–1960. He was a member of the House Staff of Methodist Hospital, Le Bonheur Hospital, and St. Joseph Hospital. He led continuing education programs and professional clinics for local, district, and state dental societies in an area covering ten states. His portrait was presented to the University of Tennessee College of Dentistry to commemorate the establishment of the "Lloyd C. Templeton Memorial Oral Surgery Clinic" in the U.T. College of Dentistry's Dunn Clinical Building in 1977.[11,15,23]

In October of 1948, James J. Vaughn, D.D.S. was elected President of the American Association of Dental Examiners. In April of 1951 Dr. Vaughn was elected President of the Pierre Fauchard Academy, an international dental organization.[15]

Cary Middlecoff is undoubtedly the most distinguished professional golfer that Memphis has produced. He comes from a family long identified with dentistry in the State of Tennessee. His father, Herman Farris Middlecoff, was an early graduate of the U.T. College of Dentistry, obtaining his D.D.S. degree in 1918. Herman's brother, Charnell W. Middlecoff, graduated later from the U.T. College of Dentistry, receiving his D.D.S. degree in 1923. Both of these brothers were famous as general practicing dentists in Memphis. Emmet Cary Middlecoff was born January 6, 1921 in Memphis and attended the University of Mississippi for his pre-professional work from 1938–1941. He then obtained his D.D.S. degree from the U.T. College of Dentistry in 1944. Dr. Cary Middlecoff is shown in Figure 101, being interviewed after winning the 1949 U.S. Open Golf Championship. Cary Middlecoff won many golf tournaments over his illustrious career in sports; the more famous ones were: the U.S. Open Golf Championship in 1949 and

1956; the Masters Golf Tournament in 1955—always held at the Bobby Jones Course in Augusta, Georgia; and the Western Open Golf Championship in 1955.[15,23]

In 1926, after 15 years as Shelby County Health Officer, Dr. T. C. Graves resigned this position, and Dr. L. M. Graves, who was a young physician and County Health Officer for Williamson County, Tennessee, replaced him. Lloyd Myers Graves was born in 1895 in Crystal Springs, Copiah County, Mississippi. He obtained his M.D. degree in 1921 from Vanderbilt University and interned at the Protestant Hospital in Nashville. He served as County Health Officer for Williamson County, Tennessee from 1922–1926; he served one year (1926–1927) as the County Health Officer for Shelby County, Tennessee. When Watkins Overton was elected as Mayor of Memphis in November of 1927, he offered the position of City Superintendent of Health to Dr. L. M. Graves, who accepted this position with the City of Memphis and served in that capacity as its Health Officer from 1928–1942. There was a long period of haggling over the idea of combining the Memphis and Shelby County Health Department as a single unit. This merger was finally accomplished in 1942, and the combined Memphis and Shelby County Health Department was moved from the County Courthouse basement to 879 Madison Avenue, which was originally Lindsley Hall of the University of Tennessee. Dr. Graves served as Director of this combined Memphis and Shelby County Health Department from 1942 until his death in 1964. The Memphis and Shelby County Health Department moved again in 1959 to its new building at 814 Jefferson Avenue, which is now named L. M. Graves Health Building, to commemorate the long, distinguished service of Dr. Graves to his City and County.

From 1928–1964, Dr. L. M. Graves was a member of the U.T. College of Medicine faculty. He moved successively through the ranks from Assistant Professor to full Professor at U.T. Memphis. In contrast to most private physicians, who rarely spoke out on public matters, Dr. Graves made health pronouncements about most events of the day. He warned that colds, grippe, or even "flu" (influenza) were likely to be the result of excessive flagpole sitting. He also pronounced against girls wearing rolled-up socks or garters that were too tight, stating that the degree of restriction of blood circulation is the health-determining factor. He advised Memphis citizens each summer about the heat—"Keep your temper and avoid heat prostration".[26] The other things that he cited to be avoided at all costs in coping with the terrific Memphis heat and humidity were hard liquor, too many soft drinks, meat, and the direct rays of the sun. One was advised to drink plenty of water, but not ice water and not to sleep beneath a fixed electric fan.[26]

Dr. L. M. Graves was certainly one of the more famous physicians of Memphis in his day. In appearance he was the epitome of the beloved family physician, as he was tall, erect, and had distinguished snow-white hair, twinkling dark eyes, and a gentle manner (Figure 102). Throughout his life he lived his own philosophy, "The best road to happiness is service", and he

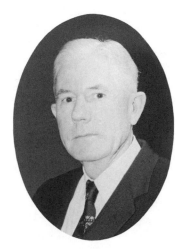

FIGURE 102. *Lloyd Myers Graves, M.D. (1895–1964) Director, Memphis & Shelby County Health Department, 1942–1964 Professor of Public Health & Preventive Medicine U.T. College of Medicine, 1928–1964 (Courtesy of Memphis & Shelby County Health Department)*

117

died from a sudden coronary occlusion in the lobby of the Hermitage Hotel in Nashville while attending a Public Health meeting in 1964. In 1958, Dr. Graves was cited as the "Citizen of the Year" by the Memphis Civitan Club. In 1965 his portrait was presented to the Memphis and Shelby County Health Department, and its building was named to honor him. The L. M. Graves Award for Outstanding Achievement in Community Health was established in 1966 to honor Dr. Graves. Since its inception, 10 of the 20 recipients of the L. M. Graves Award have been U.T. Memphis alumni and/ or faculty (these individuals are listed by year in Table 9).

The 1940's decade began with World War II and the loss of two of U.T. Memphis' most distinguished faculty (Drs. Campbell and Wittenborg), but it was the University's good fortune also to acquire in 1941 one of its greatest educators—Simon Rulin Bruesch, Ph.D., M.D.[34]

Dr. Bruesch was born July 7, 1914 in Norman, Oklahoma. He received his A.B. degree in 1935 from LaVerne College in LaVerne, California. Later, his college would award him its Alumnus of the Year in 1967 and an honorary D.Sc. degree in 1968. His interest in medicine began to develop during his junior year in college with a required biology course. The main stimulus arose from his strong, positive impressions derived from a textbook

---

Table 9

U.T. Memphis Alumni and/or Faculty Recipients of the L.M. Graves Award

1968	Phineas J. Sparer, M.D.	U.T. Department of Psychiatry
1970	Maston Kennerly Callison, M.D.	Dean, U.T. College of Medicine
1973	Bland Wilson Cannon, M.D.	U.T. Department of Neurosurgery
1975	Francis Hamilton Cole, Sr., M.D.	U.T. Department of Surgery
1978	John William Runyan, M.D.	U.T. Department of Community Medicine
1980	T. Albert Farmer, M.D.	Chancellor, U.T. Memphis
1981	Iris Annette Pearce, M.D.	U.T. Department of Medicine
1983	Louis G. Britt, M.D.	U.T. Department of Surgery
1984	Sheldon B. Korones, M.D.	U.T. Department of Pediatrics

on embryology, written by Leslie Arey of Northwestern University. He vowed to study under Arey and applied only to Northwestern Medical School.[3,30]

It was in the Spring of his second year that Simon Bruesch approached Dr. Arey with a request to do graduate work. By the mechanism of a combined medical/basic science educational program, he was able to earn an M.S. degree in 1939, an M.B. degree in 1940, a Ph.D. degree in 1940, and an M.D. degree in 1941. He served a mixed internship (1940–41) at the Passavant Memorial Hospital in Chicago.[3]

Dr. Bruesch's preference for an academic career over a clinical career is best stated in his own words: "If I hadn't come to U.T., I probably would have done a residency. However, I was very attracted to an academic career. I was enormously curious and eager to learn, and I still am. To satisfy this curiosity, one needs some leisure time to read and contemplate, to think about what one's learning means in a greater sense. It's important for individuals to learn what their strengths and weaknesses are and to find a career to stress their strengths."[30]

When Dr. Bruesch joined the U.T. College of Medicine faculty in September of 1941, there was already a beginning manpower shortage due to the possibility of war, and these shortages became greater with the wartime years. Thus, he had patient care duties to keep him busy, as well as his teaching responsibilities. His belief remains very strong that the University faculty have not only the responsibility to strive for excellence in teaching, but also to strive for excellence in scholarship. In addition to his own outstanding credentials as a nationally recognized anatomist, Dr. Bruesch is the authority on medical history in Memphis, in Tennessee, and in the South. His own excellent library is a treasure house of historical information on the healing arts' professions. He wrote 13 of the 45 chapters in the *History of Medicine in Memphis*.[26,30] Simon Bruesch was the major historical source and advisor for the Health Sciences Museum Foundation of the Memphis and Shelby County Medical Society Auxiliary in its commendable effort in establishing the Health Sciences Exhibit at the Memphis Pink Palace Museum. He also wrote the Foreword for their publication regarding this exhibit, *From Saddlebags to Science: A Century of Health Care in Memphis 1830–1930.*[12]

His honors at U.T. Memphis include: the first Goodman Professor at U.T. in 1961; the Golden Apple Award, given him by the U.T. Chapter of the Student Medical Association in 1968–1969; establishment of the S. R. Bruesch Library Endowment Fund—a gift by the 1967 U.T. College of Medicine Graduating Class; the University of Tennessee Alumni Outstanding Teacher Award in 1975; and the Faculty Recognition Award in the Basic Sciences, accorded him by the Graduating Medical Class of June, 1976, December, 1976, and June 1979. He has authored 37 papers, dealing with both scientific and historical subjects.

The greatest honor accorded to Dr. Bruesch (Figure 103) by his former University students and friends was the Simon Rulin Bruesch Alumni

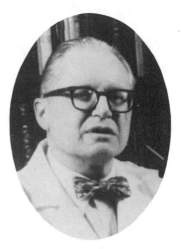

FIGURE 103. *Simon Rulin Bruesch, Ph.D., M.D. (1914–   ) Emeritus Professor of Anatomy and History of Medicine, 1983–present*

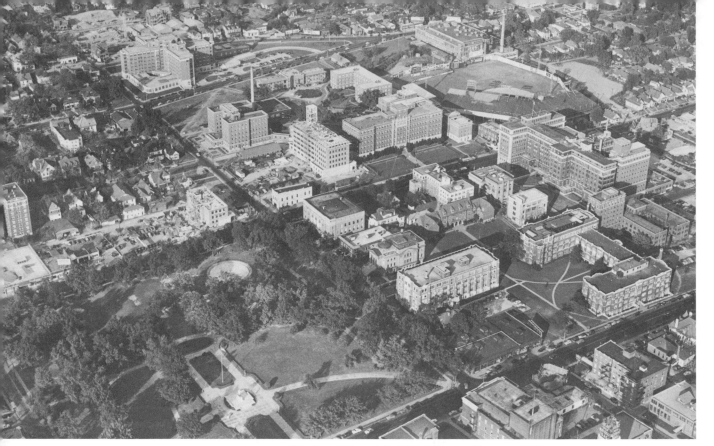

FIGURE 104. *Aerial View of the U.T. Memphis Campus, 1948*

Professorship in Anatomy, established with gifts totaling more than $1,000,000. It was the first endowed Alumni Professorship created in the U.T. College of Medicine. Dean Robert L. Summitt stated, "Never before in the history of the College of Medicine have alumni responded so generously to such urgent need". In making this announcement to the 1982 graduating classes, Chancellor James C. Hunt described Dr. Bruesch, thusly—"Dr. Bruesch is a most admired and revered member of the faculty. Throughout his tenure, he has exhibited all of those characteristics which the University would anticipate from the holder of an Academic Chair— the highest level of scholarly achievement, noteworthy contribution to the ongoing dialogue of his discipline, and significant influence on his colleagues."[30] On the plaque, which commemorates the Simon Rulin Bruesch Alumni Professorship in Anatomy, and which has been placed in the Student-Alumni Center, Dr. Bruesch responded, "Recognition of one's efforts, when unsought, is doubly pleasing. But my greatest reward is the memory of the eagerness to learn and the positive responsiveness of my many talented students over these 41 years."[30]

Although Dr. Bruesch conceded that it was a great honor to have the first Alumni Professorship named for him, his philosophy in regard to his students and as an educator is best summarized as follows: "I'm not a possessive person. I may be close to my students during the period they're in school, but I don't expect ever to see them again or hear from them. If I do, that's great, but it's not something that I expect. The reward for my efforts was having for that particular time, that association with them from which I gained something, and they gained something. That, I can remember with great pleasure and satisfaction. I feel that if they wish in any way to manifest any appreciation for what they've gained in medical school, the best way is to serve in some way themselves. I feel every time a former student of mine has done something of excellence to serve, in a way, I'm participating. I do make a serious effort to follow their career choices and professional successes. The most important thing for my students is for them to do well in their field. This is also the hardest thing that I could ask of them."[30]

Figure 104 depicts the University of Tennessee, Memphis campus as it appeared in 1948. The University was still oriented toward Dunlap Street and Madison Avenue. Old Russwood Park, home of the Memphis Chicks Baseball Team is seen in the upper right corner. Construction had commenced on the U.T. Institute of Pathology Building on Madison Avenue and the Van Vleet Building on Dunlap Street.

REFERENCES

1. A.A.O.S. —11–1, April, 1963 (p. 3–6) — ("James Spencer Speed, M.D.")
2. Asklepieion, 1966.
3. Bruesch, Simon R.: Personal Communication, 1985.
4. Crenshaw, A. Hoyt: Personal Communication, 1985.
5. Diggs, Lemuel W.: Personal Communication, 1985.
6. Etteldorf, James N.: Personal Communication, 1985.
7. Hughes, James G.: Personal Communication, 1985.
8. Hughes, James G.: Department of Pediatrics—UTCHS: 1910–1985, 1985.
9. J.B.J.S.: 63 A, Oct., 1981 (p. 1351–1352) — ("Harold Buhalts Boyd, M.D.").
10. Jones, Madison: History of the Tennessee State Dental Association, (Tennessee Dental Association: Memphis, TN.), 1958.
11. Justis, Sr., E. Jeff: Personal Communication, 1985.
12. LaPointe, Patricia M.: From Saddlebags to Science, (The Health Sciences Museum Foundation: Memphis, TN.), 1984.
13. Lollar, Michael: Commercial Appeal Mid-South Magazine, May, 1984.
14. McKnight, James P.: Personal Communication, 1985.
15. Medical Accomplishments: U.T. College of Dentistry.
16. Medical Accomplishments: U.T. College of Nursing.
17. Medical Accomplishments: U.T. College of Pharmacy.
18. Montgomery, F. June: Personal Communication, 1985.
19. Montgomery, J. R., Folmsbee, S.J., and Greene, L.S.: To Foster Knowledge: A History of the University of Tennessee 1794–1970, (The University of Tennessee Press: Knoxville, TN.), 1984.
20. Morris, Joe Hall: Personal Communication, 1985.
21. Murry, Ruth Neil: Personal Communication, 1985.
22. Neely, Charles L.: Personal Communication, 1985.
23. Reynolds, Richard J.: Personal Communication, 1985.
24. Sprunt, Douglas H. and Crocker, Robert A.: History of the Department of Pathology of the University of Tennessee, (Private Printing), 1965.
25. Stewart, Marcus J.: Personal Communication, 1985.

26. Stewart, Marcus J. and Black, William T., Jr.: *History of Medicine in Memphis,* (McCowat-Mercer Press, Inc.: Jackson, TN.), 1971.

27. Summitt, Robert L.: Personal Communication, 1985.

28. Tennessee Medical Alumnus: (Spring, 1977—Dr. James G. Hughes).

29. Tennessee Medical Alumnus: (Summer, 1978—Dr. Harwell Wilson).

30. Tennessee Medical Alumnus: (Winter, 1982—Dr. Simon R. Bruesch).

31. Tennessee Medical Alumnus: (Summer, 1983–Dr. James N. Etteldorf).

32. University Center-Grams: Oct., 1950 ("Dr. Richard D. Dean").

33. University Center-Grams: August, 1960 ("Dr. Frank Thomas Mitchell").

34. University of Tennessee, Memphis—Bulletins (1940–1949).

35. Wooten, Nina E. and Williams, Golden: *A History of the Tennessee State Nurses Association,* (Tennessee Nurses Association: Nashville, TN.), 1955.

CHAPTER SIX
1950–1959

*T*HE decade of the Golden Fifties witnessed a rapid increase in student enrollment for all of the U.T. Memphis Colleges, with the exception of the School of Nursing, which remained fairly constant (Table 10). When one compares the mean ($\bar{x}$) enrollment statistics in Table 7 (the 1940's) with those figures of Table 10 (1950's), the increase is even more dramatic: increases of 48% for Medicine, 64% for Dentistry, 55% for Pharmacy, 4% for Nursing, and 55% for Biological Sciences (Table 11). It was an era typified by a national surge forward in all areas of health professional manpower.

Table 10

The University of Tennessee, Memphis—Enrollment 1950–1959

Fall Term	College of Medicine	College of Dentistry	School of Pharmacy	School of Nursing	School of Biological Sciences
1950	473	352	220	166	41
1951	543	408	138	170	27
1952	536	468	198	163	31
1953	571	480	186	192	30
1954	604	470	172	249	35
1955	620	450	182	229	27
1956	671	442	187	229	23
1957	625	455	196	210	27
1958	639	419	189	141	24
1959	563	384	195	99	43

Table 11

Comparison of Average Enrollment 1940–1949 : 1950–1959
The University of Tennessee, Memphis

	1940–1949	1950–1959	% Increase
College of Medicine	$\bar{x} = 394$	$\bar{x} = 585$	48%
College of Dentistry	$\bar{x} = 154$	$\bar{x} = 433$	64%
School of Pharmacy	$\bar{x} = 84$	$\bar{x} = 186$	55%
School of Nursing	$\bar{x} = 178$	$\bar{x} = 185$	4%
School of Biological Sciences	$\bar{x} = 14$	$\bar{x} = 31$	55%

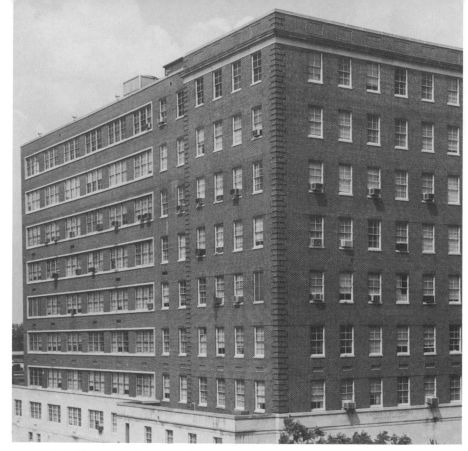

FIGURE 105. *University of Tennessee Institute of Pathology Building, 1951*

With such a rapid rise in enrollment, it was only natural that an expansion in building facilities would ensue, as supply rose to meet demand (Appendix K). The University of Tennessee Institute of Pathology Building was completed in 1951 (Figure 105), followed by the Van Vleet Memorial Cancer Center (Figure 106), also in 1951. Douglas H. Sprunt, M.D., who had become Chairman of the U.T. Department of Pathology in 1944, played a vital role in acquiring the monies needed to construct these two very important buildings. The U.T. Institute of Pathology Building housed the offices, teaching laboratories, research facilities, an auditorium for lectures, and the academic and forensic pathology morgues for the U.T. Departments of Pathology and Microbiology from 1951–1985. In 1985, the building was renovated and divided between the Department of Microbiology and the Department of Biochemistry. In 1964, the Belz-Kriger Cancer Clinic would be constructed directly in front of and connected to the Van Vleet Memorial Cancer Center.

Building expansion along Union Avenue extended the University of Tennessee's limits eastward to East Street with the completion of the T. P. Nash Building in 1955 (Figure 107). This building housed the Department of Biochemistry from 1955–1985; the U.T. Department of Physiology was moved to the Nash Building in 1955 from the Wittenborg building, and now in 1986, it occupies the entire building.[17,37]

Westward expansion along Union Avenue to South Dunlap Street was

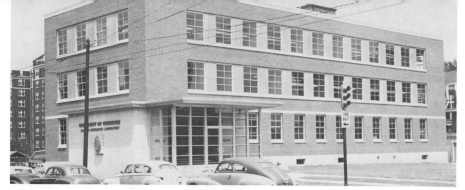

FIGURE 106. *Van Vleet Memorial Cancer Center, 1951*

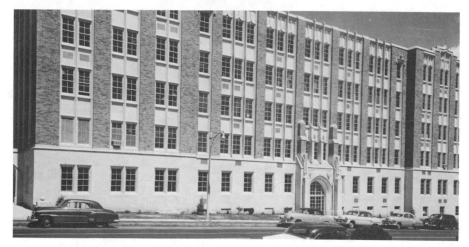

FIGURE 107. *T. P. Nash Biochemistry-Physiology Building, 1955*

marked by the O. W. Hyman Building, also completed in 1955. This building was designed for administrative activities and houses the Offices of the Chancellor, the Vice Chancellor for Financial Affairs, the Vice Chancellor for Academic and Student Affairs, the Vice Chancellor for Administration, the Vice Chancellor for Development, and the Registrar. Figure 108 shows the South Dunlap Street entrance to the Hyman Building, and Figure 109 depicts its Union Avenue entrance. A cloistered walkway (Figure 110) connects the Hyman Building with the Crowe Building along Union Avenue; further eastward, a smaller, cloistered walkway connects the Nash Building to the Crowe Building. Facing South Dunlap, an archway (Figure 111) and walls connect the Hyman Building with the U.T. College of Dentistry Building which was constructed earlier in 1949. Centered through the University of Tennessee Archway (Figure 111) is the old C. P. J. Mooney Library with the Wittenborg Building on the left. These new buildings and connecting structures completed the original architectural concept of an enclosed collegiate quadrangle (Figure 61) with certain modifications.

The University of Tennessee Memorial Hospital and Research Center in Knoxville was completed in 1956, expanded in the 1980's, and now forms a sizable portion of the University's effort to expand teaching programs and clinical clerkships for the U.T. College of Medicine statewide. Figure 112 illustrates the appearance of the U.T. Department of Operative Dentistry Clinic during the 1950's. The Bishop Gailor Hospital Annex, which was

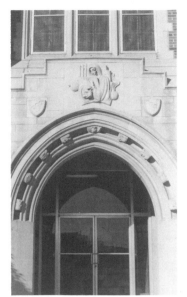

FIGURE 109. *O. W. Hyman Administration Building, 1955 Union Avenue Entrance (courtesy of James E. Hamner, III, D.D.S., Ph.D.)*

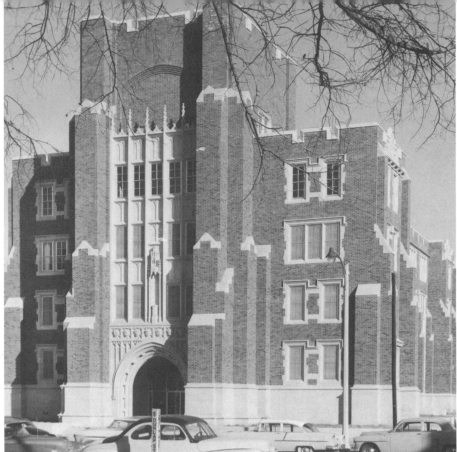

FIGURE 108. *O. W. Hyman Administration Building, 1955 South Dunlap Street Entrance*

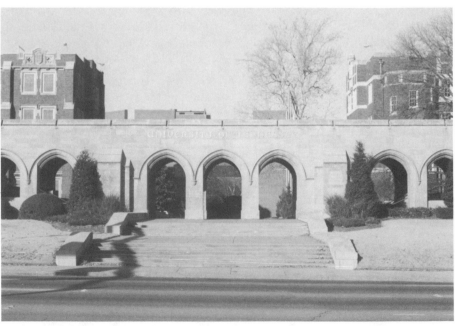

FIGURE 110. *Cloistered Walkway, Connecting the Hyman Building with the Nash Building along Union Avenue, 1955*

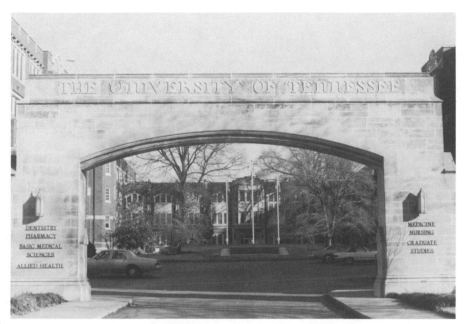

FIGURE 111. *University of Tennessee Archway, Connecting the Hyman Building with the U.T. College of Dentistry Building, 1955 (courtesy of James E. Hamner, III, D.D.S., Ph.D.)*

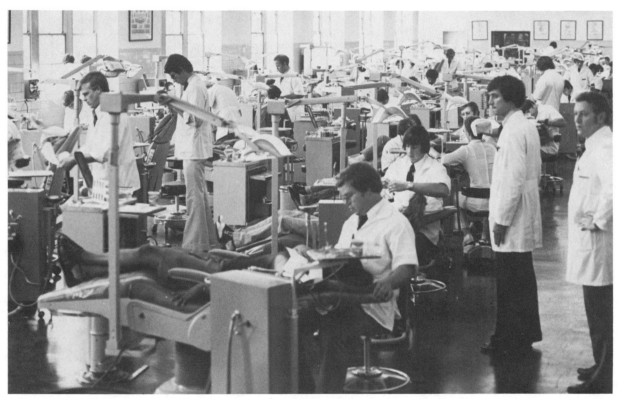

FIGURE 112. *U.T. Department of Operative Dentistry Clinic, 1950's*

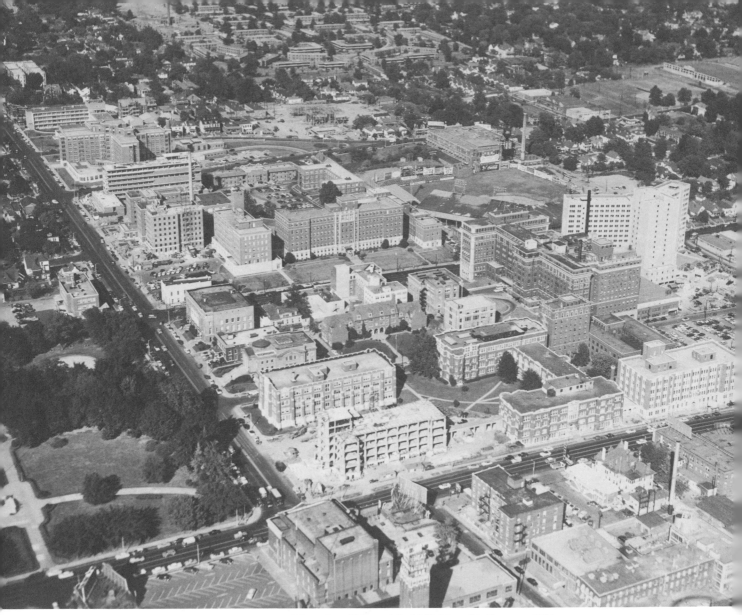

FIGURE 113. —*Aerial View of the U.T. Memphis Campus, 1954*

built to house the Medical-Surgical portions for that hospital, was also ready for occupancy in 1955. An aerial view (Figure 113) of U.T. Memphis in November of 1954 shows that the Nash Building is almost completed, the structures of the Hyman Building and connecting cloisters are up, the Medical-Surgical Building Annex to Bishop Gailor Hospital is bricked in, and the new wing of the main Baptist Hospital (facing Madison Avenue) is nearing completion.

Dr. O. W. Hyman continued as the chief administrative official for U.T. Memphis; his title from 1949–1961 was Vice President in charge of the U.T. Medical Units. Much of the credit for the huge building program of the 1950's, which greatly increased the University's physical size, was due to his foresight and supervision. In 1950, President Truman appointed him as a member (there were only 21) of the newly created National Science Foundation; it was a noteworthy compliment to the University, Tennessee, the Mid-South, and Dr. Hyman personally.

In addition to marked increases in student enrollment and building construction during the 1950's, there was a significant turnover in the various college Deanships. Dean T. P. Nash and Dean Ruth Neil Murry administered, in a commendable fashion, the School of Biological Sciences and the School of Nursing, respectively, throughout the 1950's.[14] In 1954, the certificate/diploma nursing program was dropped, and the baccalaureate nursing degree, which had been budding for several years, was instituted. U.T. Memphis and the City of Memphis Hospital in 1958 amended their old contract of 1926 in order for the University to assume full responsibility for nursing education.[19,44] Because of ill health, Richard Doggett Dean, M.D., D.D.S. retired as Dean of the U.T. College of Dentistry on July 1, 1950; he died later in October of 1950.[8,12] James Theda Ginn, D.D.S. (Figure 114), who had been Chairman of the Operative Dentistry Division since June of 1948, was appointed as Dean of the U.T. College of Dentistry by Dr. Hyman.[29] He had joined the dental faculty in January of 1946 as an Associate Professor of Oral Medicine and Surgery. Dr. Ginn was born in 1909 in Snow Hill, North Carolina, graduated from the University of North Carolina with a B.S. degree in 1934, and received his D.D.S. degree from Loyola University of New Orleans in 1939. From 1940–1942 he was a Carnegie Fellow in Dentistry at the Graduate School of the University of Rochester (New York). In 1943, he returned to Loyola University School of Dentistry in New Orleans as an Associate Professor of Histology and Pathology until 1946, when he came to U.T. Memphis. In addition to his duties as Dean, Dr. Ginn taught a course in Oral Medicine, published numerous scientific articles as well as a textbook entitled *A Review of Dentistry*, and was elected as a Fellow of the American College of Dentists in 1949. He was a member of the International Association for Dental Research, the American Association for the Advancement of Science, Sigma Xi, and was one of the founders of the R. D. and M. T. Dean Odontological Honor Society at the University of Tennessee, Memphis.[29] Dr. Ginn served as Dean of the University of Tennessee College of Dentistry until October 31, 1959 when he was suddenly struck down by a fatal coronary occlusion.[8,22,43] Dean Ginn labored long and tirelessly for the progress of Dentistry, the improvement of the U.T. College of Dentistry, and for the establishment of dental research. To commemorate his efforts, the dental faculty established the Ginn Memorial Library Fund to purchase scientific books and periodicals for use in the proposed Dental-Pharmacy Research Building, which was destined to be built in 1962. By August of 1950, the U.T. College of Dentistry was the second largest among the 42 United States dental schools, based on the number of graduates during the preceding year; New York University College of Dentistry in New York City was first.

The School of Pharmacy saw two changes in its Deanship during the 1950's. Its first vacancy was occasioned by the death of Dean Robert Latta

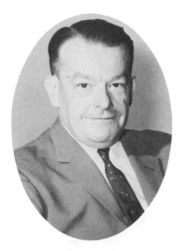

FIGURE 114. *James Theda Ginn, D.D.S. (1909–1959) Dean, U.T. College of Dentistry, 1950–1959*

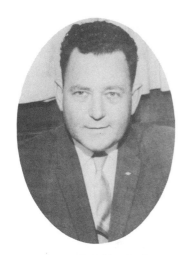

FIGURE 115. *Seldon Dick Feurt, Ph.D. (1923–1975) Dean, U.T. College of Pharmacy, 1959–1975*

Crowe on July 26, 1953. Dr. Crowe had been Dean for 17 years, serving as both a motivating and a stabilizing force in that position since 1936. Karl John Goldner, Ph.D., Professor of Pharmacy at the University of Tennessee, Memphis since 1947, was appointed by Dr. Hyman in October of 1953 as the new Dean of the U.T. School of Pharmacy. Dr. Goldner was born in Minneapolis and obtained his B.S. (in Pharmacy), his M.S., and his Ph.D. degrees from the University of Minnesota. His major was Pharmaceutical Chemistry, and his doctorate was earned in 1934. He served as an Instructor of Pharmacy at the University of Wisconsin until 1940, when he joined the faculty of the University of Tennessee, Memphis. From Assistant Professor in 1940, he advanced to Associate Professor in 1943 and full Professor in 1947. Dr. Goldner was a member of Sigma Xi and the American Association for the Advancement of Science. He served as Dean for six years until 1959, when he stepped down from this position. Dr. Goldner remained with the University as a Professor of Medicinal Chemistry for many years until his retirement.[15,38,43]

On March 1, 1959 at age 36, Dr. Seldon Dick Feurt (Figure 115) assumed his duties as Dean of the U.T. College of Pharmacy; he was selected in October of 1958 for that position. Dr. Karl Goldner, the previous Dean, resigned from those responsibilities to devote all of his time to teaching and research. Dr. Feurt was born in Wichita, Kansas on October 21, 1923. From October, 1942 through November, 1945 he served as a Pharmacist Mate 1st Class, U.S.N. with the 4th Marine Battalion in the South Pacific Theatre during World War II and was commissioned an Ensign, U.S. Navy after the War. His undergraduate B.S. degree in Pharmacy was obtained in 1949 from Loyola University in New Orleans. From 1949–1953, Dick Feurt attended the University of Florida and earned both the M.S. and Ph.D. degrees in Pharmacology. He was an Associate Professor of Pharmacology at the University of Georgia from 1953–1958 and was named Professor of Pharmacology at the same school from 1958–1959, when he came to Memphis. Dr. Feurt was described by his University of Tennessee faculty colleagues as "a young man, full of vigor, energetic, aggressive, bold, and seething with ideals."[15] He was a member of Sigma Xi and the American Association for the Advancement of Science, a Fellow of the American College of Apothecaries, author of 17 scientific articles and one book, recipient of "Pharmacist of the Year for the State of Tennessee" award in 1965, and performed significant research in perfecting the animal capture gun.[21] From 1959–1975 Dean Feurt, until his untimely death on January 19, 1975, following major surgery for lung carcinoma, led the School of Pharmacy during the era that it was renamed the University of Tennessee College of Pharmacy in 1959.[15,16,43]

It was announced in February of 1958 that Maston Kennerly Callison, M.D., an Associate Professor of Medicine at the University of Tennessee College of Medicine and Chief-of-Staff of the City of Memphis Hospitals, would succeed Dr. O. W. Hyman as Dean of the U.T. College of Medicine.[42] Dr. Hyman retained his position as Vice President of the U.T.

Medical Units; separation of the two Offices was the natural result of rapid growth by U.T. Memphis, causing even heavier burdens of responsibility for Dr. Hyman to oversee the expanding Colleges.[16]

Maston Callison was born on January 14, 1917 in Knoxville, Tennessee, and in a special program he obtained two degrees from the University of Tennessee: a B.S. in 1937 and an M.D. in 1939.[1] He interned at the Knoxville General Hospital and served his residency in Internal Medicine at the John Gaston Hospital from 1942–1944. During 1944–1947, he was a Captain (MC) U.S. Army during the closing years of World War II. Dr. Callison returned to Memphis after his service discharge, joined the U.T. College of Medicine faculty, and advanced from Instructor to Associate Professor in the U.T. Department of Medicine during 1947–1958. Dr. Callison is a well-respected internist among his medical colleagues. During his tenure as Dean, he supervised the establishment of the University-oriented, teaching hospital—the William F. Bowld Hospital—and the James K. Dobbs Research Center, directly associated with this hospital. Figure 116 depicts Dean Callison at his desk in 1966.

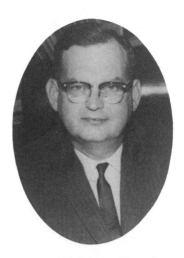

FIGURE 116. *Maston Kennerly Callison, M.D. (1917–) Dean, U.T. College of Medicine, 1957–1970*

The medical accomplishments and recognition awards for Dr. Callison's labors have been numerous: recipient, L. M. Graves Memorial Health Award for Outstanding Service to Memphis and the Mid-South, 1970; recipient, Distinguished Service Award of the Tennessee Medical Association, 1970; recipient, First Distinguished Service Award of the University of Tennessee Chapter of Alpha Omega Alpha, 1970; member, Alpha Omega Alpha; member, Sigma Xi; Diplomate, American Board of Internal Medicine; and Fellow, American College of Physicians.[1,16,42] Dr. Callison's portrait now hangs in the Coleman College of Medicine Building. He continues a very active private practice of Internal Medicine as well as serving his University as a Clinical Professor of Medicine in the U.T. Department of Medicine.

One of the most significant events during the 1950's decade was the Korean War, which commenced on June 25, 1950 with an unprovoked attack by North Korean Forces across the 38th Parallel into South Korea. This War ended July 27, 1953. During the 1950's, four University of Tennessee, Memphis graduates were killed.

Ralph Lee Borum, a 1st Lieutenant in the U.S. Air Force, received his B.S. degree in Pharmacy from the University of Tennessee in 1949, flew 50 missions over Europe as a Flying Fortress Navigator during World War II, and was killed October 14, 1951 in a B-29 crash landing near Tokyo, as his plane returned from an air raid over North Korea.

Bert Nelson Coers, M.D. was a Lieutenant Colonel (MC) U.S. Army. He received his M.D. degree from the University of Tennessee in 1937. Lieutenant Colonel Coers was assigned to duty in Korea as a regimental surgeon in the Second Division of the U.S. Eighth Army. He was wounded by artillery fire and captured December 1, 1950, and died on August 22, 1953 in a North Korean prisoner of war camp.

In September of 1950, 1st Lieutenant Clarence L. Anderson arrived in

131

Korea as a combat surgeon; he received his M.D. degree from the U.T. College of Medicine in 1948. On November 2, 1950 his regiment was ambushed and practically destoyed. Dr. Anderson was listed as missing in action, but fortunately he did survive as a prisoner of war. In that capacity, Dr. Anderson treated the wounded Americans and allied soldiers while he served as a prisoner in a Chinese Communist prisoner of war camp; he survived the War and returned to the United States after the armistice was signed.

William Lindsey Wallace, Jr. received his M.D. degree from the University of Tennessee College of Medicine in 1932. While in medical school, the needs of the sick in foreign countries weighed heavily upon him, and in 1935 he made the decision to become a Baptist medical missionary and was assigned to serve in Wuchow, China. His medical skill, patience, and compassion were known to all of the Chinese in his district; their esteem for him became even more pronounced after the Japanese invaded China. His hospital was bombed during the air raid on Suchow, but he remained to serve those injured persons in need. Communist domination after the Chinese Civil War, following World War II, presented new threats for him. Dr. Wallace decided to continue his work and remain in China despite the hindrance of the Communists, but it was his undoing. Their false propaganda about this "wicked American" could not stand against his living example. He was jailed by the Chinese Communists on the fake charge of possession of a pistol, and was killed by them in his prison cell on February 9, 1951. His U.T. medical school classmates of 1932 set up a Memorial Book Collection in the Mooney Library of the University of Tennessee, Memphis as a memorial for Dr. Wallace. Drs. O. W. Hyman, Battle Malone, and Hugh Smith served as the steering committee for this memorial. It continues today in 1986 as a living tribute to his courage and dedication to alleviate the suffering of others (see Appendix J). The Wallace Collection now contains 255 books.[13,30]

James M. Thayer, Jr. was a Captain (MC) U.S. Air Force. He received his M.D. degree from the University of Tennessee College of Medicine in 1954 and was killed on February 15, 1958 when his troop transport plane crashed into Mt. Vesuvius, Italy. He was returning home from overseas duty.[3]

There were numerous, important events affecting the growth and development of the University of Tennessee, Memphis during the 1950's. In June of 1951, the name of Wittenborg was carved in the white stone above the Monroe Street entrance to the ivy-covered Anatomy Building in the heart of the Memphis Medical Center. The Anatomy Building was named to honor August Hermsmeier Wittenborg, M.D., the German-born anatomist, who was one of the University's greatest teachers. Countless physicians, who began their study of medicine under him, have summed up his greatness as an educator in these words: "He was more interested in his students than anything else."[31]

On July 21, 1951 the U.T. Cancer Research Laboratory, located in the

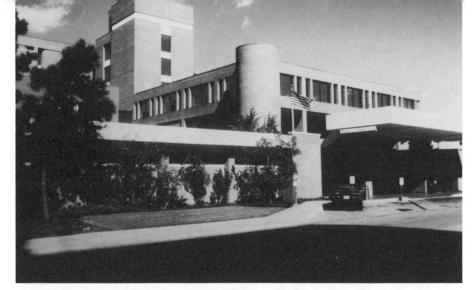

FIGURE 117. *Le Bonheur Children's Hospital, 1952*

newly built Van Vleet Memorial Cancer Center, was opened with facilities unparalleled in the South for cancer research. This building and its $53,425 for laboratory equipment were made possible by a grant from the National Cancer Institute of the U.S. Public Health Service. Individual laboratories were designed to enable University of Tennessee scientists to take full research advantage of the radioactive isotopes from Oak Ridge, Tennessee, and offer vastly improved facilities for fighting cancer, the second leading cause of death in the United States. This building was designed not as a hospital to treat cancer patients, but to perform basic research in cancer.[32]

In October of 1951 to commemorate Dr. Harry Schmeisser's 30 years of service with the U.T. Department of Pathology, a life-sized portrait was hung on the wall of the U.T. Pathology Institute auditorium. The portrait was a gift of his wife and was presented by Dr. E. W. Goodpasture, the world famous Professor and Chairman of the Department of Pathology at Vanderbilt University and a former classmate of Dr. Schmeisser's at the Johns Hopkins University. Dr. O. W. Hyman, in accepting the portrait, praised Dr. Schmeisser for his extreme loyalty and faithfulness throughout his 30 years of service to the University of Tennessee.[33]

In 1952 a private hospital, Le Bonheur Children's Hospital (Figure 117), long the dream of the Le Bonheur women's social and welfare organization, was opened. This small hospital for children has developed into a comprehensive medical center for the diagnosis and treatment of children's diseases, disorders, and injuries. It also functions as the principal teaching hospital for both pediatrics and pedodontics for the U.T. Colleges of Medicine and Dentistry, respectively. The Medical Director of Le Bonheur Children's Medical Center also wears the hat of Professor and Chairman of the U.T. College of Medicine's Department of Pediatrics.[13] This hospital is situated along the east side of Dunlap Street between Adams and Washington Streets. Its construction was a significant leap forward because it provided the special equipment, special hospital facilities, and laboratory expertise which permitted the treatment of children with unusual or life-

133

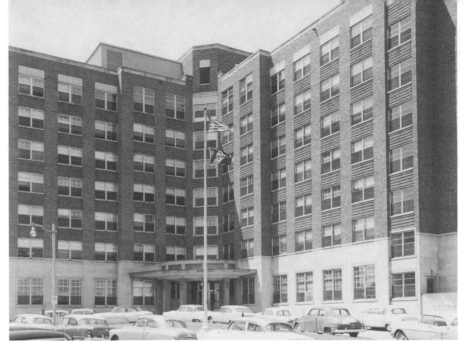

FIGURE 118. *West Tennessee State Tuberculosis Hospital, 1948*

threatening diseases; heretofore, these patients were referred to St. Louis, Chicago, New York, Baltimore, or Philadelphia medical facilities by Memphis pediatricians. Also, research space was provided for a five year period for U.T. faculty and postdoctoral fellows in nephrology, endocrinology, cardiology, and hematology.[3,5,6]

Two other hospitals along Dunlap Street, which are not owned by the University of Tennessee, but which have played important roles in the clinical education of medical students and residents, are the West Tennessee State Tuberculosis Hospital and the E. H. Crump Hospital. The former one, also known as the "Chest Hospital", is located between Adams and Jefferson Streets facing Dunlap Street. Dr. O. W. Hyman represented the U.T. College of Medicine on the Tennessee Tuberculosis Hospital Commission from 1945–1948 and was instrumental in having the hospital built in Memphis in 1948. It was used for the treatment of chest diseases, and with the closure of the old John Gaston Hospital as a functioning hospital, it became the main City Hospital (Figure 118) until 1985.

The E. H. Crump Memorial Hospital was built in 1955 and was named for the famous Memphis Mayor and political leader, Edward Hull Crump. When the old maternity wing of John Gaston Hospital was closed, the Crump Hospital became the primary maternity hospital for the City of Memphis. It also houses the University of Tennessee Newborn Center, which will be discussed in more detail later.

National rankings of health professional schools in 1953 revealed that the U.T. Colleges of Medicine and Dentistry were in the top echelon. The University of Tennessee Colleges of Medicine and Dentistry were the only such schools in the United States that operated on an individual quarter system, accepting and graduating classes of students four times a year. Medicine admitted 50 students, and Dentistry admitted 35 students every 3 months. In a 1953 issue of the *Journal of the American Medical Association*, figures giving total enrollment from July 1, 1952 through June 30, 1953 listed the University of Tennessee as training more medical students than any other University in the United States. The U.T. College of Medicine was first with 713 students, the University of Michigan with 683 students was second, and the University of Illinois with 678 students third. The *American Dental Association's Dental Students Register* gave statistics on students registered in school on October 15, 1952. By adding the number of students who were admitted to each school during the next 12 months, the results showed the University of Tennessee to be the third largest in enrollment. New York University was first with 609 students, the University of Pennsylvania second with 542 students, and the University of Tennessee College of Dentistry third with 517 students.[39]

Beginning with the class of September, 1953, the College of Medicine required three years of premedical training. The first class selected under this new requirement entered the U.T. College of Medicine in January of 1953. This change complied with accrediting requirements by the A.M.A.'s Council on Medical Education.

The L. G. Noel Memorial Foundation was established in 1954 as the philanthropic arm of the Tennessee State Dental Association. The three primary objectives of the foundation have always been:

(1) to support dental health care education;
(2) to encourage and support dental research programs; and
(3) to provide educational loans for junior and senior dental students.

As a memorial tribute, the Foundation was named for Llewwellyn Garnet Noel, M.D., D.D.S. (Figure 23) of Nashville, who was one of Tennessee's earliest and most distinguished dental educators and practitioners. Dr. Noel served as President of the Tennessee State Dental Association in 1878 as well as the American Dental Association in 1903.[7] Dr. Noel began the movement to establish the American Dental Association Relief Fund, which now provides monthly financial assistance to dentists who are no longer self-supporting due to illness, accident, age, or other disabling conditions. The L. G. Noel Memorial Foundation has a proud heritage and has received nationwide recognition for its services.[11,12]

The installation of a chapter of the Society of Sigma Xi on May 17, 1956 at the University of Tennessee, Memphis reflected, in large measure, the high caliber of medical research conducted by members of the faculty staff in all Schools and Colleges. To qualify for chapter status, an institution must meet rigid standards, both as to the extent of research activity and the quality. Before the national organization of Sigma Xi would approve formation of a chapter at the University of Tennessee, the petitioners had to show all of the contributions they had made to the scientific literature during the previous five years. The purpose of the Sigma Xi Society, the first chapter of which was organized at Cornell University in 1886, is "the encouragement of original investigation in science, pure and applied." Its motto is,

"Companions in zealous research."[1,21,40] The chapter in Memphis was designated as the University of Tennessee Medical Units Chapter; however, its membership as charter members included scientists at Buckeye Cotton Oil Company, Memphis State College (now Memphis State University), Southwestern College (now Rhodes College), Kennedy Veteran's Hospital, the old Veteran's Hospital on Crump Boulevard, and the Buckman Laboratories.[40] There were originally 83 Charter Members and 11 Associate Charter Members in the Memphis chapter. Even though this list is lengthy, it is of historical importance to include the names of these charter members, because they represent the core of scientific research in the Memphis area in the mid-1950's. The original charter members were: Drs. Roland H. Alden, John W. Appling, George Barlow, Abraham Bass, Eldon A. Behr, Levi E. Bigenheimer, Jr., Robert T. Bliekenstaff, Daniel A. Brody, Carl D. Brown, Simon R. Bruesch, Stanley J. Buckman, Bland W. Cannon, William C. Chaney, Sidney A. Cohn, Clark E. Corliss, Edward Doody, James S. Davis, Arthur M. Dowell, Jr., Charles V. Dowling, Anna D. Dulaney, Wolcott B. Dunham, Donald F. Durso, James N. Etteldorf, Don E. Eyles, Robert L. Fischer, Elton Fischer, Laurence R. Fitzgerald, Aaron Ganz, Colvin L. Gibson, Karl J. Goldner, Marvin I. Gottlieb, William M. Hale, Clarence R. Houck, Orren W. Hyman, William E. Jefferson, Jr., Arthur F. Johnson, Raburn W. Johnson, Helen H. Kaltenborn, Howard S. Kaltenborn, Roger E. Koeppe, Norman D. Lee, Frederick W. Lengemann, Alys H. Lipscomb, Hortense S. Louckes, Marion L. MacQueen, Clement H. Marshall, Pasquale Martignoni, Esther L. McCandless, Israel D. Michelson, Martin L. Minthorn, Manuel F. Moose, Dempsie Morrison, William A. Mueller, Thomas P. Nash, Jr., Carl E. Nurnburger, Richard R. Overman, Henry Packer, Kenneth Pearce, Jesse D. Perkinson, Jr., John P. Quigley, Robert C. Rendtorff, Peyton N. Rhodes, Frank L. Roberts, George G. Robertson, Charles A. Rosenberg, Douglas A. Ross, Altheus S. Rudolf, Jack U. Russell, Frank S. Schlenker, Arlo I. Smith, Edward H. Storer, Wheelan D. Sutliff, Hall S. Tacket, Henry B. Turner, Arliss H. Tuttle, Raymond T. Vaughn, William J. von Lackum, James L. A. Webb, Harry H. Wilcox, Edward F. Williams, Jr., John L. Wood, Robert A. Woodbury, and Donald B. Zilversmit.

The Charter Associate Members were: Drs. Otto A. Alderks, Merlie W. Buckman, Rocco A. Calandruccio, Weddie H. Hassler, Charles J. Lilly, John P. Milnor, Jr., Amy W. Moore, Albert H. Musick, Raymond L. Tanner, Lester van Middlesworth, and Thomas L. Waring.

In 1957 the former pediatric wing of John Gaston Hospital was rebuilt, adding two floors and excavating the ground floor to house laboratories. It was named for the late Mayor Frank Tobey, who was very much interested in this expansion for the University of Tennessee Pediatric Research Laboratory. The laboratory was devoted exclusively to special patient studies and research into children's diseases, making it one of the few such facilities of its kind in the United States. The University of Tennessee provided money for personnel and equipment for the Pediatric Research Laboratory, and space was provided by the City of Memphis Hospitals. Dr. James Etteldorf conducted research in leukemia, kidney diseases (nephrology), disturbances in body fluids and electrolyte balance, in diabetic ketoacidosis, diarrhea of infancy and childhood, and metabolic disturbances.[3,5,6] Assistant Professor A. H. Tuttle carried out research in oncology and blood dyscrasias (leukemias and anemias). Work was also done on convulsions and muscular dystrophy. The late Dr. M. J. Sweeney was highly involved with pediatric clinical research activities and worked closely with Dr. Jim Etteldorf.[3,5,6,41] Dr. Lorin Ainger conducted research in cardiophysiology and in the diagnosis and treatment of congenital and acquired heart disease. This laboratory served to prepare postdoctoral fellows for careers in academic medicine. As has been mentioned previously, this Pediatric Research Laboratory received long-range funding from the National Institutes of Health.[3]

Herbert Thomas Brooks, M.D. was the first Chairman of the U.T. Department of Pathology from 1912–1918, as well as Dean of the U.T. College of Medicine from 1912–1917. Edgar Matthias Medlar, M.D. served as the second Chairman from 1917–1921. Dr. Harry Christian Schmeisser, who served from 1921–1944, was an outstanding third Chairman, whose medical achievements have been discussed previously in Chapter 3 (Figure 71). The fourth Chairman of the Pathology Department was Douglas Hamilton Sprunt, M.D., who served from 1944–1968, which was the longest tenure.[13,43]

Dr. Sprunt (Figure 119) was born August 2, 1900 in Wilmington, North Carolina. He received an excellent undergraduate education at the University of Virginia and obtained his B.S. degree in 1922. Leaving Charlottesville, he attended medical school at Yale University and obtained his medical degree in 1927. He was an Instructor at the Yale University School of Medicine from 1927–1929 and also did graduate work, receiving an M.S. degree from Yale University in 1929. He began his pathology training at Yale in 1927, was a Sterling Research Fellow from 1929–1930, and completed his residency at the Rockefeller Institute for Medical Research in 1932. From 1932–1934, he was an Associate Professor of Pathology at the Duke University School of Medicine. From 1944, when he was appointed Professor and Chairman of the U.T. Department of Pathology, he also assumed the responsibilities as Chief of Laboratories for the City of Memphis Hospitals.[23,43]

Dr. Douglas Sprunt's medical accomplishments were numerous. It has already been mentioned that he was strongly instrumental in obtaining construction grant funds from the National Institutes of Health to build the University of Tennessee Institute of Pathology and the Van Vleet Memorial Cancer Center in 1951. He was appointed as a member of the Cancer Control Advisory Committee of the National Cancer Institute, N.I.H. from 1955–1962. Within the American Society of Clinical Pathologists, Dr. Sprunt was a Member of the Council from 1955–1962, Vice President in 1959, President in 1960, and Secretary in 1961. He was a Diplomate of the American Board of Pathology, a Fellow of the American College

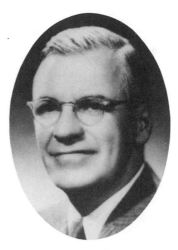

FIGURE 119. *Douglas Hamilton Sprunt, M.D. (1900–1983) Professor and Chairman, U.T. Department of Pathology, 1944–1968*

137

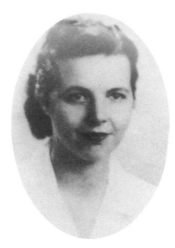

FIGURE 120. *Alys Harris Lipscomb, M.D. (1915–) First Director of the U.T. Radioisotope Unit, 1948*

of Physicians, a Fellow of the College of American Pathologists, a Member of the International Academy of Pathology, and Chairman of the National Research Council Coordinating Committee for the International Intersociety Committee on Pathology in 1959. Dr. Sprunt played a vital role in the acquisition of over $2,000,000 in grants for the Papanicolaou Cervical Smear Cytology Program, which was conducted by the University's Department of Pathology in the 1950's. This very important medical accomplishment will be discussed later. He published 101 articles in scientific journals, and by taking advantage of N.I.H. health manpower grants, he instigated residency programs and productive M.S. and Ph.D. postgraduate programs in pathology and microbiology, which still bear fruit today in such contributing faculty members as: Doctors Sid Coleman, Jerry Francisco, Bill Jennings, Harry Mincer, Willie R. Phillips, Morris Robbins, and Roy Smith. He had the honor of being elected a member of the prestigious Cosmos Club in Washington, D.C. It is composed of men who have done meritorious original work in science, literature, and the arts, who are well-known and cultivated in one or more of these fields. The only other person affiliated with the University of Tennessee, Memphis, who has also been so honored is James E. Hamner, III, D.D.S., Ph.D. (D'55). Dr. Sprunt retired in 1968 and was honored as an Emeritus Professor of Pathology until his death in 1983.[13,23]

For four years after her graduation from the University of Tennessee in Knoxville, Miss Alys Harris Lipscomb was employed as a chemist in the University's Hospital. Her interest in medicine grew with each year of her employment, and in the fall of 1940 she entered the U.T. School of Biological Sciences, as a graduate student in physiology, and continued through 1941. She entered the U.T. College of Medicine in 1942 and continued her graduate work in physiology, receiving an M.S. degree in 1944. Her performance in medical school was so outstanding that when she received her M.D. degree in 1945, she was awarded a three-year fellowship at the Cleveland Clinic in Ohio. The William E. Lower Prize, given each year for the most outstanding thesis among third year fellowship students at the Cleveland Clinic, was awarded to Dr. Lipscomb.

Dr. Alys Lipscomb (Figure 120), in collaboration with Dr. Carl Nurnberger—a U.T. radiation physicist, pioneered the planning and implementation necessary for diagnostic and therapeutic application of radio-nuclides in Memphis. The inception of the University of Tennessee's Radioisotope Unit occurred in 1948, and the first therapeutic dose of I^{131} (for the treatment of hyperthyroidism) was administered by Dr. Lipscomb in 1950. For many years, private physicians locally and throughout the Mid-South referred their patients to the University of Tennessee for diagnosis and treatment of thyroid disease and hematologic disorders.[13,19]

Initially, the Radioisotope Unit did not have departmental attachment, and Dr. Lipscomb, who was an Instructor in both Medicine and Clinical Pathology in Dr. Lemuel Diggs' Department of Medical Laboratories, was drafted to head the Unit because of her clinical experience at the Cleveland

Clinic, prior to returning to Memphis in October of 1948. This assignment was given in addition to her duties as Instructor in Medicine and Clinical Pathology. She had no budget; a desk, chair, and file cabinet were borrowed from Dr. Diggs; a microscope was loaned by the U.T. Department of Pathology; and her technician was paid from a research grant.[2,13] It was not until later when radiology residents were required to have a background in Nuclear Medicine as a requisite for qualification for the American Board of Radiology, that Dr. David Carroll, then Chairman, created a Section of Nuclear Medicine in the U.T. Department of Radiology. This recognition occurred at the time the Chandler Building was constructed; Dr. Lipscomb continued to head this unit until 1965. Also, Dr. Lipscomb determined the blood volume in patients with sickle cell anemia during times of crisis as well as stabilized periods, using radioisotope techniques.[2,13,19]

The University of Tennessee College of Dentisty commenced a course in Dental Hygiene in the late 1920's, and this course continued until 1942 when it was discontinued because of a lack of teaching personnel. In February of 1950, Dean Richard D. Dean announced that the Dental Hygiene Program would recommence in the Fall Quarter (September) of 1950, and it would be located on the fifth floor of the new College of Dentistry Building. Thirty-two students would be accepted for each class; the program would cover six consecutive quarters of academic and clinical work. At graduation a Certificate in Dental Hygiene would be issued. Miss Sarah E. Hill, who had graduated from the University of Tennessee Dental Hygiene Program in 1934, was appointed as Director of the reinstated U.T. Dental Hygiene Program in 1950. She was installed as President of the American Dental Hygienists' Association in December of 1954.[11,12]

The *American Surgeon*, a professional publication of surgery, dedicated its April, 1952 issue to Robert L. Sanders, M.D., who was Professor of Surgery at the University of Tennessee, Memphis. The occasion was his seventieth birthday, April 7, 1952. Dr. Sanders was a member and past President of the Southeastern Surgical Congress. In the dedication page in the *American Surgeon*, it stated of Dr. Sanders: "Over a period of 40 years, he has used his talents and efforts to improve surgical practice through the advancement of surgical knowledge. His contribution to scientific literature would fill volumes." In 1951, the American Cancer Society presented Dr. Robert L. Sanders the Distinguished Service Award for outstanding cancer control in Tennessee.[34]

Daniel Anthony Brody was born on June 9, 1915 in Youngstown, Ohio. In 1932, he won a four-year scholarship at the Case Institute of Technology, receiving a B.S. degree from that school in 1936. Following his father's footsteps, he attended Western Reserve, and in 1940 he received his M.D. degree. As a medical student, he had performed some experiments under the guidance of Dr. J. P. Quigley, Professor of Physiology. His interest in biophysical phenomena became evident with his publication of two papers, one on intraluminal pressure in the digestive tract, and the other paper on the mechanics of gastric evacuation; both of these papers

"They that wait upon the Lord shall renew their strength. They shall mount up with wings as eagles. They shall run and not be weary; and they shall walk and not faint."

Isaiah 40:32

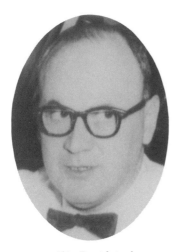

FIGURE 121. *Daniel Anthony Brody, M.D. (1915–1975) Professor, U.T. Department of Medicine, and Professor, U.T. Department of Physiology and Biophysics*

were written before or soon after his graduation from medical school.

At the completion of his internship and residency in Medicine in 1943, he joined the U.S. Army Air Corps. He requested a transfer to the line Army and served with the 3rd Armored Division in the European Theatre of operations during World War II, until he was separated from the Army in 1946 with the rank of Major. After the War, Dr. Brody decided to settle in Memphis, influenced in his decision by Dr. Quigley, who in the interim had become Chief of the Division of Pharmacology and Physiology at the University of Tennessee. Initially, he was given a part-time position in Dr. Quigley's Department, while maintaining a private medical practice. In 1953, he abandoned his private practice and became a full-time Associate Professor of Medicine, rapidly advancing to full Professorship in both Medicine and in Physiology and Biophysics (Figure 121).

After 1952, Dr. Brody's interests were transferred permanently from physiology of the gastrointestinal tract to electrophysiology of the heart. His many contributions in basic medical research were recognized by his becoming one of the earliest recipients of a Research Career Award from the National Heart Institute, N.I.H. in 1962. Dr. Brody was concerned with the effect on body surface electrocardiographic leads of electrical inhomogeneities of the conducting media of the body. In 1956 he described a theoretical model which extended Lord Kelvin's physical concept of electrical images to the biologic system. He concluded from his idealized model that blood in the cavities of the heart augmented the effective strength of components of the myocardial doublets normal to the endocardial surface and reduced the effective strength of tangential components. This phenomenon has since come to be known as the "Brody effect."[9]

The overall conclusion of his many experiments and basic research regarding electrocardiographic signals was that, with normal intraventricular conduction, the early and late portions of ventricular activation were essentially dipolar, but the middle portion contained a very considerable proportion of non-dipolar elements. The T-wave, on the other hand, was generated by an essentially immobile equivalent dipole.

His extensive bibliography of 92 scientific papers and 64 abstracts in the field of fundamental cardiac electrophysiology and instrumentation were a significant contribution to the medical literature. At age 42 in 1957, he suffered an initial coronary occlusion with myocardial infarction that healed. A sudden and unexpected massive heart attack occurred on September 30, 1975, while he was working at his desk on his final manuscript.[9,13]

Dr. Grover C. Bowles, Jr. has had a long and distinguished career in Pharmacy. He was born on February 15, 1920 in Piedmont, Missouri and obtained his B.S. degree in Pharmacy from the University of Tennessee School of Pharmacy in 1942. From 1942–1946 during World War II, Grover Bowles served in the U.S. Navy Hospital Corps. After his release from active duty, he completed a residency in Hospital Pharmacy at the University of Michigan Hospital in Ann Arbor, Michigan from 1946–1947. He returned to Memphis in 1947 and served as an Instructor for the University of Tennessee School of Pharmacy from 1947–1948. He was recruited by the University of Rochester School of Medicine and Dentistry in New York as an Instructor in Pharmacology and Chief Pharmacist for Strong Memorial Hospital. He served in these two capacities until 1954, when he became the Associate Administrator of Memorial Hospital Association of Kentucky for one year.[15,36]

In 1955 Dr. Bowles again returned to Memphis, where he served as Director of the Department of Pharmacy at the Baptist Memorial Hospital until 1984. During that time he was awarded an honorary Doctor of Science degree from the Philadelphia College of Pharmacy and Science in 1968. Dr. Bowles was appointed as Associate Professor in 1958 and a full Professor in 1979 at the University of Tennessee College of Pharmacy, his alma mater.[15,36]

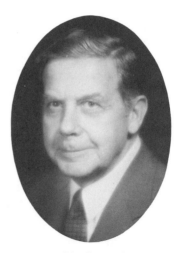

FIGURE 122. *Grover C. Bowles, Jr., D.Sc. (1920–   ) Professor, U.T. College of Pharmacy President, American Pharmaceutical Association, 1965*

Grover Bowles (Figure 122) has served in positions of important responsibility in numerous pharmaceutical scientific societies. From 1952–1953 he was President of the American Society of Hospital Pharmacists. In that capacity he attended the International Congress of Hospital Pharmacists at Berne, Switzerland in October of 1952. He was President of the American Pharmaceutical Association from 1965–1966, and from 1967–1978 he also served as Treasurer of this Association. From 1982–1986 Dr. Bowles has been the President of the American Council on Pharmaceutical Education. He has also served on scientific editorial boards, being a Contributing Editor of the *American Journal of Hospital Pharmacy* from 1956–1967, and a Contributing Editor of *The Modern Hospital* from 1957–1974.[15,36]

Dr. Bowles has been the recipient of the following honors in recognition of his many contributions to Pharmacy: 1960—Man of the Year in Tennessee Pharmacy; 1962—H. A. K. Whitney Lecture Award of the American Society of Hospital Pharmacists; 1973—Remington Honor Medal of the American Pharmaceutical Association; 1977—Distinguished Service Award of the Tennessee Society of Hospital Pharmacists; 1979—the Hugo H. Schaefer Medal of the American Pharmaceutical Association; and 1979—Distinguished Service Award of the University of Tennessee College of Pharmacy.[15,36]

One of the most distinguished Tennessee graduates in organized Dentistry is E. Jeff Justis, Sr., D.D.S. who was born December 28, 1898 in Kennett, Missouri, graduated from the University of Tennessee College of Dentistry in 1923 (Charnell W. Middlecoff was one of his classmates), and entered private practice afterwards. He is a Fellow of the American College of Dentists, a Fellow of the International College of Dentists, and a member of both the Pierre Fauchard Academy and the Federation Dentaire Internationale.[7] In 1940, he served as President of the Tennessee State Dental Association (Figure 123). On behalf of his dental colleagues in Tennessee, he was presented with a silver service at the 1951 Tennessee State Dental Meeting in appreciation of his outstanding contributions to Dentistry.[22]

Dr. Jeff Justis was the first University of Tennessee graduate to be elected

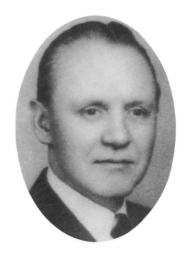

FIGURE 123. *Elvis Jeff Justis, Sr., D.D.S. (1898–   ) Trustee, American Dental Association, 1959–1965 Treasurer, American Dental Association, 1964–1967*

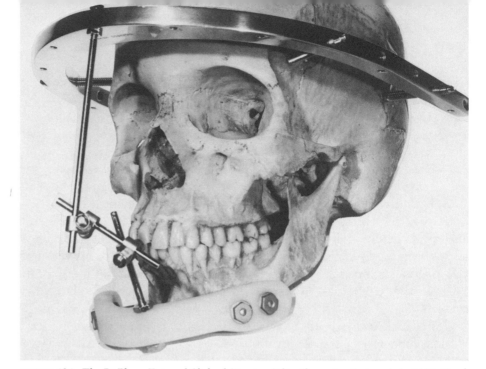

FIGURE 124. *The Bi-Phase External Skeletal Fixation Splint (lower portion) and the U.T. Head Frame (upper portion), designed by Joe Hall Morris, D.D.S., 1949*

as a national Trustee of the American Dental Association and served in that capacity from 1959–1965. He was also honored by the American Dental Association to serve as its national Treasurer from 1964–1967.[8,22] Dr. Justis is well-loved and respected by his fellow dentists in Tennessee and has long been recognized as an elder statesman and the leading authority on local dental history. His son, E. Jeff Justis, Jr., M.D. graduated from the University of Tennessee College of Medicine in December of 1956 and is a Board-certified orthopedic surgeon, specializing in hand surgery in Memphis.

One of the best clinical teachers-by-example of oral surgery was Dr. Julius Roy Bourgoyne, who was Chairman of the U.T. Department of Oral Surgery from 1948–1959. He obtained his D.D.S. degree from Loyola University School of Dentistry in 1941, and after World War II, he followed Dr. James T. Ginn from New Orleans to U.T. Memphis. His textbook, *Surgery of the Mouth and Jaws* (published in 1949), was long the standard textbook on oral surgery for U.T. College of Dentistry students.[12] Few students will forget Dr. Bourgoyne's cool exterior demeanor, his patience and understanding with beginning clinical students, and his intricate expertise as a surgeon.

The Bi-Phase External Skeletal Fixation Splint (Figure 124) was invented by Dr. Joe Hall Morris in 1947 and developed through 1949, when he first published this medical contribution in the scientific literature. Today, it is internationally utilized by the dental and medical professions alike in alignment and stabilization of skeletal components, particularly fractured bones of the face and skull. The University of Tennessee Head Frame was also developed by Dr. Morris to give skeletal fixation and angle of traction to facial bones; such positioning was most difficult to achieve before the development of this head frame.

Dr. Joe Hall Morris graduated from the University of Tennessee College of Dentistry in December of 1945. He served as a part-time faculty member in the U.T. Department of Oral Surgery during the 1950's, and after Dr. Templeton's retirement in 1966, he became Chairman of the U.T. Department of Oral Surgery. Also, he conceived the idea for the O.S.S.I. (Orthognathic Surgery Stimulating Instrument) in 1973 and refined its design through 1979. Since that time, all of the University of Tennessee orthognathic surgery utilizes the O.S.S.I. in treatment planning and pre-operative fabrication of intraoperative occlusal acrylic splints. This instrument has had a significant impact on the field of orthognathic surgery, and its importance is rapidly gaining international acclaim—the name Dr. Joe Hall Morris is paramount in the field of biomechanical engineering in the 1980's.[11,12,18]

In the late 1950's, Professor Meyer-Schwickerath of Germany startled the ophthalmologists of the world by reporting the treatment of a number of retinal conditions by the use of the Zeiss light photo-coagulator, which he devised. Dr. Ralph O. Rychener of the University of Tennessee medical faculty obtained one of these remarkable instruments in 1959 for use by Memphis ophthalmologists. It was housed in the Memphis Eye, Ear, Nose, and Throat Hospital and was probably the fifth such instrument to be used in the United States. Use of this Meyer-Schwickerath light coagulator in treating a retinal condition of a patient was reported in the *Journal of the Tennessee State Medical Association* in July of 1960 by William F. Murrah, M.D., who is a Professor of Ophthalmology in the University of Tennessee College of Medicine. This case was the first patient so treated and reported in the Mid-South area.[13] Two other University of Tennessee ophthalmologists achieved international recognition for their medical accomplishments. Dr. Roland H. Myers was President of the International Association of Secretaries of Ophthalmology and Otolaryngology Societies. Dr. Wesley McKinney served as Secretary-Treasurer of the Pan-American Association of Ophthalmology for 14 years.[13]

Dr. Moore Moore, Jr. was born in Memphis, Tennessee in 1909 and obtained his M.D. degree from the University of Tennessee College of Medicine in 1933. His training in orthopedic surgery was taken in a variety of excellent institutions: New York City Hospital, the University of Chicago Hospital, the Children's Hospital in New Orleans, Presbyterian Hospital in New York City, and the Memorial Hospital (Tumor Service) in New York City. He compiled a distinguished service record with the U.S. Navy during World War II, became a Rear Admiral (MC) U.S. Naval Reserve (Appendix H), and Chief of Orthopedic Surgery for the Methodist Hospital in Memphis, where he has made numerous contributions in that specialty of surgery.[24]

Iris A. Pearce, M.D. served as an Ensign from January, 1943 through February, 1946 in the U.S. Naval Reserve (WC). She remained on inactive duty reserve status from February of 1946 through October of 1956 as a Lieutenant (WC) U.S.N.R. She received her M.D. degree from the Uni-

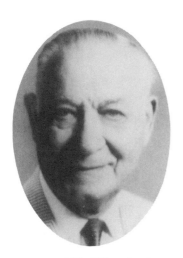

FIGURE 125. *Gilbert Joseph Levy, M.D. (1893–1975) Clinical Professor, U.T. Department of Pediatrics*

versity of Tennessee College of Medicine in September of 1950 and was the second female intern at the John Gaston Hospital in 1951. Dr. Pearce took her residency in Medicine at the John Gaston Hospital and served in a number of leadership roles in that institution, attaining the title of Chairman of the Medical Board. She was also the first female Chief-of-Staff of all the City of Memphis Hospitals. She was the first woman to receive the Distinguished Service Award of the City of Memphis Hospital Medical Staff in 1977. The U.T. National Alumni Association awarded her in 1978 the National Alumni Public Service Award. In 1981 she received the L. M. Graves Memorial Health Award (Table 9), and in 1984, Dr. Pearce received the Tennessee Hospital Association Community Service Award.[13]

Dr. Gilbert Levy was one of the most highly regarded pediatricians ever to practice in Memphis—local mothers by the hundreds swore by him. He was born in Memphis in 1893, the son of Joseph E. Levy, who was a co-founder of the Levy's Specialty Stores. In June of 1915, he earned his M.D. degree from the University of Tennessee College of Medicine. His postgraduate training in pediatrics was taken at the Memphis City Hospital, the New York Nursery and Children's Hospital, and Seaside and Bellevue Hospitals in New York. He entered the U.S. Army Medical Corps and was the first Memphis physician to land in France in World War I. At St. Aignan he was instrumental in saving the lives of many ill French civilians who had been without a physician for three years. After the Armistice he returned to Memphis to continue his medical career in pediatrics. For 30 years, he was the attending pediatrician at the Memphis General Hospital and later at the John Gaston Hospital when it replaced the old hospital in 1936. For many years he was credited with single-handedly staffing the contagious disease ward of the Hospital.[25,26]

For 50 years he was a member of the Memphis-Shelby County Medical Society and served as its President. Also, he was President of the Memphis Pediatric Society and of the Methodist Hospital Staff. When St. Jude Children's Research Hospital was established in Memphis in 1962, he served as a member of its Board of Governors for many years. Other pediatric honors include being President of the Tennessee Pediatric Association and Chairman of the Pediatric Section of the Southern Medical Association. On a national level, Dr. Levy headed the Polio Liaison Committee, served on several committees within the American Academy of Pediatrics, and served as both Chairman and Secretary of the Pediatric Section of the American Medical Association. One of his most significant awards was his selection as Tennessee's Outstanding Physician of 1971 by the Tennessee Medical Association. He also received the Service to Mankind Award from the East Memphis Sertoma Club in 1968 for his "dedication to the finest ideals of the medical profession and his unselfish service to his fellow man." He was widely recognized for his tireless and sometimes single-handed efforts in health care. Gilbert Joseph Levy, M.D. (Figure 125) was a Clinical Professor in the Department of Pediatrics at the University of Tennessee College of Medicine. He died May 28, 1975 after an active medical practice of nearly 60 years. [13,26]

Thomas D. Moore, M.D. became Chairman of the U.T. Department of Urology in the 1940's. He established approved training programs which incorporated the M.S. degree. Dr. Moore was keenly interested in clinical investigative procedures and contributed substantially to the use of radiology in urologic procedures, including intravenous contrast media. Dr. Moore was the second Memphis urologist to attain the Presidency of the American Urology Association. The first President of the A.U.A. was George Livermore, M.D. (1933); the third President (1964) was Samuel L. Raines, M.D. All of these gentlemen were closely affiliated with the University of Tennessee, Memphis. [3,13]

On July 1, 1952 the University of Tennessee, Memphis became involved in one of the largest cervical cancer surveys ever attempted up to that time. Dr. Douglas Sprunt had been busy on the initial planning of this project, and groundwork was laid more than a year previously, when the U.S. Public Health Service Cytology Laboratory was moved from Hot Springs, Arkansas to the U.T. Memphis Cancer Research Laboratory. The mass survey had two main goals—detection of cancer in women who could thus begin treatment early, and the vast accumulation of knowledge to benefit scientists in their fight against cancer. It was the start of the routine "Pap." (Papanicolaou) smear test on 200,000 women between the ages of 20 and 50 years old to determine whether they had carcinoma of the cervix. In positive cases a biopsy would be taken, and the specimen would be sent to the U.T. Institute of Pathology for final diagnosis. By the time this original study was completed, over 500,000 Pap. smears were taken by the University of Tennessee group. [1,35]

Dr. Cyrus Conrad Erickson, a Professor in the U.T. Department of Pathology, was the Chairman of the coordinating committee to manage this extensive project. Other University of Tennessee members on the Committee were Dr. Henry Gotten (U.T. Medicine 1926), who was an Associate Professor of Medicine at the University of Tennessee College of Medicine and who was also at that time President of the Memphis and Shelby County Medical Society; Dr. Frank Whitacre, who was Chief and Professor of the U.T. Department of Obstetrics and Gynecology; Dr. Phil Schreier, an Associate Professor in the U.T. Department of Obstetrics and Gynecology; and Dr. L. M. Graves, Professor in the U.T. Department of Medicine and Director of the Memphis Health Department. [35] The study was planned to continue for three years at an estimated cost of $200,000 per year and was funded by a grant from the U.S. Public Health Service.

Cyrus Conrad Erickson, M.D. (Figure 126) was born in Alexandria, Minnesota on August 18, 1909. He received his B.S. degree in 1930 and his M.D. degree in 1933 from the University of Minnesota. He served as a Lieutenant Colonel in the U.S. Army Medical Corps during World War II, and came to the University of Tennessee College of Medicine in 1949. From 1950 through 1965 he was the Associate Director of the U.T. Institute of Pathology. His very important co-authored papers on cervical cancer

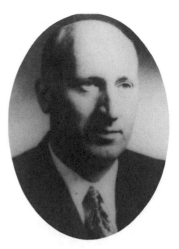

FIGURE 126. *Cyrus Conrad Erickson, M.D. (1909–   ) Professor, U.T. Department of Pathology*

145

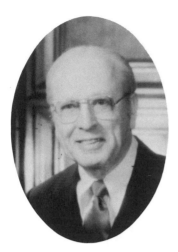

FIGURE 127. *Faustin Neff Weber, D.D.S. (1911–   ) Professor and Chairman, U.T. Department of Orthodontics, 1951–1978*

screening appeared in 1956 in the *Journal of the American Medical Association*, the *Acta Union Internationale Contre Le Cancer*, and the *Annals of the New York Academy of Science*. Dr. Erickson served as the Director of the Memphis-Shelby County Population Cancer Survey from 1952–1958 for evaluating cytology screening for early detection of uterine cancer and the study of age, specific incidence, and prevalence of intraepithelial carcinoma and invasive carcinoma. The United States Postal Service issued a 13¢ stamp honoring Dr. Papanicolaou, and at the same time a special ceremony was held in Memphis honoring the work of Dr. Cyrus Erickson and his associates in the Papanicolaou Smear Cancer Study. In 1965 Dr. Erickson received the prestigious Papanicolaou Award in New York City which was given by the Society of Cytologists for his work in directing the mass detection program carried out by the University of Tennessee, Memphis and cooperating agencies (the National Cancer Institute, N.I.H.).[1,13,35]

When one thinks of Orthodontics at the University of Tennessee, Memphis, in the State of Tennessee, in the South, or in the nation, the name Faustin Weber immediately comes to the forefront of one's mind. Dr. Weber has been in academic Orthodontics at the University of Tennessee, Memphis since 1936. He founded the advanced training programs in Orthodontics at the University of Tennessee College of Dentistry: the postgraduate course in 1947 and the graduate course in 1953. During his tenure as Chairman of the U.T. Department of Orthodontics, 152 men completed this two-year course of study in Orthodontics, leading to the M.S. degree. His graduates are located as far east as New Jersey, as far west as California, as far north as Michigan, and as far south as Florida. Some of these individuals are in academic Orthodontics; the majority of them are clinical orthodontists in private practice. One is Chairman of a Department of Orthodontics; one has served as a Trustee of the American Dental Association of Orthodontists; and two have served as President of the American Association of Orthodontists.[12]

Faustin Neff Weber, D.D.S., M.S., F.A.C.D. (Figure 127) was born November 5, 1911 in Toledo, Ohio. He attended St. John's College in Toledo from 1929–1931, at which time he was accepted into the University of Michigan School of Dentistry. He received his D.D.S. degree in 1934 and his M.S. degree (in orthodontics) from the University of Michigan in Ann Arbor in 1936. After graduation he came to Memphis, Tennessee and was appointed as an Assistant Professor of Orthodontics in the U.T. College of Dentistry. He became an Associate Professor in 1941 and a full Professor in 1951. At that time he was both Professor of Orthodontics and Chairman of that Department in charge of undergraduate and graduate programs in Orthodontics for the U.T. College of Dentistry. In 1948, he was certified as a Diplomate of the American Board of Orthodontics. Dr. Weber received the Tennessee Dental Association Fellowship Award in 1956 and the Albert H. Ketcham Memorial Award in 1980. He is a member of Omicron Kappa Upsilon and the Deans' Odontological Society (charter member). He became a Fellow of the American College of Dentists in 1948, a Fellow of the American Association for the Advancement of Science in 1956, and a Fellow of the International College of Dentists in 1975. As an orthodontic consultant, he has served on the Craniofacial Anomalies Group at the University of Tennessee Child Development Center and also as an orthodontic consultant for the Councils on Dental Education and Hospital Dental Service of the American Dental Association from 1972–1982.

Dr. Weber, over his long and illustrious career, has been identified with many professional societies. He has been an active participant in the International Association of Dental Research, the American Association of Dental Research, the American Cleft Palate Association, the American Society of Dentistry for Children, and the American Association of Orthodontists. He has directed the research projects of 152 graduate students in orthodontics for 25 years from 1953–1978 at the University of Tennessee College of Dentistry. He has also served as President of the Southern Society of Orthodontists from 1968–1969, President of the Memphis Dental Society from 1971–1972, President of the Tennessee Dental Association from 1975–1976, and Vice President of the American Association of Orthodontists from 1979–1980. During his academic career, he served on numerous committees for the American College of Dentists, the Tennessee Dental Association, the Southern Society of Orthodontists, the American Association of Orthodontists, and the University of Tennessee. Dr. Weber has presented papers before dental societies, dental alumni groups, and university audiences in 26 states, the District of Columbia, the Bahamas, and Mexico. He served as Editor of the *Journal of the Tennessee Dental Association* from 1952–1954; Editor of the *Orthodontic Section of the Dental Clinics of North America* in 1964; and was Editor of the *Orthodontic Section: Clinical Dentistry* from 1976 until 1981. He has authored over 40 scientific publications. Throughout his career, he has represented the epitome of academic excellence and proficiency.

I remember Dr. Weber in the 1950's as a serene, elegant lecturer— postgraduate orthodontics seemed another world away to awed sophomore dental students. As we sat huddled on the back rows of the lecture hall, hoping not to be called upon, his opening comment for the first lecture was, "Dental students are a gregarious lot; why don't more of you sit down front where you can hear and perhaps even learn something?" It was later, after some maturity in school, that we began to appreciate what an outstanding teacher Dr. Weber was. He is, indeed, a nationally recognized, eminent leader in Orthodontics and has been one of the greatest academic assets for the University of Tennessee College of Dentistry. Dr. Weber continues to serve today as a Professor Emeritus for the University of Tennessee Department of Orthodontics.

One of the well-remembered Chairmen of the U.T. Department of Obstetrics and Gynecology was Phillip Charles Schreier, M.D. (Figure 128). Dr. Schreier came to Memphis in 1924, when he joined the University of Tennessee, Memphis medical faculty and opened an office for private practice. He received his B.S. degree from the University of Mississippi and

"You cannot separate passion from pathology any more than you can separate a person's spirit from his body."

Richard Selzer, M.D.

147

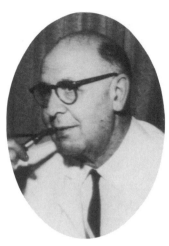

FIGURE 128. *Phillip Charles Schreier, M.D. (1897–   ) Professor and Chairman, U.T. Department of Obstetrics and Gynecology, 1954–1966*

his M.D. degree from the University of Pennsylvania. His obstetrical and gynecological training was taken at the University of Pennsylvania Hospital, prior to his arrival in Memphis. He served on the University of Tennessee College of Medicine faculty for many years, and from 1954–1966, he served as Professor and Chairman of the Department of Obstetrics and Gynecology.

On November 18, 1961, a portrait of Dr. Phil Schreier was given by his former residents to the University of Tennessee, Memphis. The occasion for this presentation was the sixth annual meeting of the WaS Society, an organization of former residents who had received their training under Dr. Frank Whitacre, former Chairman of the U.T. Department of Obstetrics and Gynecology, and Dr. Schreier who was then Chairman of that Department. This society numbered 80 obstetricians in December of 1961.[13,16] When the University of Tennessee Student-Alumni Center was built in 1969, Dr. Phillip C. Schreier donated the portion that now comprises the Schreier Auditorium within this structure. It was given in memory of his parents: Mr. and Mrs. Sam Schreier and his brother, Paul Schreier.[13,16]

One of the best-known physicians in Memphis, both nationally and internationally, is John Joseph Shea, Jr., M.D. (Figure 129). Perhaps Dr. Shea could best be described by the profile that Kenneth Neill wrote about him in the 1980's:

"Maverick. Visionary. Egomaniac. Miracle worker. These are just a few of the epithets that have been applied to John Shea during the long and distinguished medical career that has brought him a generous share of both fame and fortune. During the late 1950's, he pioneered and developed a surgical technique that has quite literally revolutionized otology. The procedure earned Shea a place in the *London Times'* list of '1,000 Makers of the 20th Century.'"[20]

John Shea was born on September 4, 1924 in Memphis, Tennessee. His father, John Joseph Shea, Sr., M.D. (1889–1952), was a distinguished otolaryngologist in Memphis for many years and served with valor in World War I. John Shea, Jr. received his B.S. degree from the University of Notre Dame in 1945 and his M.D. degree from the Harvard Medical School in 1947. He interned at Bellevue Hospital in New York City from July 1947–June 1948. He spent an additional year at the Harvard Medical School, learning the basic sciences related to otolaryngology, and then served a residency in otolaryngology at the Massachusetts Eye and Ear Infirmary in Boston, Massachusetts. He joined the Naval Reserve Program at the University of Notre Dame in 1942 and served six months on active duty in the Navy from July through December 1943. He was called to active duty in 1950 and served as a Lieutenant (jg), (MC), USNR with the U.S. Marine Corps during the Korean War. During the winter of 1954, he worked in the autopsy room of the Pathology Department in a hospital in Vienna, Austria, dissecting thousands of ears, trying to work out in his own mind a possible cure for otosclerosis. In the words of Dr. Shea, "I worked in a room in the basement, where there was no heat; it was 54°, and I always had to wear my overcoat. I worked day and night, Saturdays, Sundays, week in, week out."[20]

At the conclusion of his individual studies on the ear in Vienna, Austria, it occurred to him in a flash what heretofore had not been so obvious: it would be necessary to recreate the sound-conducting mechanism by creating an artificial stapes. Otosclerosis is the pathological formation of excessive bone on the stapes, one of the three tiny bones (incus, stapes, and malleus) which conduct sound within the middle ear. In his first efforts, Dr. Shea used bone grafts as replacement tissues in the first stapedectomies he performed; with these he obtained mixed results, because in most cases the same calcium deposits that immobilized the original stapes bone formed again on the replacement bone graft. In a collaborative effort with Harry Treace of Richards Medical Manufacturing Company in Memphis, Dr. Shea was able to reproduce the structure and characteristics of the stapes, which was only a few millimeters in size, with an artificial structure made of Teflon. In May of 1956 at the Baptist Memorial Hospital, Dr. Shea performed a stapedectomy in which he replaced the bone with a Teflon stapes, and it was successful. That same year he presented the paper at a meeting of the American Otological Association in Montreal on his original work, but, unexpectedly, his reception was lukewarm. At that time "stapedectomy" was a dirty word among otolaryngologists and possessed all of the archaic connotations of a word such as "blood letting." He continued to operate in Memphis and to refine his technique, so that by 1958 when he again addressed the same professional group in Montreal, his successful results spoke for themselves. Of the 88 patients on whom he had performed this operation, 50% had their hearing fully restored, while the majority of the others showed dramatic degrees of improvement in their hearing. Otosclerosis had been conquered, and now this operation is a standard procedure throughout the otolaryngology world.

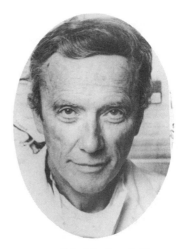

FIGURE 129. *John Joseph Shea, Jr., M.D. (1924–   ) Clinical Professor, U.T. Department of Otolaryngology and Maxillofacial Surgery*

The Shea operation is a very delicate one that requires the precision of a watchmaker and the steadiness of a diamond-cutter, since the entire operating area is no larger than a medium-sized shirt button, and the replacement stapes occupies only a small fragment on the face of a penny. Dr. Shea has now performed thousands of these operations, and people from all over the nation and the world travel to the Shea Clinic in Memphis, which he founded as an otolaryngology clinic. Dr. Shea was certified as a Diplomate of the American Board of Otolaryngology in 1951 and was elected as a Fellow of the American College of Surgeons in 1955. He is a Clinical Professor for the University of Tennessee Department of Otolaryngology and Maxillofacial Surgery.[13,20]

Dr. Phineas J. (Jack) Sparer was born in Vienna, Austria, in 1899 and came to the United States as a child in 1910. He attended Tulane University, both the College and Medical School, where he obtained his B.S. and M.D. degrees, the latter in 1932. He interned at Touro Infirmary in New Orleans and took further training at Sydenham Hospital and Johns Hopkins University in Baltimore. In 1934, he was appointed Director of the Bureau

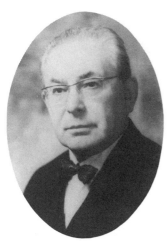

FIGURE 130. *Phineas J. Sparer, M.D. (1899–1977) Professor, U.T. Department of Psychiatry, and Professor, U.T. Department of Preventive Medicine*

of Tuberculosis for the City of Baltimore. Continuing in the field of chest diseases, he joined the U.S. Public Health Service in 1940, then switched to the U.S. Army Medical Corps from 1943 to 1946, attaining the rank of Major by the end of World War II. While serving in the Army, he was stationed in Denver, Colorado, and pursued courses in psychology and psychiatry at the University of Colorado College of Medicine. He completed his psychiatry and neurology residency in Chicago and was Board-certified in 1951.[13,27]

Dr. Sparer was unique in the fact that he had an illustrious career in two fields—chest diseases and psychiatry. He came to Memphis in 1951 to serve as the Chief of Intensive Care Psychiatry at the Kennedy Veteran's Administration Hospital; later he became Chief of Psychiatry at the old Veteran's Administration Hospital #88. His experiences in chest diseases and psychiatry led in 1956 to a Symposium which he organized and the publication of its proceedings, *Personality, Stress, and Tuberculosis.* Dr. Sparer became a member of the medical faculty for the University of Tennessee College of Medicine in 1956 and made many teaching contributions to the University. He organized a special course, entitled "Industrial Psychology and Mental Hygiene for Executives," in the U.T. Department of Preventive Medicine. This course continued for 12 years and was attended by leaders in the financial, legal, business, medical, and theological communities of Memphis.[13,27]

Dr. Jack Sparer was extremely active in other community activities in Memphis, becoming the first psychiatric consultant to the Juvenile Court. In recognition of his outstanding contributions to the civic health of Memphis, he was awarded the L. M. Graves Award in 1968 (Figure 130). He was the President of the Tennessee District of the American Psychiatric Association, a Fellow of the Southern Psychiatric Association, and a Fellow of the College of Chest Physicians.[13]

The influence of Dr. Jack Sparer did not end with his death in 1977. Through generous gifts from Dr. Sparer's widow, Mrs. Florence Sparer, and many of his University of Tennessee friends and colleagues, the Sparer Distinguished Visiting Professorship was established at the University of Tennessee, Memphis on July 31, 1979 to commemorate the good works of her late husband. This Professorship continues to spread the teachings and philosophy of this gentle physician, who enriched the lives of all who were fortunate enough to have known him. The Phineas J. Sparer Distinguished Visiting Professorship was the first of its kind at the U.T. College of Medicine. There are now four additional Distinguished Visiting Professorships which will be discussed later.[13]

In the fall of 1937, a U.T. sophomore medical student stood before a professor, asking him where he could find enough money to support his wife and young son, and to pay his medical tuition. "Why don't you write your father?" asked the professor. "No, he's dead," the medical student responded. That Professor and former Acting Dean of the University of Tennessee College of Medicine, August H. Wittenborg, M.D., was so moved by the student's desperate plight, that he assured him that a loan could be arranged from the Ladies' Auxiliary to the Memphis and Shelby County Medical Society. That young student, for whom Dr. Wittenborg showed compassion, was Charles Coleman Verstandig, M.D., who did graduate from the University of Tennessee College of Medicine in 1939.[28]

Dr. Verstandig was born in Opelika, Alabama in 1908. After he graduated from high school, he joined the military, and in 1930 he entered the Alabama Poly Technic Institute (which today is known as Auburn University). He graduated during the difficult days of 1934, and with the encouragement of his physics professor, he applied to the University of Tennessee Medical School and was accepted. Even with the Auxiliary's loan, Charlie Verstandig's time in medical school was extremely difficult. He worked part-time at Plough's Drug Store on Beale Street, the original Piggly Wiggly Grocery Store, and elsewhere. His wife, Mary Elizabeth Lovely, worked as a medical librarian at the Baptist Memorial Hospital, where she was known as "Mary Lovely," since the couple decided that Verstandig's marital status should not be advertised. As Dr. Verstandig said, "In those days they didn't like their medical students to be married." So, very few people even knew that he was married. "I think Pinkie Hyman (Dr. Hyman was Dean of the U.T. College of Medicine at that time) knew right from the beginning, but he never said a word about it to me," Verstandig stated. His financial worries continued right up to the end of medical school. Two days before he was due to graduate, he was contacted by the financial office and was informed that unless he could pay a diploma fee of $25, he would not be allowed to graduate. He asked his wife to call Dr. Henry G. Rudner, who was in charge of the Baptist Memorial Hospital blood bank service, to arrange for him to be a blood donor the next day. "That patient no more needed a blood transfusion than you or I, but Dr. Rudner paid me the $25 right then and there, and I paid for my diploma," Verstandig stated.[28]

During World War II, Dr. Verstandig served as a Colonel, (MC) U.S. Army and remained in the Army for five years. His last assignment took him to New Haven, Connecticut where he worked in the Yale University Army Tactical Training Command Air Corps Hospital as a radiologist. He continued to practice radiology in New Haven and became a nationally recognized radiologist. In 1984 Dr. Verstandig was honored by the University of Tennessee by receiving the Distinguished Alumni Award. He was the recipient of many other awards for his services to mankind, including the Presidential Citation for Care of the Aged by President Reagan and the Distinguished Service Award from the American Medical Association.[13,28]

Upon his return to Memphis briefly after World War II, he visited Dr. Hyman and asked how he could help repay the University for all that it had done for him. Dr. Hyman suggested that funds could be set aside for a student who experienced significant financial worries during his course in medical school. Since 1952, when the Charles C. Verstandig Award was first established, it has been given to the graduating University of Tennessee medical student who, in the opinion of his classmates, has overcome the

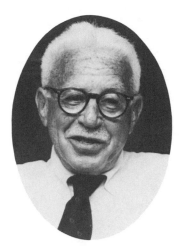

FIGURE 131. *Charles Coleman Verstandig, M.D. (1908–1985)*

151

greatest difficulties in obtaining the M.D. degree. On July 31, 1979 Charles C. Verstandig, M.D. established at the University of Tennessee, Memphis the Charles C. and Mary Elizabeth Lovely Verstandig Endowment Fund; income from this fund provides annual money for the Verstandig Distinguished Visiting Professorship in honor of his wife, who died in an automobile accident in 1965. Dr. Verstandig is depicted in Figure 131. By his gratitude and generosity as a devoted alumnus, Dr. Charles Verstandig repaid the University multifold for his education. He was a member of the U.T. College of Medicine Alumni Council and the Heritage Society, which recognizes those individuals who have donated $50,000 or more to the University. His son, Lee L. Verstandig, is the Under Secretary for the U.S. Department of Housing and Urban Development in Washington, D.C.[13,28]

Dr. Donald Berthold Zilversmit joined the University of Tennessee Department of Physiology as an Instructor in 1949, after receiving his Ph.D. in Physiology from the University of California in 1948. In collaboration with Dr. van Handle, he published in 1954 a method for phospholipid analysis which has been the third most referenced scientific paper in all of the biochemical literature, up to approximately 1980. In 1959 he was the founder and first Editor of the *Journal of Lipid Research*, which is still a major scientific journal. In 1959, Dr. Zilversmit was awarded one of the first Career Investigator Awards as a lifetime career support mechanism ($30,000 per annum) from the American Heart Association. He was the seventh such individual to be selected for this prestigious award and was the first one in the South.[4,13]

Dr. Zilversmit was one of the favorite lecturers among the U.T. students. He always arrived precisely on time for his scheduled lecture, and with a dramatic entrance, he slammed the door after him—no student ever dared enter the closed lecture hall afterwards. The old doors in the Wittenborg Building lecture rooms had frosted glass panels in the upper portion. Every time he slammed the door violently and launched rapidly into his lecture, the glass in the door would quiver and shake—students always expected the glass to shatter one day, but it never did, as he evidently knew exactly the amount of force to use. One of his more famous quotes that remained with his old students years afterwards dealt with his lecture on the male reproductive system, specifically spermatozoa, which he compared to college students aspiring to enter medical school—"many are called, but few are chosen."

Lester van Middlesworth was born in 1919, and received two degrees from the University of Virginia (a B.S. in 1940, and an M.S. in Chemistry in 1942). His Ph.D. degree in Physiology was completed at the University of California (Berkeley) in 1946. He came to U.T. Memphis in 1946 as an Instructor in the Department of Physiology and also entered the University of Tennessee College of Medicine, receiving his M.D. in 1954.[4] Dr. van Middlesworth has continually taught physiology classes to medical and/or dental students each year since October of 1946. In 1967 he received the first U.T. Alumni Association's Outstanding Teacher Award. His extensive research activities have concentrated on the thyroid gland. In 1954 Dr. van Middlesworth made the very important discovery that the thyroid gland tended to store radioactive iodine. In 1960 he reported his results of studying several thousand thyroid glands from cattle on four continents, noting the increase in radioactive iodine levels after atomic bomb testing. This original concept provided an important, easily measurable method for determining the amount of radioactive fallout throughout the world after atomic or hydrogen bomb testing. Beginning in 1965, he received a Career Research Award from the National Institutes of Health, and this award has continued annually from 1965 to the present.[4,13]

Richard R. Overman, Ph.D. (Figure 132) has been one of the most productive researchers and most renowned teachers in the U.T. Department of Physiology in his 35 years of affiliation with the University. He was born on November 10, 1916 in Richmond, Indiana, and attained his A.B. degree with a major in Zoology from DePauw University in 1939. From 1939–1940 he worked as a Research Assistant in Biology at Harvard University, then was selected as a Francis H. Maule Fellow in Biology at Princeton University for 1940–1941. He was a John DeWitt Sterry Fellow in Biology from 1942–1943, receiving his M.A. degree in 1942 and his Ph.D. degree in 1943 from Princeton University. He accepted an appointment as Instructor in Physiology at the College of Physicians and Surgeons of Columbia University in New York City from 1943–1945.[21]

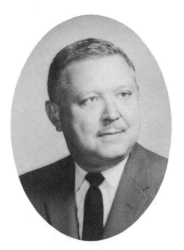

FIGURE 132. *Richard R. Overman, Ph.D. (1916–) Professor, U.T. Department of Physiology, 1954–1980, and First Distinguished Professor of The University of Tennessee, Memphis, 1975*

Dr. Dick Overman came to the University of Tennessee College of Medicine in 1945 as an Instructor in the Department of Physiology. He has held responsible positions in teaching and administration and has made significant scientific contributions in medical research. He published the first scientific paper on the use of flame photometry for sodium and potassium determination in biological fluids, and he introduced this method into local clinical investigative efforts. He was also instrumental in introducing infrared absorption spectroscopy and atomic absorption spectrometry to clinical studies. In addition, the first blood, extra-cellular fluid, and total body water measurement on patients was performed in his laboratory at the University of Tennessee, Memphis. After being trained for six months in the handling of radioactive materials at Oak Ridge, Tennessee, Dr. Dick Overman was the first researcher in Memphis to utilize radioactive materials.[21] He was almost singularly responsible for the early functional integration that occurred between the basic and clinical sciences at U.T. Memphis. In 1952 Dr. Overman was responsible for the establishment of the Institute of Clinical Investigation, which was physically located in the old Institute of Pathology and housed in the Division of Clinical Physiology, the Division of Clinical Chemistry, and the Division of Experimental Surgery. His further efforts in collaboration with other investigators led to the establishment of the Clinical Investigative Unit for Internal Medicine and the Clinical Investigative Laboratory, which served as the forerunner to the present University of Tennessee Clinical Research Center. In addition, basic sciences were integrated with radiology in the design and establishment of the Division of Radiation Biology, where significant contributions were made in studying whole body radiation. During the process of his research endeavors, approximately $20,000,000 in grant and construction funds were secured by him from outside the State of Tennessee,[21] and nearly 100 scientific publications were produced by Dr. Overman in national and international journals.[10,13,21]

For much of his 35 years with the University of Tennessee, Memphis, Dr. Overman taught all or portions of the Physiology course to nursing, pharmacy, medical, and dental students, instructing approximately 4,000 to 5,000 students in his career, both at the University of Tennessee, Memphis and at the College of Physicians and Surgeons of Columbia University. He served for four years as a member of the Cardiovascular Study Section, one year as a member of the General Medical Sciences Section, one year as a member of the Cardiovascular Training Committee, and three years as a member of the Committee on Radiological Health, all associated with the National Institutes of Health in Bethesda, Maryland. The Division of Clinical Physiology, under Dr. Overman's guidance, mounted a large graduate program (5 M.S. and 16 Ph.D. degrees) for basic science students.[21] The unique character of this particular training program was that it was performed in an atmosphere of clinical or applied research, rather than in pure basic science isolation.[13] Among his more important administrative positions held at the University of Tennessee College of Medicine are the following: Assistant Dean for Research and Grant Affairs, 1964–1966; Associate Dean of the College of Medicine, 1966–1970; Acting Dean of the College of Medicine, 1970–1972; Vice Chancellor for Academic Affairs, 1972–1974; and Vice Chancellor for Research and Support Services, 1974–1980. As part of his international scientific activities, Dr. Overman established the Rockefeller Foundation Program for collaborative teaching and research between the University of Tennessee, Memphis and the Universidad del Valle in Cali, Colombia from 1960–1972. During that time 14 Colombian physicians earned Ph.D. degrees in the United States and returned to Colombia to establish modern basic science departments there and also to found the first Graduate School of Medical Science in South America.[13,21]

In 1975 Richard R. Overman, Ph.D. was designated as the first Distinguished Professor of the University of Tennessee, Memphis by Chancellor Al Farmer because of his many accomplishments in the U.T. Departments of Physiology, Medicine, Radiology, Obstetrics/Gynecology, and Psychiatry.[21] He was also named as Emeritus Professor within the U.T. Department of Physiology in 1980.[13]

Mention will be made in detail of their specific medical accomplishments in subsequent chapters, but a significant number of U.T. Memphis graduates in the brief span of time from March through September of 1955 reached national prominence in varied ways: Dr. Louis Britt—an outstanding general surgeon, respected clinical teacher, and developer of the University of Tennessee Kidney Transplant Program; Dr. Dee Canale—one of the distinguished neurosurgeons in the Mid-South area and President of the Memphis and Shelby County Medical Society, 1985–1986; Dr. Winfield Dunn—Governor of the State of Tennessee, 1971–1975; Dr. Jim Enoch—Rear Admiral (DC) U.S. Navy and Chief of the U.S. Navy Dental Corps; Dr. Jim Hamner—Associate Director of the National Cancer Institute, National Institutes of Health, a noted researcher in Pathology, and textbook author of *The Management of Head and Neck Cancer*; Dr. Malcolm Lynch—Associate Dean of the University of Pennsylvania School of Dentistry and textbook author of *Oral Medicine*; Dr. Mike Overbey—Brigadier General (DC) U.S. Army Reserve; and Dr. Bob Summitt—Dean of the U.T. College of Medicine, a noted researcher in Genetics, and Rear Admiral (MC) U.S. Naval Reserve.

REFERENCES

1. Bruesch, Simon R.: Personal Communication, 1985.

2. Diggs, Lemuel W.: Personal Communication, 1985.

3. Etteldorf, James N.: Personal Communication, 1985.

4. Ginski, John M.: *History of the Department of Physiology 1879–1984, U.T. College of Medicine*, (Private Printing: Memphis, TN.), 1984.

5. Hughes, James G.: Personal Communication, 1985.

6. Hughes, James G.: *Department of Pediatrics—UTCHS: 1910–1985*, 1985.

7. Jones, Madison: *History of the Tennessee State Dental Association*, (Tennessee Dental Association: Memphis, TN.), 1958.

8. Justis, Sr., E. Jeff: Personal Communication, 1985.

9. Kossmann, Charles E.: "Daniel Anthony Brody: 1915–1975", *Transactions of the Assoc. of Amer. Physicians* 89:15–17, 1976.

10. Lollar, Michael: *Commercial Appeal Mid-South Magazine*, May, 1984.

11. McKnight, James P.: Personal Communication, 1985.

12. Medical Accomplishments: U.T. College of Dentistry.

13. Medical Accomplishments: U.T. College of Medicine.

14. Medical Accomplishments: U.T. College of Nursing.

15. Medical Accomplishments: U.T. College of Pharmacy.

16. Montgomery, F. June: Personal Communication, 1985.

17. Montgomery, J. R. Folmsbee, S. J., and Greene, L. S.: *To Foster Knowledge: A History of the University of Tennessee 1794–1970*, (The University of Tennessee Press: Knoxville, TN.), 1984.

18. Morris, Joe Hall: Personal Communication, 1985.

19. Murry, Ruth Neil: Personal Communication, 1985.

20. Neill, Kenneth: "Profile: Dr. John Shea", (Private Printing: Memphis, TN.), 1984.

21. Overman, Richard R.: Personal Communication, 1985.

22. Reynolds, Richard J.: Personal Communication, 1985.

23. Sprunt, Douglas H. and Crocker, Robert A.: *History of the Department of Pathology of the University of Tennessee*, (Private Printing), 1965.

24. Stewart, Marcus J.: Personal Communication, 1985.

25. Stewart, Marcus J. and Black, William T., Jr.: *History of Medicine in Memphis*, (McCowat-Mercer Press, Inc.: Jackson, TN., 1971.

26. Tennessee Medical Alumnus: (Fall, 1975—Dr. Gilbert J. Levy).

27. Tennessee Medical Alumnus: (Fall, 1979—Dr. Phineas J. Sparer).

28. Tennessee Medical Alumnus: (Winter, 1984—Dr. Charles C. Verstandig).

29. University Center-Grams: April, 1950 ("Dr. James T. Ginn").

30. University Center-Grams: Feb., 1951 ("Dr. William L. Wallace").

31. University Center-Grams: June, 1951 ("Dr. August H. Wittenborg).

32. University Center-Grams: Aug., 1951 (U.T. Cancer Research Laboratory").

33. University Center-Grams: Oct., 1951 ("Dr. Harry Schmeisser").

34. University Center-Grams: June, 1952 ("Dr. Robert L. Sanders").

35. University Center-Grams: Aug., 1952 ("Dr. C.C. Erickson").

36. University Center-Grams: Oct., 1952 ("Dr. Grover Bowles").

37. University Center-Grams: April, 1953 ("U.T. Building Programs").

38. University Center-Grams: Oct., 1953 ("Dr. Karl Goldner").

39. University Center-Grams: Dec., 1953 (U.T. Ranking").

40. University Center-Grams: April, 1956 ("Sigma Xi").

41. University Center-Grams: Aug., 1957 ("Pediatric Research Lab" & "Dr. Jesse D. Perkinson").

42. University Center-Grams: Feb., 1958 ("Dr. Maston Callison").

43. University of Tennessee, Memphis: Bulletins (1950–1959).

44. Wooten, Nina E. and Williams, Golden: *A History of the Tennessee State Nurses Association*, (Tennessee Nurses Association: Tennessee, TN.), 1955.

156

CHAPTER SEVEN
1960–1969

*T*HE 1960's were a troubled, perplexing decade for the entire United States, and the academic world felt its deleterious effects most acutely. The upsurge of national enthusiasm and confidence, which followed John F. Kennedy's narrow, closely contested victory for the Presidency in 1960, was shattered by his assassination on November 22, 1963. Vice President Lyndon B. Johnson was inaugurated as President immediately after this tragedy and rapidly proceeded to pass an immense legislative program through the Congress, much of it affecting both health care and health manpower.

American military advisors were first sent to South Viet Nam in 1962 by President Kennedy—by the end of 1963 there were over 15,000 U.S. servicemen there. On August 2, 1964 North Vietnamese ships attacked two U.S. destroyers in international waters, and on August 7, 1964 Congress passed the Gulf of Tonkin Resolution, which authorized active military intervention in Viet Nam by the President. An initial amphibious landing by the Third Marine Regiment, Third Marine Division escalated into a full-scale extensive war, which finally ended with the total withdrawal of U.S. Forces in April of 1975.

As the battle casualties increased and the fighting continued for years without a clear-cut victory, there was much discontent and unrest during these unsettled times in the United States—this frustration was especially manifested among college undergraduates and even health professional students. The University of Tennessee, Memphis had many medical, dental, and nursing graduates in the Armed Forces who were directly involved in caring for the wounded in this War. Karl Edmond Shenep, M.D., who was a Captain (MC) U.S. Army, received his medical degree from the U.T. College of Medicine in 1964. He was killed in action on April 16, 1967 by enemy ground fire, while flying on a rescue helicopter mission in Viet Nam (Appendix I).

Important leadership changes occurred during the 1960's at U.T. Memphis, the most significant one being the retirement of Orren W. Hyman, Ph.D. on June 30, 1961. "Pinkie" Hyman devoted 48 years of his life to the University of Tennessee, Memphis—and for 40 of those 48 years he led our University—and he led it exceptionally well. There was unprecedented growth of the U.T. Medical Units during his tenure, and he retired with justifiable recognition as one of the nation's leading health education administrators, having stood his watch well. Dr. Hyman was honored at a testimonial dinner on May 23, 1961 at the Memphis Country Club by University of Tennessee faculty, his former U.T. students, and

"Religious or philosophical commitment is not an optional extra in the practice of Medicine; it has a fundamental bearing on the way the work is done."

Dame Cicely M. Saunders, M.D.

157

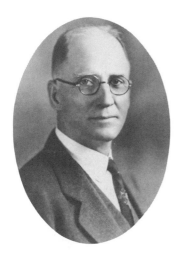

FIGURE 133. *Harcourt A. Morgan, B.S., A.M., LL.D. (1867–1950), President, University of Tennessee, 1919–1933*

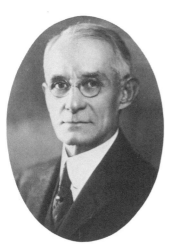

FIGURE 134. *James D. Hoskins, B.S., A.M., LL.B., LL.D. (1870–1960), President, University of Tennessee, 1933–1946*

his many friends. Earlier on May 17, 1961 the Tennessee State Dental Association paid special tribute to Dr. O. W. Hyman for his many services to dentistry in Tennessee and the Mid-South by presenting Mrs. Hyman and him with a silver platter, appropriately engraved for the occasion.[17,18]

With the death in 1919 of President Brown Ayres, who had been President of the University of Tennessee for 15 years and who had manipulated the entire merger that formed U.T. Memphis from 1911–1913, he was succeeded by three distinguished gentlemen before the 1960's. Harcourt A. Morgan, B.S., A.M., LL.D. (Figure 133) was President for 14 years (1919–1933), at which time he was appointed by President Franklin D. Roosevelt to be the first Chairman of the Tennessee Valley Authority (T.V.A.) in 1933. During the severe Depression years of the 1930's through the end of World War II, the University of Tennessee was in the capable hands of James D. Hoskins, B.S., A.M., LL.B., LL.D. (Figure 134), who served 13 years as President from 1933–1946. He, in turn, was succeeded by President C. E. Brehm, B.S., LL.D. (Figure 135), who also served 13 years from 1946–1959.[4,29]

Andrew D. Holt, Ph.D., LL.D. became the sixteenth President of the University of Tennessee on July 1, 1959. Dr. Holt was one the most outstanding Presidents in the University's proud history (Figure 136). He was born in Milan, Tennessee in 1904 and earned his B.A. degree from Emory University in Atlanta. Afterwards, he completed his graduate studies at Columbia University in New York, obtaining both his M.S. and Ph.D. degrees. Union University granted him an honorary Doctor of Legal Letters degree in recognition of his long-time service to education. Dr. Holt was familiar with U.T. Memphis, having served as Principal of the Training School at Memphis State University, a Professor on the M.S.U. faculty, and High School Supervisor for West Tennessee. Before joining the University of Tennessee in Knoxville as the Administrative Assistant to President C. E. Brehm in 1950, he was the Executive Secretary of the Tennessee Education Association. He later was appointed as Vice President of the University of Tennessee, then President. Dr. Holt was given an honorary life membership in the Tennessee State Dental Association—being the only layman so honored—for his interest in the dental profession. Dr. Andy Holt led the huge building program of the University of Tennessee from 1959–1970.[29]

President Holt best summarized Dr. Hyman's life, character, and numerous contributions by his famous one-sentence introduction of Pinkie Hyman to the Memphis Rotary Club in 1961:

"No University has ever had a Vice President who was able to squeeze more and better education out of a tax dollar, no faculty has ever had a leader who fought harder for their welfare or who left less doubt about where he stood on the problems they brought to him, no student body has ever had a Dean more grimly determined that they shall not be shortchanged in their education, no President has ever had a Vice President who more effectively keeps his boss' chestnuts out of the fire, no head of an institution has been more soundly cussed but more universally loved and respected by his alumni, no vicious critic of U.T.'s mighty Vols has ever backed into a sharper buzz saw, no salesman has ever encountered a customer less inclined to accept a wooden nickel, no city has ever had a citizen with fewer inhibitions about bragging on his home town from its Cotton Carnival to its mighty Mississippi, no Rotary Club has ever had a member who more faithfully practices in everything he does the ideal of service above self, no man of 30 has ever had a more youthful spirit, contagious enthusiasm or limitless vision, no duck has ever dodged a more deadly hunter, no homelier guy ever married a lovelier wife, and no person in this audience has ever known a nicer guy than O. W. Hyman."

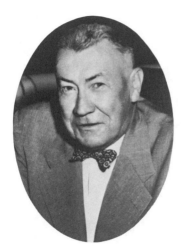

FIGURE 135. *C. E. Brehm,*
B.S., LL.D. (1889–1971)
President, University of
Tennessee, 1946–1959

The successor to Dr. O. W. Hyman, as Vice President and Chancellor of the U.T. Medical Units, was Dr. Homer F. Marsh. He was born in Terre Haute, Indiana in 1909, received his B.S. in Chemistry in 1927 from Indiana Teacher's College, received his M.S. degree in Bacteriology from Purdue University in 1932, and obtained his Ph.D. degree in Bacteriology from Ohio State in 1941. Following his graduation from Ohio State in 1941, Dr. Marsh joined the faculty of the University of Oklahoma School of Medicine in its Department of Bacteriology; in 1946 he became Chairman of that Department. Also, he served as Associate Dean of Student Affairs at the Oklahoma School of Medicine from 1947–1952. At that time, he moved to the University of Miami to assist in the organization of the University of Miami's new School of Medicine. For 10 years he served as its Dean and guided it to become the focus of an international medical center. Dr. Marsh held memberships in numerous professional organizations, including the Society of American Bacteriologists and Sigma Xi. He was also the author of numerous scientific articles. (Figure 137) Dr. Homer Marsh performed the arduous task of guiding the University of Tennessee, Memphis through the turbulent times of the 1960's decade in an exceptionally fine fashion. He was responsible for an additional extensive building program which will be discussed later.[18]

Dr. Maston Callison, as mentioned in Chapter Six, remained as Dean of the University of Tennessee College of Medicine from 1957–1970.[18]

With the sudden death of Dr. James T. Ginn from an acute coronary occlusion on October 31, 1959, William Herbert Jolley, D.D.S. was appointed by Dr. Hyman as Acting Dean for the U.T. College of Dentistry on November 2, 1959 (Appendix C). He served in this capacity until July of 1961 (Figure 138). Earlier, he attended Lambuth College and Memphis State University prior to receiving his D.D.S. from the University of Tennessee, Memphis in 1941. During World War II, Dr. Jolley was a Major in the U.S. Army Dental Corps. He served in the U.S. Army Reserve's 330th General Hospital Unit as a Colonel and commanded the Dental Section. After his service discharge, he conducted a successful private practice in Paris, Tennessee for ten years, then returned to the U.T. College of Dentistry in July of 1956 as an Assistant Professor in the Oral Medicine and Surgery Department. Dr. Jolley was appointed Associate Professor and Clinical Director of the U.T. College of Dentistry in July of 1958.[16,17]

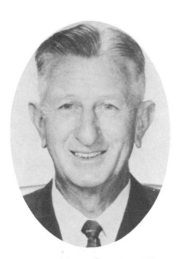

FIGURE 136. *Andrew D. Holt,*
A.B., M.S., Ph.D., LL.D.
(1904–   ), President,
University of Tennessee,
1959–1970

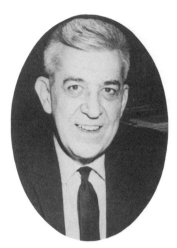

FIGURE 137. *Homer F.
Marsh, Ph.D. (1909–   )
Vice President and Chancellor,
U.T. Medical Units,
1961–1970*

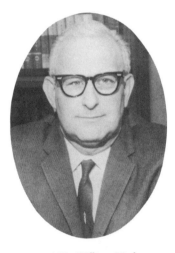

FIGURE 138. *William Herbert
Jolley, D.D.S. (1916–   )
Acting Dean, U.T. College of
Dentistry, October, 1959—
July, 1961 and February,
1969—August, 1970*

After an extensive national search, Shailer A. Peterson, Ph.D. was selected as the new permanent Dean of the University of Tennessee College of Dentistry in February of 1961. Dr. Peterson (Figure 139) was a nationally known dental educator, who had served previously as Secretary of the Council on Dental Education for the American Dental Association since 1948. By being directly involved with the accrediting agency for all American dental schools, he brought a wealth of broad knowledge and national experience to his new position at U.T.[17,22]

Dr. Shailer Peterson was born in 1909, received a B.A. and an M.A. from the University of Oregon, and obtained his Ph.D. in Education from the University of Minnesota. He was a member of 22 professional organizations, published over 200 articles and reviews for professional journals, and participated in many national conferences which dealt with dental education.[16]

There were no administrative changes in either the College of Pharmacy or the College of Nursing during the 1960's decade. Dr. Dick Feurt remained as Dean of the U.T. College of Pharmacy from 1959–1975. Ruth Neil Murry remained as Dean of the U.T. College of Nursing from 1949–1977.[19,20]

The year 1960 witnessed the retirement of Thomas Palmer Nash, Ph.D. as Dean of the School of Biological Sciences, which he had led so adroitly since 1928. Dr. Nash was honored by his many friends and University of Tennessee faculty colleagues with a retirement dinner at the Memphis Country Club on May 24, 1960. Laudatory remarks were made by President Andrew Holt, Vice President O. W. Hyman, and Dr. Roland H. Alden, who succeeded Dr. Nash as Dean of the School of Biological Sciences. This School had a humble beginning with only a few graduate students; however, with persistent nourishment and demanding leadership, Dr. Nash saw it mature significantly, having grown to an annual enrollment of 65 students at the time of his retirement in 1960 (Table 12). Along with the previously

Table 12
The University of Tennessee, Memphis—Enrollment 1960–1969

Fall Term	College of Medicine	College of Dentistry	School of Pharmacy	School of Nursing	School of Biological Sciences
1960	568	370	253	72	65
1961	581	352	269	65	80
1962	546	362	267	58	81
1963	535	369	252	72	97
1964	527	387	241	100	106
1965	471	366	254	123	114
1966	517	388	268	122	106
1967	502	374	279	155	98
1968	545	397	307	144	99
1969	560	399	307	139	109

mentioned retirement of Dr. Pinkie Hyman on June 30, 1961, the University of Tennessee, Memphis lost two of its educational and administrative "giants" with the departure of Drs. Hyman and Nash. The 1960's ushered in a new era of different leadership, which was indeed fortunate to have such a solid base on which to build.[4,27]

Roland Herrick Alden, Ph.D. was extremely well-qualified to become the new Dean (Figure 140). He was born on February 4, 1914 in Champaign, Illinois, received his A.B. degree from Stanford University in 1936 with honors, and obtained his Ph.D. degree with a major in Zoology and a minor in Anatomy from Yale University in 1941.[29] After a year as an Instructor in Zoology at Yale University, he joined the U.T. Memphis faculty as an Instructor in the Department of Anatomy, originally planning to stay only two years.[27]

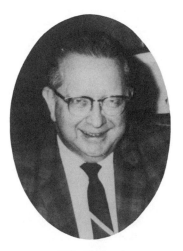

FIGURE 139. *Shailer A. Peterson, Ph.D. (1908–1978) Dean, U.T. College of Dentistry, 1961–1969*

The expected two years stretched into thirty-seven years, during which time Dr. Alden served through the academic ranks to become a Professor of Anatomy (1949), Head of the Department of Microscopic Anatomy (1949–1951), Chief of the Division of Anatomy (1951–1961), Associate Dean of the Graduate School of Medical Sciences (1960–1968), Dean of the School of Basic Medical Sciences (1968–1979), and Acting Chancellor of the University of Tennessee, Memphis (November of 1970).[4]

Dr. Roland Alden was appointed on January 1, 1960 to the position of Associate Dean of the Graduate School of Medical Sciences, which was newly created by the University of Tennessee Board of Trustees. While retaining his position as Chief of the Division of Anatomy, he relieved part of the academic burden from Dr. Nash's shoulders, who remained as Dean of the School of Biological Sciences until his retirement in 1961. At that time the positions were merged, and Dr. Alden became Dean of the renamed "College of Basic Medical Sciences" (see Appendix G) and remained in that position through June 30, 1979.[29]

Dr. Alden was heavily involved with the American Association of Anatomists, serving as a member of the Committee on Educational Affairs from 1962–1968, a member of the Executive Committee from 1967–1968, and as its President from 1969–1970. He held membership in many professional societies and published 27 significant scholarly articles in the scientific literature. On a national level, he served as a member of the Anatomy Test Committee for the National Board of Medical Examiners (1959–1962); he was Chairman of the Board of Directors of the Les Passees Treatment Center for Cerebral-Palsied Children and served as its Director from 1950–1952; he was President of the Memphis and Shelby County Chapter of the Tennessee Society for Crippled Children and Adults; he was Chairman of the U.S. Public Health Service Anatomical Services Training Committee from 1960–1964; and he was a Member of the Board of Directors of the Associated Pathologist Foundation from 1970–1976. Also, it should be remembered that he was one of the Founding Members of the University of Tennessee, Memphis Chapter of Sigma Xi.[29]

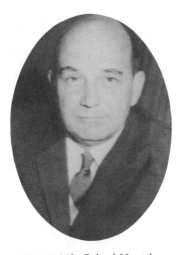

FIGURE 140. *Roland Herrick Alden, Ph.D. (1914–   ) Dean, College of Basic Medical Sciences, 1961–1979*

In his 37 years of commitment and contribution to U.T. Memphis,

Roland Alden exerted a cumulative, intellectual impact on the University, and he was greatly admired by his colleagues as both a scholar and a humanist.[4,27] As a student, I recall Dr. Alden as a professor who was highly regarded and universally respected by students from all of the Colleges. He was dedicated to a high sense of principle and scholastic excellence—and he led by example, which is the best form of leadership. He was an outstanding teacher of Head and Neck Anatomy. When we, as freshmen in anatomy, tried frantically to scribble down each of his words during one of the initial lectures, he paused and stated to the class, "You cannot possibly copy every word that I utter—just listen and absorb it; this information will make you intelligent doctors, not just trained technicians." His friends, faculty colleagues, and students donated generously to commission a portrait of Dr. Alden, and it now hangs in the office of the Vice Chancellor for Academic Affairs at the University of Tennessee, Memphis.

Student enrollment for the U.T. College of Medicine remained fairly constant in the 1960's decade, commencing with 568 students in 1960 and ending with 560 students in 1969 (Table 12). It never reached the 600+ mark, as it had five out of the ten years during the 1950's decade. The U.T. College of Dentistry followed a similar pattern: 370 students in 1960 and 399 students in 1969. During the 1950's, eight out of the ten years carried a class enrollment of over 400 students in this College, reaching a high of 480 in 1953, in contrast to a high mark in the 1960's of 399 students in 1969. The U.T. College of Pharmacy continued its rise in enrollment, growing from 253 students in 1960 to 307 students in 1969. Likewise, the U.T. College of Nursing enrollment rose from 72 nursing students in 1960 to 139 nursing students in 1969. This figure was a rise of almost 100%. The School of Biological Sciences' enrollment rose dramatically and almost doubled during the 1960's decade, enlarging from 65 students in 1960 to 109 students in 1969. (Table 12).

An ambitious building surge forward was accomplished by the University of Tennessee, Memphis and the hospitals with which it was closely allied during the 1960's. The Baptist Memorial Hospital was enlarged and modernized, completing the Madison Avenue Wing in 1960 (Figure 141). The old, trackless trolley buses can be seen in the lower portion of this illustration. Figure 142 depicts the entire current Baptist Memorial Hospital with the Union Avenue Wing facing the heliport and front lawn area. It was completed in February of 1968. This photograph was taken in 1985, as evidenced by the new University of Tennessee, Memphis Library, which was completed and dedicated in 1985, just to the left of the new hospital wings and the old Physicians and Surgeons Office Building. These additions created a total of just over 2,000 beds, making Baptist Memorial Hospital the largest private hospital in the world. U.T. medical students receive clinical training in the Baptist Memorial Hospital, and in 1986 the Departments of Pathology for U.T. Memphis and Baptist Memorial Hospital are planned to be merged and quartered within the Baptist Memorial Hospital.

The year 1962 saw the completion of the Chandler Clinical Services

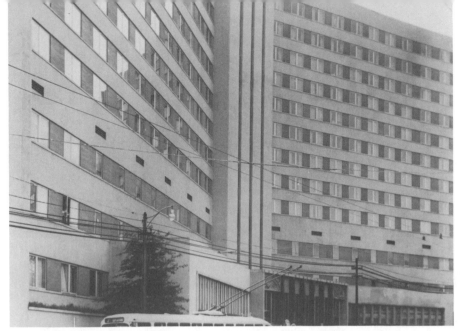

FIGURE 141. *Baptist Memorial Hospital Madison Avenue Wing, 1960*

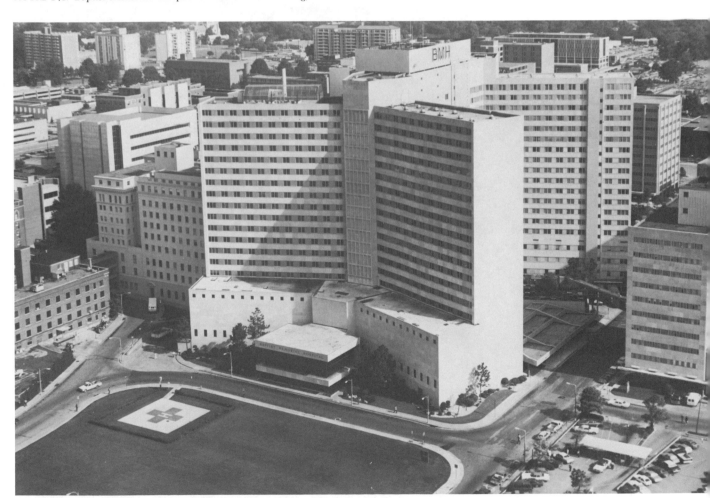

FIGURE 142. *Baptist Memorial Hospital Union Avenue Wing, 1968*

163

Center, which was named for former Memphis Mayor Walter Chandler. The construction of a five-story Dental-Pharmacy Research Building (Figure 143) was also finished in 1962. Originally this building was used for research purposes by both the U.T. Colleges of Dentistry and Pharmacy faculty. Today, it is occupied totally by the College of Pharmacy. This building was renamed the Seldon D. Feurt Memorial Building in 1975 to honor and commemorate Dr. Feurt, who was Dean of the U.T. College of Pharmacy from 1959 until his death in 1975.[20]

The Memphis Mental Health Institute (Figure 144) was constructed and opened in 1962; it is located at the southeastern corner of Dunlap and Poplar, facing Poplar Avenue. As the first fully-accredited psychiatric hospital in the State, it serves as a short-term intensive treatment center for Memphis area residents. The Alcohol Rehabilitation Research Center, started by David H. Knott, M.D., Ph.D. and James D. Beard, Ph.D., was the first of its kind in Tennessee, and this program has evolved into an Alcohol and Drug Abuse Center and a Methadone Maintenance Program. Its Alcohol Research Project has gained national recognition. The Children's Unit, which was opened in 1967, includes a residential center that offers treatment to mentally disturbed children through age 12, while the Adolescent Unit offers treatment to persons up to age 18 years.

The Institute has emphasized training and research since its inception. It has participated in the education and training of psychiatric residents, psychologists, social workers, nurses, and pharmacists from the University of Tennessee, Memphis and Memphis State University, as well as other institutions in the Mid-South area. Also, the Memphis Mental Health Institute has a partial hospitalization unit, a crisis intervention program, and an aftercare follow-up system in both the Institute *per se* and in community mental health centers. Full collaboration with the University of Tennessee was accomplished in 1974 with a merger which entailed the appointment of the Memphis Mental Health Institute's Superintendent as Chairman of the University of Tennessee College of Medicine's Department of Psychiatry. Its average daily bed occupancy rate in 1976 was 118; this figure has risen to 212 in 1986. The Memphis Mental Health Institute and the U.T. Department of Psychiatry are ably administered by Neil B. Edwards, M.D., who is the current Chairman.[1]

In June of 1968, Sheldon B. Korones, M.D. relinquished his private practice in pediatrics to join the University of Tennessee, Memphis faculty on a full-time basis. His major objective was to combat the high infant mortality rate in Memphis, Shelby County, and the surrounding counties. There was an urgent need for adequately trained personnel in sufficient numbers to care for "high-risk" infants and modern monitoring equipment to care for the newborn ill. In 1967 the considered acceptable mortality rate in the United States was 18.3 per 1,000 births. The infant mortality rate in Memphis-Shelby County was 30.4 per 1,000 births. Thus, the University of Tennessee Newborn Center began in a small space within the John Gaston Hospital's Maternity Wing.[18]

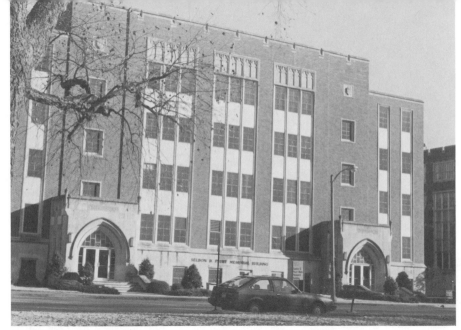

FIGURE 143. *Dental-Pharmacy Research Building, 1962 (Renamed the Seldon D. Feurt Memorial Building in 1975)*

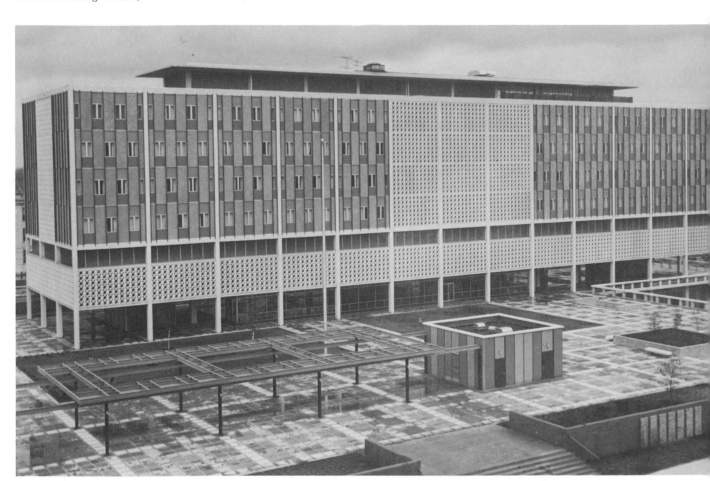

FIGURE 144. *Memphis Mental Health Institute, 1962*

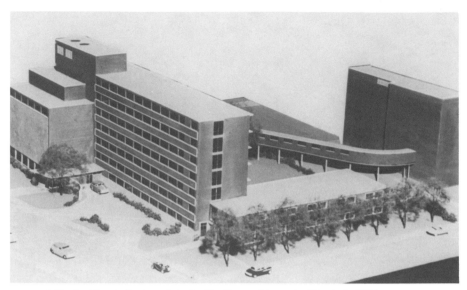

FIGURE 145. *Architect's Design of the E. H. Crump Maternity Hospital, 1955*

In 1971, the City of Memphis and the U.T. Department of Pediatrics cooperated in a joint program to enlarge and renovate the original, restricted, minimally prepared space occupied by the Newborn Center. The renovated unit was occupied on November 14, 1971. After a series of growth spurts, dictated by pressing need, in six years it evolved into the current U.T. Newborn Center, occupying an entire floor of the Edward Hull Crump Maternity Hospital (Figure 145). To this outstanding University of Tennessee, Memphis facility, 1,300 critically ill or tiny infants are admitted annually for total newborn care by a dedicated, compassionate health professional staff. The U.T. Newborn Center in Memphis is one of the largest of its kind in the United States and has served as an excellent example for the establishment of similar-type newborn centers elsewhere. In addition, it has contributed greatly to the nation by training many health care professionals in this subspecialty of pediatrics.[11]

Dr. Sheldon B. Korones was born April 26, 1924 in New York City. He completed his undergraduate training at the University of Tennessee in Knoxville and received his B.S. degree in 1944. His M.D. degree was also obtained from the University of Tennessee, Memphis in 1947. After a year's internship at the Boston City Hospital from 1948–1949, he completed a four-year residency in pediatrics at the Babies Hospital in New York City in 1954. In addition to his pediatric training, Dr. Korones also spent one year in Pathology at the Children's Medical Center in Boston. He is a Diplomate of the American Board of Pediatrics (1954) with a Sub-Board Specialty in Neonatal/Perinatal Medicine (1977). His professional society memberships include the Southern Society for Pediatric Research, the American Academy of Pediatrics, the Tennessee Pediatric Society, the Memphis Pediatric Society, Sigma Xi, and an Associate Fellow, American College of Obstetricians and Gynecologists. His other activities include: Board Examiner for Oral Exams for Maternal and Fetal Medicine, American Board of OB/GYN, consultant for the United States Department of Justice, and Director of Newborn Service at the University of Tennessee College of Medicine. Honors and commendations for Dr. Korones have been extensive. He was a member of the Board of Directors for the Memphis Symphony Orchestra from 1961–1970; he was Citizen of the Year, Newspaper Guild of Memphis in 1974; he was given the Myrtle Wreath Award for Humanitarian Service for the Hadassah Organization in 1976; he was commended for his contributions to Perinatal Medicine by the Commissioner of Public Health for the State of Tennessee in 1978; and he was awarded the prestigious L. M. Graves Award in 1984 (Table 9). Figure 146 depicts Dr. Korones and one of his nurse attendants caring for a tiny infant in the U.T. Newborn Center.[29]

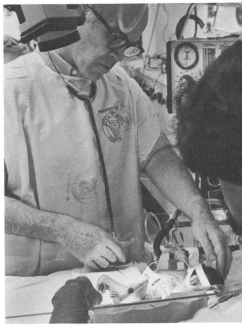

FIGURE 146. *Seldon B. Korones, M.D. (1924–   ) Professor, U.T. Department of Pediatrics, 1971-present Director, U.T. Newborn Center, 1968-present*

In addition to Le Bonheur Children's Medical Center, which has been previously described in Chapter Six, Memphis has witnessed an immense amount of growth and positive transformation in the field of pediatric medicine during the past three decades. The 1960's decade witnessed the coming to fruition of two other pediatric oriented institutions: the Child Development Center and St. Jude Children's Research Hospital, in addition to the Newborn Center which was just described. The Child Development Center was originally called the Mental Retardation Clinic, and it was established in 1957 through a grant to the University of Tennessee, Memphis by the United States Children's Bureau. With a skeleton staff of only three health professionals—a pediatrician, a social worker, and a psychologist—it was originally located in the Le Bonheur Children's Medical Center. It offered limited out-patient clinical services to retarded children and their families in the Mid-South area. In March of 1966, the U.S. Public Health Service awarded a construction grant to establish a University-affiliated Mental Retardation Training Center in the University of Tennessee, Memphis. Thus, in 1966, the C.D.C.'s primary focus was redesigned from service to training. Matching funds were provided by the Tennessee Department of Public Health, the University of Tennessee, the United Cerebral Palsy Association of Memphis and Shelby County, the Goodman Foundation, Cer-Pals, and the National Council of Jewish Women, Memphis Section. The Child Development Center and its staff were designated as the nucleus of this professional training program and became a separate unit of U.T. Memphis. The primary mission of the C.D.C. was to develop an interdisciplinary training program in mental retardation for students from various disciplines that served retarded children. In addition to the training and service aims, other goals of the Child Development Center were defined as: to participate in community and regional activities, to serve as an information and referral source, to recruit professional trainees, and to conduct research. The Child Development Center (Figure 147) handles approximately 2,000 students per year engaged in learning experiences. The program involves over 12 disciplines which includes medical specialties such as pediatric, psychiatric, and non-medical

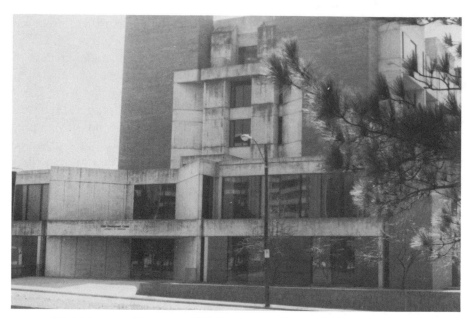

FIGURE 147. *University of Tennessee Child Development Center, 1966*

specialties such as psychology, nutrition, and speech pathology. Its general purpose is to provide service for retarded children and to allow students and hospital residents an opportunity to familiarize themselves with mental retardation and other developmental and learning disorders of child hood, as they affect the patient, the family, the physician, and the community. Medical specialties represented on the staff of the C.D.C. include pediatrics, neurology, psychiatry, genetics, otolaryngology, and ophthalmology.[18]

St. Jude Children's Research Hospital first opened its doors in 1962—the fulfillment of the promise made by its founder and major fund raiser, Danny Thomas, to build a shrine for the comfort and care of the poor, the helpless, and the hopeless. It is a children's hospital and research center dedicated to oncologic research and devoted to the care of children afflicted with the most devastating types of childhood diseases such as: acute lymphocytic leukemia, Hodgkin's disease, and other childhood cancers; infantile malnutrition; muscular diseases; sickle cell anemia; and numerous other severe maladies that afflict children. St. Jude Hospital has reached both national and international fame for its excellent, compassionate care of these extremely ill children. Its patients arrive from all over the world, as well as the United States, and locally. A major bond exists between the people of Memphis and St. Jude Children's Research Hospital, as witnessed by the love, support, and pride that each feels in the other. The University of Tennessee, Memphis and St. Jude Children's Research Hospital have recently entered into extensive research agreements and commitments to enhance the oncologic aspects of pediatric medicine, with the prime goal of keeping both institutions in the forefront of pediatric oncologic research. St. Jude Children's Research Hospital is depicted in Figure 148. The original

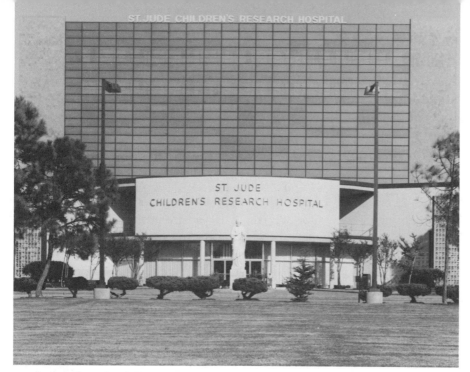

FIGURE 148. *St. Jude Children's Research Hospital, 1962*

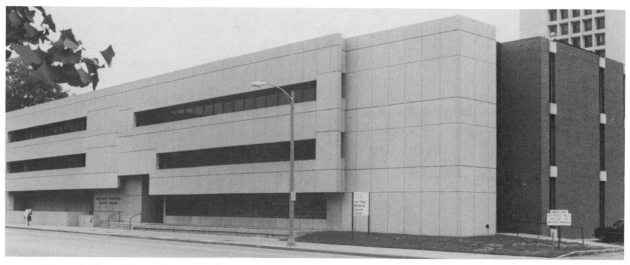

FIGURE 149. *Belz-Kriger Cancer Clinic, 1964*

Director of St. Jude Hospital was Donald Pinkel, M.D., followed by Alvin M. Mauer, M.D., who is currently Chief of Hematology and Director of the Comprehensive Cancer Center for the University of Tennessee, Memphis. The current Director of St. Jude Hospital is Joseph V. Simone, M.D. who continues to lead this hospital forward in research, and also serves as a member of the Executive Committee of the University of Tennessee and as a Trustee of the Crippled Children's Hospital Foundation Forum on Child Health, which is administered by the University of Tennessee, Memphis.

The Belz-Kriger Building, which housed the West Tennessee Cancer Clinic from 1964–1977, is an integral part of the Van Vleet Memorial

169

Cancer Center (Figure 149), which continues the public service tradition begun by the Belz and Kriger families. The building was dedicated in 1964 in loving memory of Rose Belz Kriger, Paul H. Belz, and Leslie A. Belz.

U.T. Memphis acquired the former West Tennessee Chest Disease Hospital from the Tennessee Department of Public Health in 1975. In January of 1980, the William F. Bowld Hospital was obtained by U.T. Memphis from Shelby County under a 40 year lease, as a result of a swap of hospital facilities between the University and the City of Memphis Hospital. The Bowld Hospital (named for William F. Bowld in gratitude for his untiring efforts and dedicated service for 15 years [1947–1962] as Chairman of the Board of Trustees of the City of Memphis Hospitals) was completed in 1965. The 162-bed facility is operated under the auspices of the U.T. College of Medicine and is where University physicians provide the most up-to-date treatment to their private patients. Approximately 300 physicians have staff privileges at this full-service hospital. It has the highest (best) nurse-patient ratio of any hospital in Memphis.[18]

Founded in February of 1964, the Clinical Research Center of the University of Tennessee Medical Center is one of 75 such centers located in teaching hospitals throughout the United States which are funded by the National Institutes of Health, Division of Research Resources, for the purpose of providing facilities for clinical study of various disease entities. The Center is housed on the third floor of the University of Tennessee Medical Center's William F. Bowld Hospital; it includes six in-patient beds and newly renovated out-patient facilities. The Center is dedicated to investigating the pathophysiology of diseases and improving diagnostic and therapeutic techniques through research in human subjects. Adjacent to the CRC is a seven-bed Specialized Care Unit (SCU) for private patients with third-party pay, who require careful monitoring of various biologic and metabolic measurements. Located within the Clinical Research Center is the Core Laboratory which contains highly sophisticated equipment and innovative methodology to provide the physician investigator in the CRC with state of the art diagnostic support. A Metabolic Research Kitchen is also an integral part of the Clinical Research Center and is staffed by two dietitians, who assist in research protocols which require strict dietary control. A computerized system of record-keeping and retrieval (CLINFO) permits statistical evaluation of all experimental data generated by the clinical investigators. Overall administrative responsibility for the Clinical Research Center is vested in Robert L. Summitt, M.D., Dean of the U.T. College of Medicine. Program direction is provided by Abbas E. Kitabchi, Ph.D., M.D., Professor of Medicine and Biochemistry, and Director of the Division of Endocrinology and Metabolism. The medical staff of the CRC is composed of physicians who hold faculty positions within the University of Tennessee College of Medicine. Patients who are admitted to the Center are given a complete orientation, and upon completion of the research study, patients are returned to their referring physicians. Current research projects conducted within the CRC include among others: studies of all

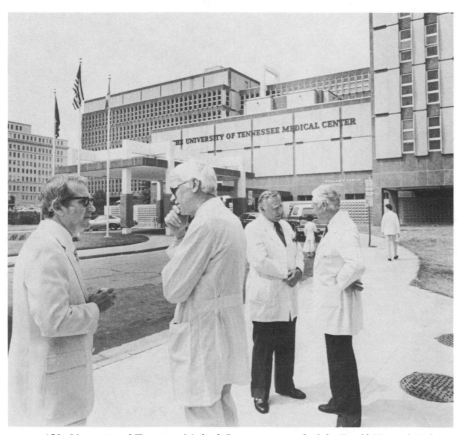

FIGURE 150. *University of Tennessee Medical Center, composed of the Bowld Hospital (right) and the Dobbs Research Institute (left). In the foreground are: Dean James C. Hunt and Drs. Clair E. Cox, II, Gene H. Stollerman, and James W. Pate*

phases of diabetes mellitus; the role of dietary sodium in the management and pathogenesis of essential hypertension; muscular dystrophy; cholesterol and fat metabolism; osteoporosis; Reye's syndrome; sexual disorders; problems of reproduction; liver disease; and liver transplantation. Approximately 60 full-time faculty members in the basic and clinical sciences of the University of Tennessee, Memphis are involved in these investigations.[18]

The Dobbs Research Institute, named for Memphis businessman and philanthropist, James K. Dobbs (1894–1966), was also built in 1965 by the generosity of the Dobbs Family through the Dobbs Foundation. It houses both the U.T. Department of Radiology and other basic/clinical research activities (such as the Cardiac Catheterization Laboratory, Endocrinology and Metabolism, Nephrology, Renal Metabolic Laboratory, and Gastroenterology) for the University of Tennessee College of Medicine. Figure 150 shows (from left to right) Dean James C. Hunt, M.D., Clair E. Cox, II, M.D., Gene H. Stollerman, M.D. and James W. Pate, M.D. in 1980, standing in front of the U.T. Medical Center.

The new Veterans Administration Hospital (Figure 151) was opened in 1967 at 1030 Jefferson Avenue. The old VA Hospital was located in a

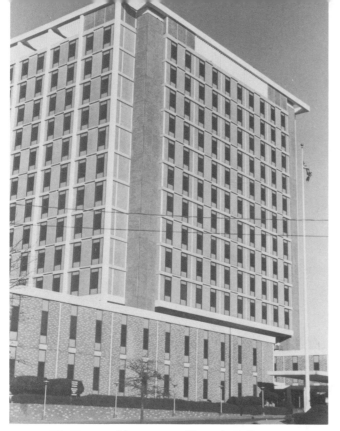

FIGURE 151. *Veterans Administration Hospital, 1967*

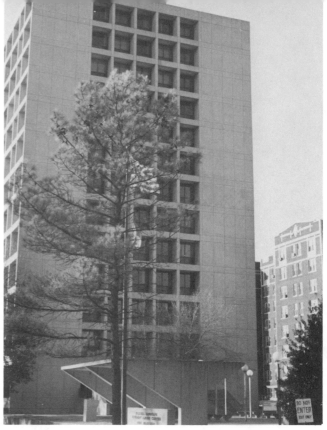

FIGURE 152. *Wassell Randolph Student-Alumni Center, 1969 (courtesy of James E. Hamner, III, D.D.S., Ph.D.)*

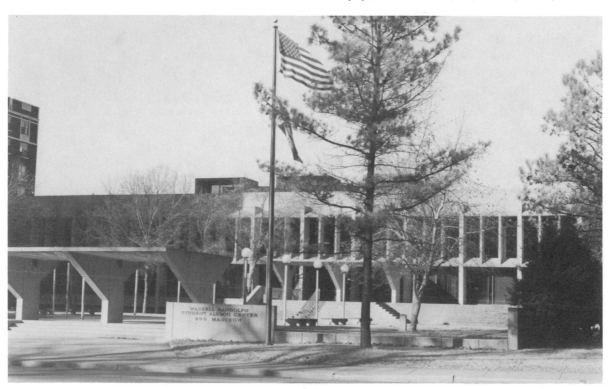

FIGURE 153. *Randolph Dormitory, 1969 (courtesy of James E. Hamner, III, D.D.S., Ph.D.)*

spread-out complex of multiple, small buildings and wards, located at Park and Getwell in East Memphis. The current VA Hospital is closely affiliated with the University of Tennessee, Memphis, since many of its medical staff have joint University staff appointments, and students/residents utilize it for a variety of clinical training experiences.

The Wassell Randolph Student-Alumni Center at 800 Madison Avenue (Figure 152) was occupied in 1969. Its excellent modern facilities replaced the old University Student Center, which stood at the southeast corner of Dunlap and Madison and had been used by the University since 1933. The S.A.C. provides a large cafeteria and private dining rooms, a movie lounge, a television lounge, a reception area, and an office on the first floor. The second floor houses many University offices related to student affairs, meeting rooms, the Sam Houston Sanders Dining Room, and a large reception/dining room. The basement area contains the U.T. Post Office, the University Book Store, the Schreier Auditorium, a small snack lounge, and game rooms. The posterior connecting wing of the Student-Alumni Center provides excellent athletic facilities: handball and racquetball courts, a large gymnasium for basketball, a weight-room, exercise/aerobics areas, locker rooms, and an Olympic-sized swimming pool. The S.A.C. is managed in a capable, friendly manner by Mr. O. D. Larry, who has served the University faithfully and well for 45 years, knowing former students, their children, and their grandchildren.

Both the Student-Alumni Center and the Randolph Dormitory (Figure 153) were named for Wassell Randolph in honor of his long and dedicated service as a University of Tennessee Trustee. The Randolph Dormitory is a 13-story modern dormitory for men and women students in all the U.T. Memphis Colleges. To the right of the Randolph Dormitory, one can see the old Goodman House Dormitory, which was originally called the Forrest Park Apartments when it was built in 1926; it was later acquired by U.T. Memphis in 1948 and renamed as the Goodman House. Figure 154 depicts the Randolph Dormitory, rising behind the statue of Lieutenant General Nathan Bedford Forrest, the famous Confederate cavalry leader from Memphis. In 1838, the State of Tennessee authorized the building of a brick hospital on this same site, chiefly for the benefit of Mississippi River boatmen and travelers. In 1873, it was acquired by the City and renamed as the Memphis City Hospital. Perhaps one of its more famous patients was the brother of Mark Twain, who visited his sick brother in this hospital, and was so pleased with the excellent care that his brother received, that he dubbed Memphis, "The City of Mercy". It was razed after 1898, and the location became Forrest Park.

The University of Tennessee, Memphis has been a pioneer in the field of Forensic Medicine. Beginning as early as 1944, Dr. Douglas H. Sprunt, as Chairman of the U.T. Department of Pathology, arranged for medicolegal autopsies to be performed. The autopsy/morgue portion of the U.T. Institute of Pathology (Figure 105) was specifically designed to have a Forensic Pathology component, as well as the Anatomical Pathology,

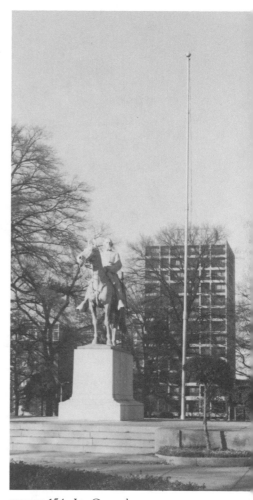

FIGURE 154. *Lt. General Nathan Bedford Forrest, C.S.A. (1821–1877). Forrest Park was the site of the first City Hospital in 1836*

173

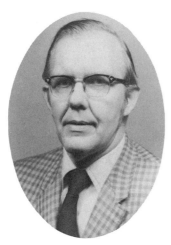

FIGURE 155. *Jerry T.*
Francisco, M.D.
(1932–   ) Professor, U.T.
Department of Pathology,
1967-present Chief Medical
Examiner, State of Tennessee,
1970-present

Teaching Amphitheatre and Museum components. In 1957, a formal contract between Shelby County and the University of Tennessee, Memphis was signed, providing for the U.T. Department of Pathology to render certain scientific services to all law enforcement agencies in Shelby County. A state-wide law by the Tennessee Legislature created the County Medical Examiner System in 1961.[7,21]

Jerry T. Francisco, M.D. (Figure 155) is the Shelby County Medical Examiner, the Medical Examiner for the State of Tennessee, and a Professor of Pathology at the University of Tennessee, Memphis. The Medical Examiner's Office in Shelby County also covers the other West Tennessee Counties. Dr. Francisco and his staff investigate approximately 3,000 cases per year. The extent of this investigation varies from a minimum telephone request to the maximum—a complete autopsy (an average of 500 autopsies are performed annually by Forensic Pathology).[7] As the Chief Medical Examiner for Tennessee, his Office has three major functions: education, consultation, and record maintenance. One of Forensic Pathology's most important support facilities is the Toxicology Laboratory, which performs a variety of analyses, including determination of alcohols, barbiturates, tranquilizers, metals, carbon monoxide, sedatives, and industrial poisons. Since the Forensic Pathology staff work very closely with Tennessee Law Enforcement Agencies, they are frequently involved as experts or consultants in legal cases.[7,28]

Dr. Francisco was born in 1932 in Huntington, Tennessee, attended Lambuth College and U.T. Knoxville, and received his M.D. degree from U.T. Memphis in June of 1955. His internship and pathology residency were also taken at U.T. Memphis with an interruption of two years of active duty as a physician with the U.S. Navy. He served as a consultant to numerous law enforcement agencies and was commended by the Federal Bureau of Investigation for a training series in Forensic Pathology for new F.B.I. agents from 1982–1984; this series was a unique training program that had not been given anywhere else throughout the United States.[29]

The University of Tennessee Dental Alumni Association was founded in 1960 by D. Dunn Clark, D.D.S., Robert P. Denny, D.D.S., William H. Jolley, D.D.S., William V. Lashley, D.D.S., Mr. F. June Montgomery, and Justin D. Towner, IV, D.D.S. The first President of this organization, which has contributed greatly to the University of Tennessee, Memphis, was William V. (Gus) Lashley, D.D.S., who graduated from the U.T. College of Dentistry in 1954. Dr. Justin D. Towner, IV is the grandson of Dr. Justin Dewey Towner who was the co-organizer and Dean of the University of Memphis College of Dentistry. Following in the footsteps of his famous grandfather, Justin Towner is also a specialist in periodontia in Memphis today.[17]

The U.T. Materials Science Toxicology Laboratory (MSTL) was established in 1968 by Dr. John Autian, a Professor of Dentistry and a Professor of Pharmacy. Prior to accepting an appointment at the University of Tennessee, Memphis, he was Director of the Drug-Plastic Research and Toxicology Laboratory at the University of Texas and was responsible for developing it into a national and international center for drug-plastic interaction studies and on various aspects of toxicology related to biomaterials. The MSTL in a brief time became a nationally recognized toxicology laboratory, specializing in dental and biomedical materials and studies dealing with fire toxicology. As it grew, Dr. Autian appointed Dr. W. H. Lawrence as Assistant Director. Additional University of Tennessee, Memphis faculty became associated with the research group, including Dr. James Turner (College of Dentistry), Dr. E. O. Dillingham (College of Pharmacy), Dr. R. Gollamudi (College of Pharmacy), and Dr. Loys Nunez (College of Dentistry). Over 30 graduate students have participated in the research activities of the Laboratory; approximately 30 postdoctorates and visiting scientists from the United States and abroad have studied in the Laboratory or conducted research jointly with faculty members of the Laboratory. Through the U.T. College of Pharmacy, it became the first College of Pharmacy in the United States to receive an N.I.H. (National Institutes of Health) graduate training grant in Toxicology. Original contributions by the research group of the U.T. Materials Science Toxicology Laboratory have led to a number of biological tests which are now used in industry to evaluate the safety of a new item or a new biomedical material.[2,3]

Dr. John Autian (Figure 156) was born August 20, 1924 in Philadelphia, Pennsylvania. He obtained his B.S. degree in Pharmacy from Temple University in Philadelphia in 1950. Continuing his postgraduate education, he received an M.S. in Pharmacy (1952) and a Ph.D. in Pharmacy and Pharmacology (1954) from the University of Maryland. From 1954 through 1967 he was a faculty member at the following universities: Temple University, the University of Maryland, the University of Michigan, and the University of Texas.[29]

Dr. Autian joined the University of Tennessee, Memphis faculty in 1967 as a Professor in the College of Pharmacy and the College of Dentistry, as well as Director of the Materials Science Toxicology Laboratory. He served as Coordinator of Dental Research for the U.T. College of Dentistry from 1970–1972, was President of the U.T. Memphis Faculty Senate from 1972–1973, and was Chairman of the Department of Molecular Biology in the U.T. College of Pharmacy from 1974–1975. At that time Dr. Autian was appointed Dean of the U.T. College of Pharmacy and led that College through 1982 (Appendix D). He was also Dean of the Graduate School of Medical Sciences from 1982–1985 (Appendix G). In 1982 he was appointed by Chancellor James C. Hunt to the newly created position of Vice Chancellor for Research and served in that capacity until 1985. Dr. Autian was the originator and editor of *Newsletter: Forum for the Advancement of Toxicology*, has contributed to 16 books, and has published 205 scientific articles. He has been a member of many national scientific committees and organizations. Dr. Autian was also the first recipient of the University of Tennessee Alumni Public Service Award in 1973. In international affairs,

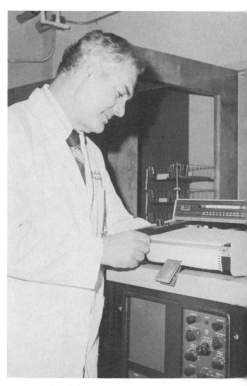

FIGURE 156. *John Autian, Ph.D. (1924–) Dean, U.T. College of Pharmacy, 1975–1982 Dean, U.T. Graduate School of Medical Sciences, 1982–1985 Vice Chancellor for Research, 1982–1985*

175

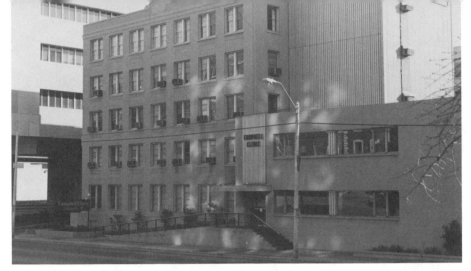

FIGURE 157. *The Campbell Clinic (constructed as one-story in 1920), as it appears in 1986 (courtesy of James E. Hamner, III, D.D.S., Ph.D.)*

he has been an invited speaker for scientific meetings in 20 foreign nations and has been a toxicology consultant for the World Health Organization.[29]

One of the medical accomplishments for which Dr. John Autian will best be remembered is his original idea for the creation of a Biomedical Research Zone in Memphis in 1983. This topic will be discussed more thoroughly in Chapter 9.

The Willis C. Campbell Clinic was originally built in 1920 at 869 Madison Avenue. This one-story building provided space for a waiting room, business office, eight examining rooms, a physical therapy department, and a brace shop. Four additional stories were added later, which served as the beginning of a fully-equipped, 80-bed orthopedic hospital for the care of private patients and for the training of orthopedic residents. This building (Figure 157) served as both in-patient and out-patient facilities until 1967, when in-patient care and operating facilities were moved to the Baptist Memorial Hospital, where they occupy an entire floor of 800 beds. As the orthopedic practice grew, new staff members were gradually taken into the private group practice; in 1986 there are currently 20 staff members. Dr. Harold B. Boyd served as Chief-of-Staff for most of the 1960's decade (1962–1971). In 1924, the Fellowship Program was begun with four residents in training as orthopedic surgeons; this number gradually expanded to the present 24 residents. After Dr. Campbell's death in 1941, the staff purchased the Clinic from his estate, and in 1946 they chartered the Campbell Foundation, as the resident training branch of the Campbell Clinic. The program became officially known as the Campbell Foundation-University of Tennessee Resident Program in the mid-1960's. Approximately 250 orthopedic surgeons from the United States, Canada, South America, and Europe have received their formal orthopedic education in this program.[5,25,26]

Dr. Andrew Hoyt Crenshaw was born July 21, 1920 in Martin, Georgia. He obtained his undergraduate B.S. degree in 1941 from Presbyterian College and his M.D. degree from Emory University School of Medicine in Atlanta in 1944. Both his surgical internship and surgical residency were taken at Grady Memorial Hospital in Atlanta from 1944–1945 and 1947–1948. From July of 1948 to July of 1951 he was awarded a Fellowship at the Campbell Clinic in Orthopedic Surgery. During the intervening years of July 1945 to January of 1947, Dr. Crenshaw served as a Captain (MC) U.S. Army. Completing his postgraduate fellowship at the University of Tennessee in July of 1951, he obtained an M.S. degree in Orthopedic Surgery.

His teaching appointments at the University of Tennessee College of Medicine rose from Assistant in Orthopedic Surgery in 1952 to Associate Professor of Orthopedic Surgery in 1970. Dr. Crenshaw was certified as a Diplomate of the American Board of Orthopedic Surgery in 1954. He is a member of numerous professional associates, including the American Academy of Orthopedic Surgeons for which he served as Librarian-Historian from 1965–1970. He was honored by the American Orthopedic Association with an award for a traveling fellowship to Great Britain in 1959. In addition to his clinical and teaching skills, Dr. Crenshaw is best known for his scholarly work in the field of publishing. He has authored 20 scientific publications, and he has served as the Associate Editor of the *Journal of Bone and Joint Surgery* from 1963–1971 and as Associate Editor from 1970–1975 for the *American Academy of Orthopedic Surgeon Bulletin*. His greatest accomplishment is the tremendous scholarly, arduous effort required to serve as Editor of Editions Four, Five, and Six of the world-famous *Campbell's Operative Orthopaedics*. Dr. Hoyt Crenshaw is depicted in Figure 158.[5,29]

The first Director of the U.T. Clinical Research Center was Dr. Frank Tullis (Figure 159). Frank Tullis was born on June 17, 1917 in McComb, Mississippi and received both his B.S. and M.D. degrees from the University of Tennessee, Memphis in 1939. His internship and residency in Medicine were taken at the John Gaston Hospital within the University of Tennessee Medical Center. He completed his residency in June of 1948, after service in the U.S. Army from 1942–1946 during World War II, when he was Chief of Field Party, Institute of Inter-American Affairs, Honduras, Central America. He maintained a private practice of medicine, as well as serving on the U.T. College of Medicine faculty for many years. He became Chairman of the Department of Medicine for the University of Tennessee College of Medicine in 1954 and continued in that role until 1964. At that time he became Director of the Clinical Research Center for the University of Tennessee. He left this position in 1971 and practiced internal medicine at the Sanders Clinic from 1971–1976. As Dr. Tullis stated, "Before the C.R.C., we had plenty of patients and plenty of physicians interested in research, but no environment to conduct clinical investigations under controlled conditions."

Dr. James R. Givens was the Assistant Director of the Clinical Research Center under Dr. Tullis. He led the research efforts in hirsutism. Among the other outstanding research projects that helped build a national reputation for the C.R.C. was the research done in sickle cell anemia, led by Dr. Lemuel Diggs and the husband and wife team of Drs. Lorraine and Alfred

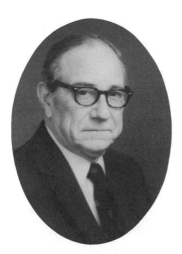

FIGURE 158. *Andrew Hoyt Crenshaw, M.D. (1920–) Editor, 4th, 5th, and 6th Editions of* Campbell's Operative Orthopaedics

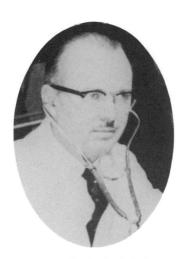

FIGURE 159. *I. Frank Tullis, M.D. (1917–) Professor and Chairman, U.T. Department of Medicine, 1954–1964 Director, Clinical Research Center, 1965–1971*

177

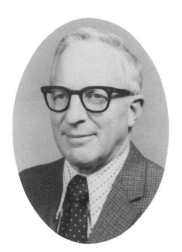

FIGURE 160. *Sidney A. Cohn, Ph.D. (1918–   ) Professor, U.T. Department of Anatomy, 1966–1985 Acting Chairman, 1980–1982, Chairman, 1982–1983*

Kraus. In 1966 they discovered a new, abnormal hemoglobin named "Hemoglobin Memphis". Another original contribution in the sickle cell anemia disease area was the work done by Dr. John Morrison, who demonstrated that replacement transfusion reduced maternal mortality and morbidity. Hemoglobin C-C crystals were described by Dr. Lem Diggs, Dr. Alfred Kraus, Dr. D. B. Morrison, and Dr. R. T. Rudnicki. Hemoglobin S-C crystals were identified by Dr. Lem Diggs and Miss Ann Bell. Another contribution from the Sickle Cell Center was the discovery that patients with pulmonary emboli revealed in their blood smears evidence of membrane injury. Therapeutic trials were conducted by Dr. Alfred Kraus and the Sickle Cell Anemia Research Staff. The pathogenesis of thrombotic thrombocytopenic purpura (Upshaw-Shulman Syndrome) was defined by Dr. J. D. Upshaw. The leader in diabetes mellitus research is Dr. Abbas Kitabchi, who transferred from the Veterans Administration Medical Center in 1968 to become Director of the C.R.C.[6,15] Dr. Kitabchi's work and medical accomplishments will be described in the next chapter.

One individual in the University of Tennessee's long line of outstanding educators for the Department of Anatomy is Sidney A. Cohn, Ph.D. (Figure 160). After obtaining his B.S. degree from the University of Connecticut in 1940, he served with distinction as an officer in the U.S. Army (Infantry Officer 1940–43 and U.S. Army Air Corps Pilot 1943–46) during World War II, being honorably discharged in 1946 as a Captain. His M.S. degree was obtained also from the University of Connecticut in 1948; then, he completed his Ph.D. degree in Anatomy at Brown University in 1951.[29]

Dr. Cohn rose steadily in academic rank from Instructor in 1951 to Professor in 1966 at the University of Tennessee, Memphis. He was always a popular and well-respected anatomy teacher, both by dental and medical students and by his faculty peers. Sid Cohn specialized in head and neck anatomy and became a very strong contributor and supporter of dental research, being one of the few basic science faculty members who were heavily involved with meetings and presentations before the International Association for Dental Research. He served as a faculty member on numerous University committees and contributed to the graduate training of 16 graduate students in the U.T. College of Dentistry, as well as compiling 43 scientific publications.[4,29]

Dr. Cohn holds membership also in the American Association of Anatomists, Omicron Kappa Upsilon, and Sigma Xi. He was selected as Chairman of the Section on Anatomical Sciences for the American Association of Dental Schools in 1948. In 1972 he was honored as the recipient of the University of Tennessee Outstanding Teaching Award, and in 1977 he received a Special Award by the Tennessee State Dental Association. In 1983 he was named the Alumni Distinguished Service Professor by the University of Tennessee. He has been Acting Chairman twice, Deputy Chairman twice, and Chairman (1982–1983) of the U.T. Department of Anatomy. After chairing the search committee, which brought Dr. Steve Kitai from Michigan State University to chair the U.T. Department of

Anatomy, Dr. Cohn retired September 4, 1985 and was named by Chancellor James C. Hunt as an Emeritus Professor. Two other anatomy teachers, who dedicated their careers to excellence in anatomical education and who were also appointed to be Emeritus Professors, were Harry H. Wilcox (1983) and Clark E. Corliss (1985).[4,29]

The interest in periodontal disease, which had been such an integral, strong part of the University of Tennessee College of Dentistry's program in its early days when under the direction of Dr. Justin D. Towner, Sr., was revived in the 1960's by Dr. Billy M. Pennel. As related by Dr. Kenneth O. King, who was engaged in clinical research with Dr. Pennel, "the attitude that prevailed at that time, instilled by Dr. Pennel to all of the staff, was a need for the Department to do something which would have the effect of putting it on the map. Since the University of Tennessee College of Dentistry did not have a strong basic science research area, nor did it have the facilities or money required for basic research, the only way he felt we could do something significant was with clinical research. Some of the projects were well thought-out and well-designed, such as the study on bone loss after tooth grinding, but others such as the free gingival graft just happened spontaneously. These spontaneous happenings occurred because of an attitude that Dr. Pennel instilled in all of us to be thinking positively in our clinical work."[12]

Billy M. "Buck" Pennel (Figure 161) played football at Ole Miss before World War II, was commissioned as a Naval officer during the War, and afterwards obtained his baccalaureate degree from the University of Virginia. He graduated from the U.T. College of Dentistry in 1951. His postgraduate work in Periodontia was taken at Ohio State University, and he returned full-time to the University in 1955. He served as Professor and Chairman of the U.T. Department of Periodontia through 1968, when he went to the School of Dentistry of the Medical College of Georgia to head their Department of Periodontia. During the 1960's Dr. Pennel, along with Dr. Kenneth O. King and other faculty members in the Department of Periodontia, were involved in clinical research that led to the first free gingival graft. This procedure was originally described by them before the Philadelphia Society of Periodontology in April of 1964, followed by later publications in the *Journal of Periodontology* in 1965 and 1969. This treatment procedure has become one of the standard ones in periodontia in the treatment of mucogingival defects. In 1965 and 1967, Dr. Pennel and other departmental faculty published additional results of their clinical research in related mucogingival areas. These contributions included the development of standardized intra-oral photographic techniques for evaluating surgical treatment results, the response and repair of bone following mucoperiosteal flap and osseous surgery, and the clinical appearance and histologic repair of tissue involved in mucogingival surgery. These clinical research activities provided important, pertinent information about this area of periodontal treatment and have been recognized nationally and internationally as valuable contributions to the early understanding and treatment of

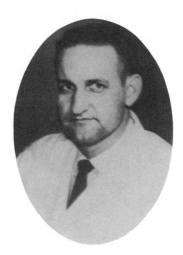

FIGURE 161. *Billy M. Pennel, D.D.S. (1924–1980) Professor and Chairman, U.T. Department of Periodontia, 1955–1968*

179

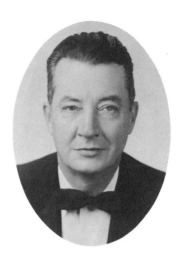

FIGURE 162. *Marion L. Fuller, D.D.S. (1903–1966) Professor, U.T. Department of Operative Dentistry, 1948–1966*

mucogingival defects in periodontal disease. They serve as the basis for treatment techniques that are currently used in periodontia. It was a tragic loss when Dr. Buck Pennel died in 1980 from a sudden massive heart attack after running.[12,16,17]

One of the most universally liked and respected professors in the U.T. College of Dentistry was Marion L. Fuller, D.D.S. (Figure 162). Over his many contributing years as a clinical teacher *par excellence*, he held faculty appointments in both the Department of Operative Dentistry and the Department of Prosthetics. His trenchant wit and humor made even the most trying of circumstances bearable and the most hopeless of situations salvageable. He always worked diligently with the students on the clinical floors and was never too busy to help someone who really needed it. When some young dental student in the laboratory would present an operative dentistry preparation that had been cut on an ivorine model tooth, far beyond the proper outline margins, he would shake his head, sigh, and say with a satiric smile, "Boy, if you do that poorly on a human tooth, you're going to find out quickly that you don't have any 'put'em back chisel' in your bag of tricks. Better learn now to do it right."[8]

Dr. Fuller was born in 1903, attended Auburn University, and graduated with honors in 1925 from St. Louis University School of Dentistry. After 23 years of private practice, he accepted an appointment at the U.T. College of Dentistry in 1948. Prior to his untimely death in 1966, he was a Professor of both Operative Dentistry and Prosthetics. The 1966 *Asklepieion* contained the following memorial to Dr. Marion L. Fuller:

"There is no way we can possibly express this great loss to the University of Tennessee College of Dentistry. Dr. Fuller was loved by all students for his understanding and for his appreciation of good education. His rich character and vast knowledge of prosthetics will be missed by all who knew him."[30]

Jerry R. McGhee, Ph.D., who graduated from the University of Tennessee Department of Microbiology in 1969, is a Professor of Microbiology at the University of Alabama School of Medicine in Birmingham. He is the author of the widely used textbook, *Oral Microbiology*. In 1967, L. Howard Moss, III received his Ph.D. degree from the U.T. Department of Microbiology and Immunology. A year previously, in 1966, his wife, Rebecca Kristin Moss, obtained her M.D. degree from the University of Tennessee College of Medicine. Presently, they own and operate the largest clinical viral diagnostic laboratory in the Mid-West.[18]

Dr. John Lewis Wood has made numerous contributions to the University of Tennessee, Memphis, both in his role as Professor of Biochemistry and in his activities with the U.T. Graduate School. He was born on August 7, 1912 in Homer, Illinois. After obtaining his B.S. degree in Chemistry from the University of Illinois in 1934, he continued his postgraduate studies at the University of Virginia and was awarded his Ph.D. degree in Chemistry in 1937. During the intervening nine years before he joined the University of Tennessee in 1946, Dr. Wood was a faculty member at the University of

Virginia, the George Washington University Medical School, Cornell Medical College, Harvard University, and the United States Food and Drug Administration. From Associate Professor in 1946, he became a full Professor in 1950 and Chairman of the Department of Biochemistry at the University of Tennessee, Memphis in 1952. He served as Chairman of the Department of Biochemistry until 1968, at which time he returned to full-time teaching. His excellent record of scholarship in Biochemistry has included selection for a Distinguished Guggenheim Fellowship in 1954. He served as a consultant to the Medical Division of the Oak Ridge Institute of Nuclear Studies from 1949–1965; also, he was a member of the Board of Directors for this Institute from 1959–1967. He was a member of a select committee assigned to review food additives for the U.S. Food and Drug Administration from 1971–1976. His other professional and scholarly activities have included a special research fellowship in the Department of Chemistry at the University of Rome from 1965–1966 and his participation in a National Academy of Sciences exchange program with the School of Medicine in Krakow, Poland in 1970.[18]

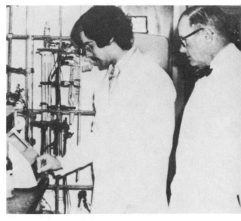

FIGURE 163. *John Lewis Wood, Ph.D. (1912–   ) Professor and Chairman, U.T. Department of Biochemistry, 1952–1968 Acting Dean, U.T. Graduate School of Medical Sciences, 1979–1980 (on right)*

Dr. John Wood has served as mentor for numerous graduate students in the U.T. Department of Biochemistry (Figure 163). From 1979–1980, he was named Acting Dean of the U.T. Graduate School of Medical Sciences by Chancellor T. Albert Farmer, Jr. Dr. Wood held this position for one year until he retired on December 31, 1980 and was appointed as an Emeritus Professor. His research interests included studies on the carcinogenic properties of hydrocarbons, and he authored 84 scientific publications in the Biochemistry field. His professional societies include: the American Chemical Society, the American Association for Cancer Research, the Society for Experimental Biology and Medicine, Tennessee Academy of Sciences, and Sigma Xi. In 1971, Dr. John Wood was honored as a University of Tennessee Alumni Distinguished Service Professor.[29]

In 1945, John Paul Quigley, a Ph.D. graduate of the University of Chicago and a faculty member of Western Reserve University, joined the University of Tennessee, Memphis faculty. Shortly thereafter, he made a lateral move as Chairman of the U.T. Department of Pharmacology to become Chairman of the U.T. Department of Physiology and Biophysics (Figure 164). It should be remembered that it was Dr. Quigley, who stimulated a deep and abiding interest in basic research in the mind of young Daniel Anthony Brody, M.D. (Figure 121), when he was a medical student at Western Reserve University.[9,13]

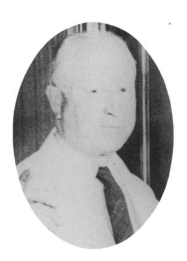

FIGURE 164. *John Paul Quigley, Ph.D. (1896–1967) Professor and Chairman, U.T. Department of Physiology and Biophysics, 1947–1964*

During the Quigley era (1947–1964), the Department of Physiology and Biophysics quadrupled its faculty size and developed a vital graduate program (17 Ph.D.'s and 11 M.S. degrees). The first doctoral degree in Physiology at the University of Tennessee, Memphis was awarded in 1949 to James Albert Richardson, who afterwards became a Professor of Pharmacology at the Medical College of South Carolina. It was a golden era academically for the Department of Physiology and Biophysics with excellent teachers and recognized, accomplished researchers, such as Drs. J. P. Quigley, C. R.

181

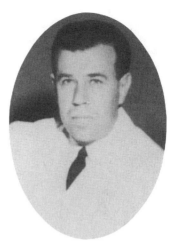

FIGURE 165. *Andrew Lasslo, Ph.D. (1922–)* *Chairman, U.T. Department of Medicinal Chemistry, 1960-present*

Houck, Richard R. Overman, Donald B. Zilversmit, and Lester van Middlesworth. Dr. Paul Quigley was the first individual to demonstrate that chyme passes through the pyloric sphincter, driven by gastric mobility; the pyloric sphincter is rhythmically opened and shut. He and Dr. Daniel A. Brody invented the inductograph, which enabled them to measure the motility of the pylorus in-situ. Dr. Quigley retired in 1964, was appointed as Emeritus Professor of Physiology in 1965, and died in 1967.[9,21]

Andrew Lasslo, Ph.D. (Figure 165) has been an extremely productive, contributing faculty member of the University of Tennessee College of Pharmacy since 1960. He was born on August 24, 1922 in Mukacevo, Czechoslovakia and obtained his degree in Pharmacy from Charles' University in Prague in 1946. Becoming an American citizen, he attended the University of Illinois, receiving an M.S. degree in 1948 and a Ph.D. degree in 1952; both of these degrees were in Pharmaceutical Chemistry. From 1952–1954 he worked for Monsanto Chemical Company in St. Louis, doing exploratory research in organic synthesis. He joined the academic world in July of 1954, becoming an Assistant Professor of Medicinal Chemistry at Emory University's Division of Basic Health Sciences. In 1960, he was appointed as Professor and Chairman of the Department of Pharmaceutical Chemistry in the U.T. College of Pharmacy.[20]

Dr. Lasslo has participated and/or chaired numerous University committees. He is involved with numerous professional societies including: the American Chemical Society, a Fellow of the American Association of Advancement of Science, a Fellow of the American Institute of Chemists (he was awarded an Honor Scroll by the Tennessee Institute of Chemists in 1976), the American Society for Pharmacology and Experimental Therapeutics (he served as a member of the Executive Committee from 1974–1978), and the Federation of American Societies for Experimental Biology (National Correspondent for Public Affairs Committee 1971–1974). Dr. Lasslo also served as President of the University of Tennessee, Memphis Chapter of Sigma Xi from 1976–1977. He has been involved with the writing of six books and has published numerous scientific articles in professional journals.[29]

In 1985 Dr. Lasso was elected as a Fellow of the American Pharmaceutical Association's Academy of Pharmaceutical Sciences. In 1984 a patent was issued to Drs. Andrew Lasslo, Ronald P. Quintana, Marion Dugdale, Randy W. Johnson, and Jay M. Sullivan for a group of compounds that may prove effective in preventing blood platelet aggregation, which could lead to the formation of blood clots or thrombi. The compounds have been shown to prevent platelet aggregation by strengthening the membrane of the platelet. This work could prove extremely beneficial for patients with artificial implants in contact with the blood stream. Other individuals who could benefit from the development of these compounds are patients who are exposed to biomaterials during such processes as renal dialysis, cardiopulmonary bypass procedures, and cardiac catheterization.[14]

Roger L. Hiatt, M.D. (Figure 166) was born March 8, 1929 in Mt. Airy,

North Carolina, attended Appalachian State University from 1945–1947, received an O.D. degree in 1949 from the Southern College of Optometry, finished his B.S. degree in 1953 from Brigham Young University, and completed his M.D. degree at the U.T. College of Medicine in 1958. His internship and Ophthalmology residency were taken at the Medical College of Virginia and completed in 1962. During 1963–1964 he served a special preceptorship in Pediatric Ophthalmology at the Children's Hospital of Washington, D.C.[29]

Dr. Hiatt was a Lieutenant (jg) in the Medical Service Corps (Optometric Division) of the U.S. Navy from 1950–1953. He held faculty appointments at the Medical College of Virginia and Georgetown University, prior to becoming Professor and Chairman of the Department of Ophthalmology at the University of Tennessee College of Medicine in 1964. He was the first ophthalmologist in the Mid-South area to establish and limit his subspecialty in Pediatric Ophthalmology.[18] He is a Diplomate of the American Board of Ophthalmology, a member of the select American Association for Pediatric Ophthalmology, and a Fellow of the American Academy of Ophthalmology and Otolaryngology. His research contributions have been in the areas of motility and sensorial aspects of strabismus, in which he has authored 45 scientific publications. Dr. Hiatt was honored by an Award of Merit from the Tennessee Academy of Ophthalmology in 1976 and an Honor Award by the American Academy of Ophthalmologists in 1976. In 1984, he was selected as the Outstanding Ophthalmologist in Tennessee. Dr. Hiatt has generously established a trust endowment for the U.T. Department of Ophthalmology and has been very active in our International Affairs Program.[29]

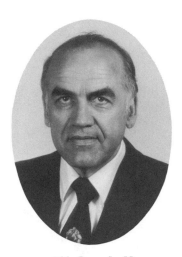

FIGURE 166. *Roger L. Hiatt, M.D. (1929–) Professor and Chairman, U.T. Department of Ophthalmology, 1964-present*

John William Runyan, Jr., M.D. (Figure 167) has made outstanding contributions, both as a health professional and as a caring citizen for the Memphis community. Bill Runyan was born on January 23, 1924 in Memphis, Tennessee, was educated at Washington and Lee University (B.A. in 1944), and obtained his M.D. degree from the Johns Hopkins University School of Medicine in 1947. After an internship year at Johns Hopkins Hospital, he spent two years in Medicine at the Albany Hospital in New York, then three additional years as a Research Fellow and Thorndike Memorial Fellow at the Boston City Hospital and Harvard Medical School.[29]

From 1953–1960 he served on the faculty of the Albany Medical College, becoming an Associate Professor in the Department of Medicine. In 1960, he joined the U.T. Department of Medicine and became a full Professor in 1964. When Dr. Henry Packer (who made national medical contributions through his efforts in screening for diabetes mellitus and glaucoma) stepped down as the Chairman of the Department of Community Medicine within the College of Medicine in 1972, Dr. Runyan was the logical choice to head it. He founded and served as Chief of the Section of Endocrinology from 1962–1972 at U.T. Memphis. Also, he developed the decentralized Clinic Network for Memphis and Shelby County (1963–1985). He is a Diplomate

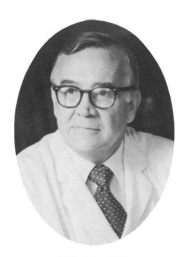

FIGURE 167. *John William Runyan, Jr., M.D. (1924–) Professor and Chairman, U.T. Department of Community Medicine, 1972-present*

of the American Board of Internal Medicine and served as an Examiner for it from 1967–1972; he is also a Fellow of the American College of Physicians and is an active member in the American Diabetes Association and the American Federation for Clinical Research, authoring 47 professional papers and a book, *Primary Care Guide*, in 1976.[23]

Dr. Bill Runyan has been an active Trustee for the Frank M. Norfleet Forum for the Advancement of Health and has been honored by numerous awards including: the Outstanding Public Service Award from the University of Tennessee National Alumni Association (1977), the John D. Rockefeller Public Service Award in Health (1977), the Award for Public Service from the Mayor of Shelby County (1977), the L. M. Graves Award for Outstanding Contributions to Community Health (1978), the Rosenthal Award from the American College of Physicians (1980), the Upjohn Award for Outstanding Physician Educator in the Field of Diabetes by the American Diabetes Association (1981), and a Special Resolution Award for "highly successful medical career filled with outstanding achievements" by the House of Representatives of the State of Tennessee (1982). The John W. Runyan, Jr. Award was initiated in his honor by the Mid-South Medical Center Council and the Nursing Council in 1979 to recognize one to two outstanding nurses each year in the Mid-South area.[23]

In 1961, a modern research laboratory was established in the basement of the Tennessee Psychiatric and Research Institute; it was sponsored jointly by the University of Tennessee and the Tennessee Department of Mental Health. It acquired some of the latest scientific research equipment available at that time. Dr. T. S. Hill, who was Chairman of the U.T. Department of Psychiatry from 1942–1963, was the key individual in the initial planning of the Tennessee Psychiatric and Research Institute, which later was renamed the Memphis Mental Health Institute. Dr. F. Christine Brown made medical contributions that received national recognition in 1968. One of her discoveries (complexes of Cyslathionase) was presented in a Symposium on Pyriodoxal Enzymes which was held in Tokyo, Japan in 1968. The University of Tennessee Department of Psychiatry, in cooperation with the Shelby County Courts, has been involved with the psychiatric evaluation of prisoners, both for competency to stand trial and for other purposes from 1942 to the present time.[1,18]

Charles Edward Kossmann, M.D. (Figure 168) was named to be the Chief of the Division of Circulatory Diseases in 1968 by Dr. Gene H. Stollerman, then Chairman of the U.T. Department of Medicine. This new Division included Sections of Cardiology, Cardiovascular Biophysics, Nephrology, and Pulmonary Medicine.[18] Under Dr. Kossmann's strong guidance over the next six years, this unit became one of the most productive ones in the University of Tennessee College of Medicine. The Division of Circulatory Diseases was reorganized in 1973 to include closer ties with the expanding cardiovascular activities in affiliated institutions, particularly the Veterans Administration Hospital, the Baptist Hospital, the Methodist Hospital, and St. Joseph's Hospital. The Sections of Nephrology, Pulmonary Medicine, and Cardiovascular Biophysics became independent entities. In 1968 this unit received a large training grant in circulatory diseases from the National Heart and Lung Institute; this grant was approved largely on the basis of the planned integrative approach to circulatory diseases. Its large level of support enabled it over a period of six years to give graduate cardiological training of either one or two years' duration to 31 physicians. The research compiled by this Division resulted in 80 publications within this six year period. In 1971, another large National Heart and Lung Institute grant to the Division of Circulatory Diseases enabled the establishment of a Specialized Center of Research in Hypertension at the University of Tennessee College of Medicine. Significant contributions in research, covering a broad spectrum from control of experimental hypertension in animals by the use of a renal medullary extract to biolateral nephrectomy and transplantation in human malignant hypertension, were carried out. Dr. Kossmann is a Diplomate of the American Board of Internal Medicine with his subspecialty Board in Cardiovascular Diseases. He has been extremely active within the American Heart Association, research activities in Sigma Xi, and editorial activities, serving on the Editorial Boards of 11 scientific publications. In April of 1982 he became the only Master of the American College of Physicians in Memphis at that time.[18,29]

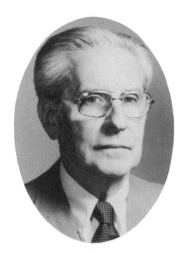

FIGURE 168. *Charles E. Kossmann, M.D. (1909–) Professor, U.T. Department of Medicine, 1967–1976*

Fred E. Hatch, M.D. is a Professor and Chief of the Division of Nephrology within the U.T. Department of Medicine. When he came to Memphis in 1961, Dr. Hatch was the first practicing nephrologist in Tennessee. He established the Section of Nephrology at the University of Tennessee in 1962; it became part of the Division of Circulatory Diseases under Dr. Kossmann in 1968, then reverted to an independent Division later. Dr. Hatch was responsible for developing the first chronic hemodialysis unit at the University of Tennessee, Memphis in the early 1970's. Along with other interested individuals, he also helped to establish the first National Kidney Foundation Chapter in Tennessee in 1971.[18]

Marion Dugdale obtained her A.B. degree from Bryn Mawr in 1950 and her M.D. degree from Harvard University Medical School in 1954. Dr. Dugdale has been an outstanding Professor in both Medicine-Hematology and Pathology, as a faculty member at the University of Tennessee, Memphis (Figure 169). She is a Diplomate of the American Board of Internal Medicine with a subspecialty Board of Hematology. Dr. Dugdale founded the first Hemophilia Clinic in Tennessee, and this Clinic currently serves 183 patients. In 1959, she established the first diagnostic laboratory for treating blood disorders and has been significantly involved in research regarding sickle cell anemia. Her main field of research is blood coagulation, and she has contributed 31 papers and chapters in two books to the scientific literature in this area. From 1974–1978 she served as a member of the National Heart, Blood, and Lung Institute Advisory Council in Bethesda, Maryland. She has received several important honors including: the Humanitarian Award, Memphis Chapter of the National Hemophilia Foundation (1977), the Gene H. Stollerman Outstanding Faculty Teaching

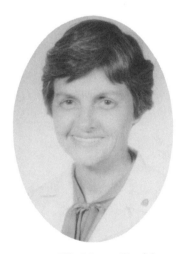

FIGURE 169. *Marion Dugdale, M.D. (1928–) Professor, Department of Medicine-Hematology, 1973-present*

Award (1981), and the U.T. Distinguished Teaching Award (1982).[18]

Jean M. Hawkes, M.D. served on the University of Tennessee College of Medicine faculty since 1947, becoming a clinical Professor of Medicine (Endocrinology). She helped to found and continues an active participation in the Tennessee Camp for Diabetic Children in Soddy, Tennessee. In 1985 she completed an explanatory book concerning diabetes mellitus for use with clinical patients.[18]

In 1966, a grant from the U.S. Public Health Service made possible the initiation of a postgraduate training program for science librarians at the University of Tennessee, Memphis under the direction of Andrew Lasslo, Ph.D., Professor and Chairman of the Department of Medicinal Chemistry in the U.T. College of Pharmacy, and Richard R. Overman, Ph.D., Associate Dean of the U.T. College of Medicine. This program initially provided training for 19 personnel, who were expected to serve as liaisons between pertinent resources of already published information and research investigators at the laboratory bench. It constituted an effective, interdisciplinary effort, which involved the participation of the University of Tennessee, Memphis Library and the Departments of Anatomy, Medicinal Chemistry, Medicine, Neurology, Operative Dentistry, Periodontia, Pharmaceutics, Physiology and Biophysics, and Surgery. These Departments represented the Colleges of Dentistry, Medicine, and Pharmacy, plus the Graduate School of Medical Sciences. A total of 33 individuals were trained and granted certificates; they came from throughout the various states of the United States and accepted appointments of similar geographic distribution. Dr. Lasslo directed this program from 1966 through 1972; then, at his request Professor Jess A. Martin, Director of the University of Tennessee, Memphis Library, assumed responsibility for the program. This particular program was unique in that the trainee spent part of his time in the laboratory itself to learn firsthand what the informational needs of the research scientist were; then he proceeded to fill those particular needs.[14]

One of the most dynamic Chairmen of the U.T. Department of Medicine was Gene H. Stollerman, M.D. He was born December 6, 1920 in New York City, graduated with an A.B. from Dartmouth College (summa cum laude) in 1941, and received his M.D. degree from the College of Physicians and Surgeons, Columbia University in 1944. After a year of internship and one year of medical residency at Mt. Sinai Hospital in New York, he served two years as a Captain (MC) U.S. Army. Returning from military duty, Dr. Stollerman completed his residency in Medicine at Mt. Sinai Hospital, plus an additional year as a Research Fellow in the Department of Microbiology of the New York University College of Medicine from 1949–1950. He served as Medical Director of Irvington House and an Instructor in Medicine at New York University from 1951–1955. At that time he became Director of the Samuel J. Sackett Laboratory for Research in Rheumatic and Infectious Diseases at Northwestern University Medical School in Chicago and remained in that position from 1955 through 1964. He became a full Professor of Medicine at Northwestern University in 1962, and left in 1965 to become Professor and Chairman of the Department of Medicine for the University of Tennessee College of Medicine (Figure 170).[18]

Dr. Stollerman remained as Professor and Chairman of the Department of Medicine at the University of Tennessee, Memphis from 1965–1981. In 1977 he was also named as a Goodman Professor at the University of Tennessee. He holds membership in many professional organizations, including: the Association of Professors of Medicine (President, 1975–1976), Infectious Diseases Society of America (Board of Directors, 1967–1970), Central Society for Clinical Research (President, 1974–1975), Fellow of the American College of Physicians (Master of the College in 1976, Regent of the College in 1978, and Vice President of the College, 1982), and from 1966–1968 he served as Chairman of the Council on Rheumatic Fever and Congenital Heart Disease for the American Heart Association. Dr. Stollerman is a Diplomate of the American Board of Internal Medicine, was Chairman of its Certifying Examination Committee 1969–1973, and was a member of its Executive Committee 1971–1973. From 1979–1982 he was a member of the National Advisory Council of the National Institute of Allergy and Infectious Diseases in Bethesda, Maryland. In addition to serving as a consultant in Medicine to the various hospitals in Memphis, Dr. Stollerman also was a consultant and member of national committees for the United States Public Health Service, the Armed Forces of the United States of America, the United States Department of State, and the World Health Organization. He served as an editor on five scientific journals and has contributed 62 articles to the medical literature.[29]

In 1981 the auxiliary medical library located in the Coleman Building at the University of Tennessee, Memphis was named the Stollerman Library in Dr. Gene Stollerman's honor. Previously, in 1978, he had been given the Maimonides Award from the State of Israel. His research interests lie in the areas of the biology of streptococci, nephritogenic strains of streptococci, and the prophylactic prevention of recurrences of rheumatic fever by the use of penicillin. Dr. Stollerman left the University of Tennessee, Memphis in 1981 to return to teaching and research as a Professor of Medicine in the Boston University School of Medicine.[29]

James Gilliam Hughes, M.D. (Figure 171) was born in Memphis, Tennessee on September 11, 1910. Both he and his twin brother, John Davis Hughes, graduated from Southwestern College in Memphis in 1932, and both received their M.D. degrees from the University of Tennessee College of Medicine with honors in 1935. John specialized in Internal Medicine, while James specialized in Pediatrics.[10]

Dr. Jim Hughes served his internship at John Gaston Hospital and his residency in Pediatrics at both the Children's Memorial Hospital in Chicago and the John Gaston Hospital in Memphis. After several months of private pediatric practice in Memphis, he was named Postgraduate Medical Instructor for the Oklahoma State Medical Association, a program funded by the Commonwealth Foundation of New York. There, he spent two years traveling around Oklahoma teaching 800 general practitioners and pediatricians

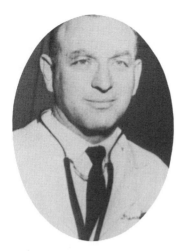

FIGURE 170. *Gene H. Stollerman, M.D. (1920–   ) Professor and Chairman, U.T. Department of Medicine, 1965–1981*

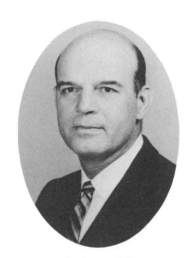

FIGURE 171. *James Gilliam Hughes, M.D. (1910–   ) Professor and Chairman, U.T. Department of Pediatrics, 1960–1976*

187

at 50 different centers. His experiences during that time resulted in his first book, *Pediatrics in General Practice*.[11]

Dr. Jim Hughes joined the U.S. Army Medical Reserve Program as a 1st Lieutenant in February of 1936 and was retired as a Brigadier General in September of 1970, a period covering 34 years of service. He served with distinction in World War II, rising from Captain in 1941 to Colonel in 1944. Colonel Hughes received numerous military decorations for his distinguished services as a hospital commander during the Italian Campaign. For many years he served as a Pediatric Consultant to the U.S. Army Surgeon General, inspecting, evaluating, and seeking to improve pediatric services in the U.S. Army both within the United States and at bases abroad. Returning to Memphis in 1946 from his duties in World War II, Dr. Jim Hughes became an Associate Professor in the U.T. Department of Pediatrics. He served on the faculty as a Professor from 1952–1960, at which time he became Professor and Chairman of the U.T. College of Medicine's Department of Pediatrics. He retired from this position in 1976 and was appointed as Emeritus Professor of Pediatrics. He became one of the principal forces in the founding of the Le Bonheur Children's Hospital, which is now renamed the Le Bonheur Children's Medical Center. Dr. Hughes was Chief-of-Staff from 1959–1960 and became the first Medical Director of Le Bonheur Children's Hospital in 1972, serving through 1976. He is a lifetime honorary member of the Center's Board. Dr. Hughes' portrait hangs in the foyer of the Le Bonheur Children's Medical Center Auditorium. In 1947 Dr. Hughes was heavily involved in the establishment of the Memphis Speech and Hearing Center, and he served as the President of its Board of Directors from 1947–1952.[11,18]

As far as it is known, Dr. James Hughes was the first pediatrician to investigate comprehensively the potential usefulness of jet injection. The first description of the use of jet injection in children was given by R. A. Hingson (a University of Tennessee Professor of Obstetrics) and James G. Hughes. These early investigations paved the way for the eventual important use of jet injection—the mass immunization of individuals by the jet injector technique. In five scientific papers between 1948–1950, Dr. Hughes delineated the various aspects of electroencephalograms (EEG) findings in newborn infants. Dr. Hughes is a Diplomate of the American Board of Pediatrics and was an official Board Examiner from 1948–1980. He served as a member of the Board of Directors from 1952–1958. He has also served as a chairman of many committees for the American Academy of Pediatrics, and was elected as President of the American Academy of Pediatrics in 1965. Dr. Hughes has published extensively in the medical literature, and he is especially well-known for serving as Editor of all six editions of *Synopsis of Pediatrics*. In 1977 the U.T. College of Medicine awarded Dr. Hughes its Outstanding Alumnus Award. As a consultant to the World Health Organization, he conducted a three-month survey of pediatric education in South and Central America. Also, as a consultant to the Rockefeller Foundation, Dr. Hughes helped plan pediatric postgraduate training in Latin America, enhanced by his ability to speak Spanish fluently. In 1980 he compiled an excellent 112 page history entitled *American Academy of Pediatrics: the First Fifty Years*. Dr. Jim Hughes continues to serve his University in many ways as a valued member of the Emeritus Faculty.[11]

It is fitting to end this decade of the 1960's with a 1969 Christmas greeting sent out to all of her University of Tennessee friends by Sara Conyers York Murray, M.D., who was the University of Tennessee, Memphis' first woman graduate in 1913—

A CHRISTMAS GIFT

(To My Beloved, Everywhere)

This is the most wonderful Christmas
That I have ever spent,
Because, by God's gracious mercy,
My 91st year was lent.
For months I have lingered
Around death's door,
That we sometimes call a gate,
At the top of a garden wall.
And oft when the gate was swinging wide
God heard and heeded my call.
Human hands too came to offer
Their kindness and their will.
But only God, who gave us life,
Can prolong it at His will.
While lingering near that gateway,
I learned a lesson old yet new,
The more you give of the best of gifts,
The more there is left for you.
So today I send you that magical gift,
That gift that we call LOVE,
Best typified by the Christ Child
And our Heavenly Father above.

Sara Conyers York Murray, M.D.
Christmas, 1969

REFERENCES

1. Aivazian, Garo: Personal Communication, 1985.

2. Autian, John and Lawrence, W. H.: "The Materials Science Toxicology Laboratories, University of Tennessee", *Medical Research Engineering*, p. 23–27, 1972.

3. Autian, John: Personal Communication, 1986.

4. Bruesch, Simon R.: Personal Communication, 1985.

5. Crenshaw, Andrew Hoyt: Personal Communication, 1986.

6. Diggs, Lemuel W.: Personal Communication, 1985.

7. Francisco, Jerry T.: Personal Communication, 1986.

8. Fuller, Pete: Personal Communication, 1986.

9. Ginski, John M.: *History of the Department of Physiology 1879–1984, U.T. College of Medicine*, (Private Printing: Memphis, TN.), 1984.

10. Hughes, James G.: Personal Communication, 1985.

11. Hughes, James G.: *Department of Pediatrics—UTCHS: 1910–1985*, 1985.

12. King, Kenneth O.: Personal Communication, 1985.

13. Kossmann, Charles E.: "Daniel Anthony Brody: 1915–1975", *Transactions of the Assoc. of Amer. Physicians* 89:15–17, 1976.

14. Lasslo, Andrew: Personal Communication, 1985.

15. Lollar, Michael: *Commercial Appeal* Mid-South Magazine, May, 1984.

16. McKnight, James P.: Personal Communication, 1985.

17. Medical Accomplishments: U.T. College of Dentistry.

18. Medical Accomplishments: U.T. College of Medicine.

19. Medical Accomplishments: U.T. College of Nursing.

20. Medical Accomplishments: U.T. College of Pharmacy.

21. Overman, Richard R.: Personal Communication, 1985.

22. Reynolds, Richard J.: Personal Communication, 1985.

23. Runyan, John W., Jr.: Personal Communication, 1985.

24. Sprunt, Douglas H. and Crocker, Robert A.: *History of the Department of Pathology of the University of Tennessee*, (Private Printing), 1965.

25. Stewart, Marcus J.: Personal Communication, 1985.

26. Stewart, Marcus J. and Black, William T., Jr.: *History of Medicine in Memphis*, (McCowat-Mercer Press, Inc.: Jackson, TN.), 1971.

27. Taylor, Robert E., Jr.: Personal Communication, 1985.

28. *Tennessee Medical Alumnus*—(Fall, 1969: Dr. Jerry T. Francisco).

29. University of Tennessee, Memphis: Personnel Records.

30. *U.T. Asklepieion*, 1966.

CHAPTER EIGHT
1970–1979

THE 1970's decade at the University of Tennessee, Memphis witnessed even more turbulent leadership changes than those which transpired in the 1960's. Between the years 1970 and 1979, five changes occurred in the Chancellorship, five in the Deanship of Medicine, two in the Deanship of Dentistry, three in the Deanship of Pharmacy, three in the Deanship of Nursing, and two in the Deanship of the Graduate School of Medical Sciences. Also, the U.T. College of Allied Health Sciences was created in 1972.[36]

In 1970, Edward J. Boling, Ed.D. (Figure 172) became the 17th President of the University of Tennessee. He was born on February 19, 1922 in Sevier County, Tennessee. Ed Boling obtained his B.S. degree in 1948 from the University of Tennessee, Knoxville, after serving in the United States Army Adjutant General's Department in the European Theatre during World War II. Afterwards, he obtained his M.S. degree in 1960 in Business Administration from the University of Tennessee, Knoxville. Continuing his graduate studies, he obtained his Ed.D. degree from the George Peabody College of Vanderbilt University in 1961. He was also awarded an LL.D. degree in 1984 from the University of Tennessee in 1970. Dr. Boling held the following positions: Instructor, College of Business Administration, the University of Tennessee, Knoxville; Research Statistician, Union Carbide Corporation; Supervisor of Source and Fissionable Materials Accounting, Union Carbide Corporation; Budget Director, State of Tennessee; Commissioner of Finance and Administration, State of Tennessee; and Vice President for Development and Administration, the University of Tennessee.[36]

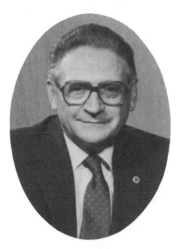

FIGURE 172. *Edward J. Boling, Ed.D. (1922–   ) President, University of Tennessee, 1970–present*

During Dr. Ed Boling's outstanding administration, the entire University of Tennessee System has expanded in quantity and quality on the Knoxville, Memphis, Martin, and Chattanooga campuses. Dr. Boling has always been a staunch supporter of the University of Tennessee, Memphis and continues to play a vital role in many of the activities on this campus.

On January 30, 1970 Chancellor Homer F. Marsh (Figure 137) completed almost nine years of service at U.T. Memphis, after having first assumed the helm in Memphis in July of 1961. He retired from the University in 1970 and accepted the position of Executive Vice President of Tranquilare Health Services, Inc. in Florida. He left behind him an impressive list of accomplishments on the U.T. Memphis campus, both from the standpoint of physical growth and expansion, as well as in concepts of quality and excellence.[2]

Dr. Homer Marsh was succeeded February 1, 1970 by Dr. Jack Kenny Williams, who was appointed Chancellor *pro tem* by the University of Tennessee President, Dr. Ed Boling, until a permanent successor could be

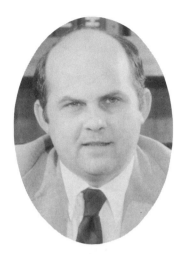

FIGURE 173. *Joseph E. Johnson, Ed.D. (1933–   ) Interim Chancellor, U.T. Memphis, December 1970–October 1971 Chancellor, U.T. Memphis and Vice President for Health Affairs, October 1971–October 1973*

selected. Jack Williams was born in Gafax, Virginia in 1920 and received a B.A. degree from Emory and Henry College in 1940; later, he also received an M.A. degree (1947) and a Ph.D. degree (1950) in American History from Emory University in Atlanta. At the time of his appointment to head temporarily the University of Tennessee, Memphis, Dr. Jack Williams was the Vice President for Academic Affairs for the entire University of Tennessee System. In addition to his U.T. duties, he was Chairman of the Commission on Colleges of the Southern Association of Colleges and Schools, and he was the Southern representative on the Federation on Regional Accrediting Commission for Higher Education. He divided his time between Memphis and Knoxville, serving the former as Chancellor *pro tem* and the latter in continuing his responsibilities in Academic Affairs for the state-wide University of Tennessee System. Dr. Williams served nine months from February through October, 1970; at that time, he left the University of Tennessee to accept the position of President of Texas A. & M. University in College Station, Texas.[35,36]

During the month of November, 1970 Dr. Roland H. Alden (Figure 140) was appointed to serve as Chancellor *pro tem*, as well as Dean of the Graduate School of Medical Sciences at U.T. Memphis. Dr. Alden carried out his duties in his usual excellent fashion for that one month in both positions. Then, President Boling decided to send Dr. Joseph E. Johnson to serve as Interim Chancellor in December of 1970 (Appendix A). He served in that capacity until October of 1971, when he was appointed permanently as Chancellor of the U.T. Medical Units and Vice President for Health Affairs, the University of Tennesseee. This appointment was the first time that the latter title came into being.[24]

Prior to his coming to Memphis to assume the duties of Interim Chancellor in December of 1970, Dr. Joe Johnson had been the Vice President for Development and Administration for the University of Tennessee System in Knoxville. Joe Johnson was born in Vernon, Alabama on July 9, 1933, received his B.A. degree from Birmingham-Southern College in 1955, and later completed his M.A. (1960) and Ed.D. (1968) degrees at the University of Tennessee, Knoxville. His former positions include: Research Associate Instructor, Department of Political Science and Bureau of Public Administration, the University of Tennessee; Director of Budget Division, State of Tennessee; Deputy Commissioner of Finance and Administration, State of Tennessee; Executive Assistant to the Governor, State of Tennessee; Vice President for Institutional Research and Executive Assistant to the President, the University of Tennessee; and Vice President for Development and Administration, the University of Tennessee. During his three years as Chancellor at the University of Tennessee, Memphis, Dr. Johnson brought a sense of stability and excellent administrative management to this segment of the University of Tennessee. Currently, Dr. Joe Johnson (Figure 173) is the Executive Vice President and Vice President for Development of the University of Tennessee System.[27]

There were many tangible accomplishments made during the Chancellorship of Dr. Johnson. State-funding support for the University of Tennessee, Memphis increased roughly twofold from a level of $6,370,000 in 1970 to approximately $12,000,000 in 1973. Enrollment in all of the Colleges was increased by 5%, along with a subsequent increase in the number of full-time faculty. The Faculty Senate was created to give the faculty more representation in the overall administration and planning of U.T. Memphis. The University's first Clinical Education Center, a Division of the College of Medicine, was established at the U.T. Memorial Research Center and Hospital in Knoxville. A long-range capital development program, which was estimated to cost over $30,000,000 projected over the next six-year period, was launched under his direction. Much of the building program in the 1970's, which will be described later, was commenced under his leadership. He established the "Chancellor's Roundtable", a group of influential business and public leaders in Memphis who agreed to serve as a continuing advisory group to the Chancellor and to U.T. Memphis in establishing mutual goals and promoting community support. Dr. Joe Johnson was most proud of an accomplishment which falls in the category of an intangible: "I think I am proudest of the fact that there seem to have emerged a new spirit of cooperation and a forward-looking attitude at the Medical Units. We may have had problems—and certainly there are many yet to be solved—but I think the campus is beginning to realize its potential for greatness. I think the Medical Units are beginning to see where they need and want to go, and how to get there."[27]

With Dr. Joe Johnson leaving the University of Tennessee, Memphis to return to Knoxville to become the Executive Vice President of the University, Dr. Edmund Daniel Pellegrino was named as the new Chancellor for U.T. Memphis. Prior to his move to Memphis to assume his duties on October 15, 1973, Dr. Pellegrino had served as Director of the Health Sciences Center at the State University of New York at Stony Brook. At that institution, he was also Vice President for Health Sciences and a Professor of Medicine in the School of Medicine.[27]

Edmund Daniel Pellegrino, M.D. (Figure 174) was born in 1920 in Newark, New Jersey. He earned his M.D. degree with honors in 1944 at the New York University School of Medicine and completed his residency in Internal Medicine, qualifying as a Diplomate of the American Board of Internal Medicine in 1956. He gained wide recognition in the United States as a dynamic contributor toward new approaches in medical education, and he held membership on more than 60 national health committees or study groups at the time of his appointment as Chancellor in 1973. Dr. Pellegrino is a Fellow of the American College of Physicians, a member of over 20 scientific and professional societies, and is widely known as an ethicist in Medicine. His excellent book on medical ethics, published in 1981 in conjunction with David C. Thomasma, *A Philosophical Basis of Medical Practice*, has been an outstanding contribution. Unfortunately, in spite of such promise as an administrative leader, Dr. Pellegrino's tenure as Chancellor, University of Tennessee, Memphis, was short-lived.[27]

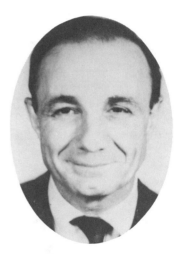

FIGURE 174. *Edmund Daniel Pellegrino, M.D. (1920–) Chancellor, U.T. Memphis and Vice President for Health Affairs, October 1973–1974*

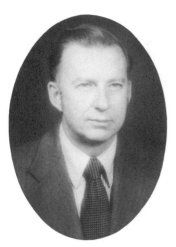

FIGURE 175. T. Albert
Farmer, Jr. M.D.
(1932–1984) Dean, U.T.
College of Medicine,
1972–1974, Chancellor, U.T.
Memphis and Vice President
for Health Affairs, 1975–1980

Significant events did transpire at the University of Tennessee, Memphis under the leadership of Dr. Edmund D. Pellegrino, despite the brevity of his tenure as Chancellor—which was a little over 14 months. The Tennessee State Legislature allocated $15,700,000 for operations at Chancellor Pellegrino's urging, and the University of Tennessee Administration and Board of Trustees approved a change in its name from the U.T. Medical Units to the U.T. Center for the Health Sciences. Working with THEC (Tennessee Higher Education Commission), he developed a plan for a state-wide multi-locational, multi-institutional system for education in the health professions. A state-wide program in Family Practice was also initiated through the U.T. College of Medicine. Dr. Pellegrino accepted the position as Chairman of the Board and Director of the Yale-New Haven Medical Center, which was effective January 1, 1975. Dr. Ed Pellegrino continues to follow the progress of the University of Tennessee, Memphis, having served as a speaker for the 1982 Frank M. Norfleet Forum for the Advancement of Health in Memphis, which is conducted annually by the University of Tennessee. He also serves on its National Advisory Board, and currently he is the John Carroll University Professor of Medicine and Medical Humanities at the Georgetown University School of Medicine in Washington, D.C.[28]

Dr. T. Albert Farmer, Jr. became Chancellor of the University of Tennessee, Memphis and Vice President for Health Affairs, the University of Tennessee on January 1, 1975, succeeding Dr. Edmond D. Pellegrino. This action had been made official by a vote of the University of Tennessee Board of Trustees on August 19, 1974, when they accepted the recommendations made by President Edward J. Boling and a special U.T. Memphis Faculty-Staff Appointment Committee that Dr. Farmer be named to the top administrative position on the Memphis campus. Prior to his appointment as Chancellor, Dr. Farmer served as Dean of the University of Tennessee College of Medicine beginning June 1, 1972. He moved to Tennessee from the University of Alabama Medical Center at Birmingham, where over a period of seven years he had previously served as Professor of Medicine and as Executive Associate Dean and Director of Undergraduate Education.[28]

T. Albert Farmer, Jr., M.D. (Figure 175) was born in Smithville, North Carolina in 1932. He attended Davidson College, obtained a B.S. degree from the University of North Carolina, and received his M.D. degree from the University of North Carolina School of Medicine. He took graduate training in Endocrinology at the University of Alabama and spent two years in the U.S. Army before entering private practice in Wilson, North Carolina. After one year, he joined the University of Alabama School of Medicine as an Associate Dean in Medical Education. Dr. Farmer was honored scholastically by membership in both Phi Beta Kappa and Alpha Omega Alpha. His specialty was Endocrinology and Metabolic Diseases, and he was a Diplomate of the American Board of Internal Medicine. As Dean of the U.T. College of Medicine, he held firmly to the belief that in order to teach health professionals, the teaching must be done by practicing physicians, and it should be performed in actual management of, or service to, patients. In his words, "In view of the rapidly changing pattern of health care support, insurance programs, etc. everyone is going to become a private patient—no longer dependent solely on large, tax-supported hospitals that primarily have served the indigent in past years. A health science center, such as ours, has no choice but to engage in the practice of medicine. If we do not, we will have no patients, and if we have no patients, we cannot teach."[28,36]

Dr. Al Farmer was an excellent Chancellor, as he previously had proved to be an excellent Dean of the U.T. College of Medicine. He served as Chancellor from 1975 through 1980. Many accomplishments were carried out during his tenure. In the words of the current Chancellor, Dr. James C. Hunt, "Although Dr. Farmer was here only about eight years, he was one of the three giants in the leadership of U.T.C.H.S.; the others are Dr. O. W. 'Pinkie' Hyman, the first U.T. Memphis Chancellor, and Dr. Joe Johnson, who is now the U.T. Executive Vice President and Vice President for Development."[3] Al Farmer was probably best known to Memphians for his role in shaping the future of the City of Memphis Hospital. During his Chancellorship, the University of Tennessee managed the City of Memphis Hospital. It was during that same period, after eight years of debate, that the Shelby County Commissioners voted to begin the $50,000,000 expansion and remodeling project which was completed in 1983. As part of that agreement in 1979, the University of Tennessee, Memphis leased the William F. Bowld Hospital from Shelby County for 40 years. In 1980, Dr. Farmer left the University of Tennessee, Memphis to become Chancellor of the University of Maryland Center for the Health Sciences in Baltimore. At a press conference announcing his resignation, Dr. Farmer stated that he received the most personal satisfaction from the following accomplishments: he raised the U.T. College of Dentistry admission standards and lowered its enrollment from 156 to 128 students per year, all U.T.C.H.S. programs were fully-accredited, the Van Vleet Memorial Cancer Center and the E. P. and Kate Coleman Medicine Building were completed, and student performance rose above the national average. It should also be remembered that it was during Dr. Farmer's tenure as Chancellor that the University of Tennessee, Memphis moved from semi-annual to annual medical school admissions (in 1963 it had changed from quarterly to semi-annual admissions), it strengthened graduate-level nursing and pharmacy programs, and it brought a modern approach to medical training. On April 9, 1984 Dr. Al Farmer died suddenly, following an acute heart attack at his home in Baltimore.[2,3,14]

With the resignation of Maston K. Callison, M.D. (Figure 116) on June 30, 1970 to enter the private practice of medicine in Memphis, Richard R. Overman, Ph.D. (Figure 132), who was an Associate Dean for the previous four years, was named as the Acting Dean of the U.T. College of Medicine, pending a decision to select a permanent Dean.[23] Dr. Overman served for two years until T. Albert Farmer, Jr., M.D. became the permanent Dean for

"Anyone, who has himself as a doctor, has a fool for a patient."

Confucius

195

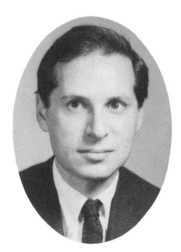

FIGURE 176. *E. William Rosenberg, M.D. (1930–) Acting Dean, U.T. College of Medicine, January-June, 1975, and 1977–1978, Professor and Chairman, U.T. Department of Dermatology, 1967–present*

the U.T. College of Medicine, effective June 1, 1972 (Figure 175). Dr. Farmer's accomplishments as Dean have been mentioned earlier in this chapter. He remained in the Deanship until he was appointed as Chancellor of the University of Tennessee, Memphis on January 1, 1975.[28]

For six months (January 1, 1975–June 30, 1975) E. William Rosenberg, M.D. (Figure 176) served as Acting Dean of the U.T. College of Medicine. He continued his previous duties as Associate Dean of Continuing and Public Education and Chief of the Section of Dermatology for the U.T. College of Medicine. Bill Rosenberg was born on March 11, 1930 in Philadelphia, Pennsylvania; he obtained his B.S. degree from Franklin and Marshall College in Lancaster, Pennsylvania in 1952. His M.D. degree was earned in 1956 from the University of Pennsylvania. His internship year was taken at the Philadelphia General Hospital in 1957; then he completed a residency in Dermatology at the Massachusetts General Hospital in 1959. Dr. Rosenberg spent an additional year of study as a U.S. Public Health Service Research Fellow at the University of Miami College of Medicine in Florida. He came to the University of Tennessee, Memphis College of Medicine in 1962 as an Assistant Professor in the Division of Dermatology. He became Professor and Chairman of the Division of Dermatology in 1967. Dr. Bill Rosenberg is a Diplomate of the American Board of Dermatology (1961) and a Fellow of the American College of Physicians. He is a member of numerous professional societies, and he has authored 37 papers related to dermatological subjects. He was given the Faculty Recognition Award by the medical class of June, 1973 for the University of Tennessee College of Medicine.[29]

Dr. Rosenberg relinquished his duties as Acting Dean of the U.T. College of Medicine June 30, 1975 with the appointment of Dr. Charles B. McCall as Dean. Again, he was called upon by Chancellor Al Farmer in July of 1977 to serve as Acting Dean for the College of Medicine for one year until Dr. James C. Hunt was appointed July 1, 1978. At that time Dr. Al Farmer stated in regard to his service, "We have been very fortunate in having Bill Rosenberg serve as Acting Dean. You could not find a more loyal or a more effective individual in keeping the College of Medicine moving ahead during this interim."[29]

The fourth Dean of the University of Tennessee College of Medicine during the 1970's decade was Charles Barnard McCall, M.D. (Figure 177). Dr. McCall's appointment as Dean held great promise, but unfortunately he remained at the University of Tennessee for only two years. He was born November 2, 1928 in Memphis, Tennessee and obtained both his B.A. degree (1950) and his M.D. degree (1953) from Vanderbilt University; he finished first in his medical class and received the Founders Medal at Vanderbilt. He interned at Vanderbilt University Hospital, served as a Clinical Associate at the National Cancer Institute, National Institutes of Health in Bethesda, Maryland (1954–1956), was Senior Assistant Resident in Medicine at the University of Alabama (1956–1957), was a Fellow in Chest Diseases, National Academy of Sciences, National Research Council

(1957–1958), and completed his residency in Medicine as Chief Resident at the University of Alabama (1958–1959). Dr. McCall first came to the University of Tennessee in 1959 as an Assistant Professor of Medicine. He was appointed as an Associate Professor of Medicine in 1964, and also that same year, he became Chief of the Section on Pulmonary Diseases within the Department of Medicine of the University of Tennessee College of Medicine. He remained in Memphis until 1969, when he accepted a position as Professor of Medicine at the University of Texas where he also had the dual responsibility of Assistant Vice Chancellor for the University of Texas. At the University of Texas Southwestern Medical School in Dallas, he served as an Associate Dean for Clinical Affairs and Director of Grants Management, before returning to U. T. Memphis the second time in 1975.[14,29]

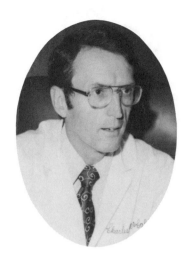

FIGURE 177. *Charles Barnard McCall, M.D. (1928–   ) Dean, U.T. College of Medicine, 1975–1977*

Dr. McCall is certified by both the American Board of Internal Medicine and the American Board of Internal Medicine in Pulmonary Diseases. He served as President of the Southern Thoracic Society in 1968–1969. He is a Fellow of both the American College of Physicians and the American College of Chest Physicians, plus holding membership in numerous professional or honorary societies, including Sigma Xi and Alpha Omega Alpha. Dr. McCall served as Dean of the University of Tennessee College of Medicine from July 1, 1975–June 1, 1977, when he resigned to accept the appointment as Dean of the Oral Roberts University College of Medicine in Tulsa, Oklahoma.[29]

The fifth Dean of the U.T. College of Medicine in the 1970's was James Calvin Hunt, M.D. (Figure 178), who assumed his duties July 1, 1978. His appointment was a fortuitous one by Chancellor Al Farmer, because it not only brought a professionally well-qualified individual into the University of Tennessee System as Dean, but by this decision U.T. Memphis acquired a well-organized visionary, who would move the University forward in giant measure during the 1980's. Dr. Jim Hunt was born September 11, 1925 in Lexington, North Carolina. During World War II he served with distinction in the U.S. Army Air Corps, flying combat missions in the European Theatre. Following his discharge from military duty in 1946, he entered Catawba College in Salisbury, North Carolina and completed his A.B. degree in 1949. He was accepted into the Bowman Gray School of Medicine of Wake Forest College and obtained his M.D. degree in 1953. Later, he obtained an M.S. degree from the University of Minnesota in 1958. Following a straight medical internship at North Carolina Baptist Hospital in Winston-Salem, he served his residency in Medicine from 1954–1957 at the Mayo Graduate School of Medicine at the Mayo Clinic in Rochester, Minnesota. From July of 1957 through June of 1958, he was a Fellow in Cardiovascular-Renal Disease, also at the Mayo Graduate School of Medicine. From 1957–1978, Dr. Hunt served as a Consultant in the Division of Cardiovascular-Renal Diseases in the Department of Medicine and in 1963 was appointed as Chairman of the Division of Nephrology, Department of Medicine, Mayo Clinic. From 1972 to 1974 he was the Associate Director

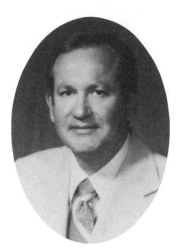

FIGURE 178. *James Calvin Hunt, M.D. (1925–   ) Dean, U.T. College of Medicine, 1978–1980*

for Clinical Educational Programs, Division of Education, Mayo Foundation. From 1974 until 1978 he was the Chairman of the Department of Medicine for the Mayo Clinic and the Mayo Medical School. During this time he also served on many committees within the Mayo Clinic and the Mayo Foundation.[31]

Dr. Hunt holds membership in numerous professional societies. He is a Diplomate of the American Board of Internal Medicine, a Fellow of the American College of Cardiology, a Fellow of the American College of Physicians, Chairman of the Renal Section of the American Society for Clinical Pharmacology and Therapeutics, a Fellow of the American Heart Association (Council on Circulation), and a member of the International Society of Hypertension, the International Society of Nephrology, the National Kidney Foundation, and the Society of Sigma Xi. In 1973 he received the distinguished Alumnus Award for the Bowman Gray School of Medicine, and from 1973–1976 he was President of the National Kidney Foundation. He was also presented with the Distinguished Service Award in 1974 from Catawba College. He has served on numerous Medical Advisory Boards and National Institutes of Health Study Sections. He was a member of the Board of Directors for the Minnesota Heart Association 1966–1970. He was on the Scientific Advisory Committee on Hypertension for the American College of Chest Physicians from 1968–1978. He has served on Study Sections for the National Heart, Lung, and Blood Institute from 1974 through the present. His research interests have been: (1) pressor and depressor substances in high blood pressure, (2) disorders of water and electrolyte metabolism, (3) disorders of renal function and renal function testing, and (4) nutrition in renal failure. He has authored over 90 scientific publications, including two textbooks on diet and nutrition related to high blood pressure (*Living With High Blood Pressure* and *Living Better: Recipes For a Healthy Heart*). Dr. Jim Hunt served well as the Dean of the University of Tennessee College of Medicine until his appointment in November of 1980 as Chancellor for the University of Tennessee, Memphis. His accomplishments as Chancellor will be covered in Chapter 9.[14,31]

The U.T. College of Dentistry witnessed two administrative changes in the 1970's decade. With the departure of Shailer A. Peterson, Ph.D. to become Dean of the newly established University of Texas at San Antonio School of Dentistry in February of 1969, Dr. Bill Jolley again served as Acting Dean from February of 1969 until August of 1970. At that time Jack E. Wells, D.D.S. was named as the permanent Dean of the U.T. College of Dentistry, and he soon became a popular and influential leader within the University of Tennessee System. His rapport with dental alumni was well-known throughout the South, and it became a model for other institutions seeking such alumni support and loyalty. Jack Wells was born January 14, 1922 in Kansas City, Kansas. From 1942–1946 he served with the U.S. Navy in Memphis, Tennessee and in the Far East Theatre, receiving his honorable discharge on January 22, 1946. His predental education was taken at the University of Kansas, and he obtained his D.D.S. degree from the University of Kansas City of Dentistry in 1951. He continued his affiliation with this school in the Department of Pedodontics and obtained an M.S.D. degree, also, in 1957. At that time he became an Associate Professor and Director of Undergraduate Pedodontics at the University of Missouri-Kansas City School of Dentistry. From 1958–1970 he was Professor and Chairman of the Department of Pedodontics at that institution. From 1960 through 1963 he was an Assistant Dean, and from 1963 through 1970 he was an Associate Dean of the University of Missouri-Kansas City School of Dentistry.[13,20]

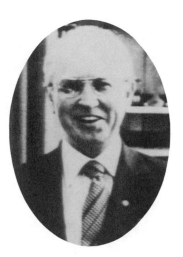

FIGURE 179. *Jack E. Wells, D.D.S. (1922–1981) Dean, U.T. College of Dentistry, 1970–1981*

Dr. Jack Wells (Figure 179) was very active in professional societies. He was a member of the American Academy of Pedodontics, a member of the American Society of Dentistry for Children, a Fellow of the International College of Dentists, a Fellow of the International Association for Dental Research, a Fellow of the American College of Dentists, a member of Omicron Kappa Upsilon, and a member of the Academy of General Practice. In organized dentistry he served as Secretary, Vice President, and President of the Johnson County Dental Association of Kansas. He organized and served as Secretary, Vice President, and President of the Kansas City Chapter of the Missouri Unit of the American Society of Dentistry for Children. He served as President of the Southern Conference of Dental Boards and Educators in 1977. During his tenure at the University of Missouri in Kansas City, Dr. Wells received numerous awards for outstanding service and teaching. He gave presentations and lectures at numerous professional society meetings, both nationally and internationally, and published over ten scientific publications. His most outstanding contribution, however, was providing the administrative leadership that the University of Tennessee College of Dentistry desperately needed at the time he became Dean. He recognized the potential of a great future for the College of Dentistry, and under his dynamic leadership, he motivated the faculty, students, and alumni toward achieving this goal. The 1970's will be remembered as a time of unparalleled successes under the 11 years of his leadership as Dean of the U.T. College of Dentistry. One of his greatest fiscal accomplishments was obtaining the new $8,000,000 Dental Clinical Building, which was named for one of the University's most distinguished alumni, Governor Winfield Dunn. This tremendous project, which was so critically needed by the College of Dentistry, was achieved without Federal funding. His motivation caused dental alumni to voluntarily contribute $600,000 to equip the new clinical facility. This building (Figure 180) stands as an appropriate memorial to the accomplishments of Dean Jack Wells.[12,13]

In addition to his many activities and responsibilities as Dean of the University of Tennessee College of Dentistry, Dr. Wells also served as President of the American Association of Dental Deans and Examiners and as a Consultant to the Council on Dental Education of the American Dental Association, while he was at the University of Tennessee. During his tenure, the dental curriculum at the University of Tennessee was changed from three to four years, and the U.T. College of Dentistry gained

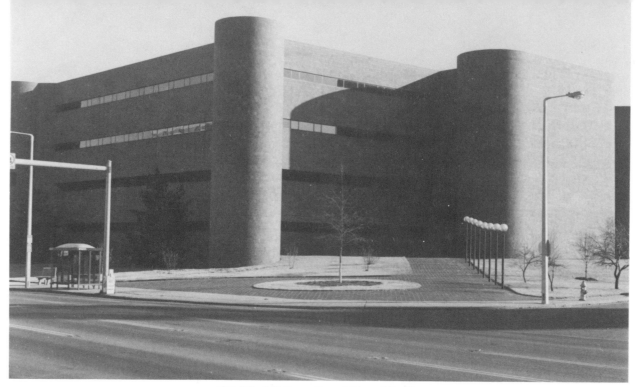

FIGURE 180. *Winfield Dunn Dental Clinical Building, 1977 (courtesy of James E. Hamner, III, D.D.S., Ph.D.)*

full accreditation by the Council on Dental Education of the American Dental Association. On March 14, 1981 Dr. Jack Wells, at age 59, suffered a coronary occlusion and died in his office at the University. Similar to Dean James T. Ginn, Dr. Wells became the second Dean of the U.T. College of Dentistry to die suddenly at a young age from a heart attack. At the time of Dr. Well's death, Dr. Edward J. Boling, President of the University of Tennessee, stated, "Without question, Jack Wells will be remembered as one of the most influential leaders in the University's history. He built one of the great dental education facilities in the country, and he guided the College to national esteem in its teaching and service programs. During his administration faculty, student, and alumni support and loyalty became the standard for other institutions." Frank P. Bowyer, D.D.S. summarized in his beautiful eulogy for Dr. Wells at his Memorial Service, which was held on March 18, 1961, "Truly, the measure of one's life is not the length of it, but the well-spending of it. This tribute to Jack Wells is not to mark merely the passage of the 59 years of life nor to list the particular events, but rather to reflect on one dynamic individual, who was dedicated to the pursuit of excellence, and who achieved his dream of excellence by strong motivation and tenacity of purpose."[1] The U.T. College of Dentistry established the Jack E. Wells, D.D.S. Memorial Student Loan Fund to aid worthy students in financial need and to honor Dean Wells.

Earlier, on January 19, 1975 the University suffered the loss of another popular, strong, and productive Dean with the death of Dr. Dick Feurt (Figure 115), Dean of the U.T. College of Pharmacy, from pulmonary carcinoma. The Dental-Pharmacy Research Building, which was built in 1962, was renamed in memory of Dean Seldon Dick Feurt in a special ceremony on November 14, 1975. Dr. Marcus Stewart, Chairman of the Medical Affairs Committee of the University of Tennessee Board of Trustees, presided. President Edward J. Boling, Executive Vice President Joseph E. Johnson, Chancellor Albert Farmer, members of the University of Tennessee faculty, and representatives of the Feurt family were present for the unveiling of a special plaque, honoring Dr. Feurt. The Seldon D. Feurt Memorial Fund was established by tripartite action of members of the Tennessee Pharmaceutical Association, the Tennessee Board of Pharmacy, and the U.T. College of Pharmacy, in cooperation with the central administration of the University of Tennessee. This endowment fund was established to be used to maintain the excellence of the College by the purchase of special equipment and the funding of scholarships, faculty awards, and research.[7,16]

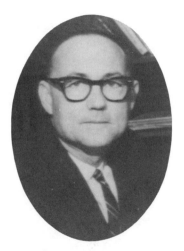

FIGURE 181. *Martin Ellis Hamner, Ph.D. (1918–) Associate Dean, U.T. College of Pharmacy, 1962–present Acting Dean, U.T. College of Pharmacy, January-July, 1975*

From January 20, 1975 through July 31, 1975, Dr. Martin Ellis Hamner, who had been Associate Dean of the U.T. College of Pharmacy since 1962, was appointed as Acting Dean for the University of Tennessee College of Pharmacy. Martin Ellis Hamner was born in Castor, Bienville Parish, Louisiana on July 28, 1918. During World War II, Martin Hamner served with the U.S. Naval Intelligence Service in the Pacific Theatre and Naval Aviation from 1942–1945. He received his B.S. degree in Pharmacy from the University of Colorado in 1949. Two years later, he received an M.S. degree from the University of Colorado; then he spent two years at the University of Florida, before completing his Ph.D. degree in 1955 at the University of Colorado. His major was Pharmacy and his minor was Biochemistry.[16]

From 1955 through 1959 Dr. Martin Hamner was an Associate Professor in Pharmacy at the Southwestern State College in Weatherford, Oklahoma. In 1959, he arrived at the University of Tennessee, Memphis to become Professor and Chairman of the Department of Pharmacy within the U.T. College of Pharmacy. In 1962 he became the Associate Dean of the U.T. College of Pharmacy, and for many years he was the Director of Admissions for that College. Dr. Hamner has been very active in numerous pharmacy professional societies, including: the American Association of Colleges of Pharmacy, the American Board of Diplomates in Pharmacy, past President of the Memphis Branch (1965 of the American Pharmaceutical Association), and Phi Delta Chi (national professional pharmaceutical society— founder and charter member—Alpha Omega Chapter 1957). He was also a member of the Rho Chi national honor pharmaceutical society and served as Secretary-Treasurer of the Tennessee Pharmaceutical Association. He served as Editor of the "Newsletter" for the Memphis and Shelby County Pharmaceutical Society from 1966 until the present time. He was also Editor of the Alumni News for the U.T. College of Pharmacy from 1969–1972. In addition to these editorial activities, Dr. Hamner has published 12 scientific articles. For this soft-spoken, mannerly man, poetry has

201

been a long-time, relaxing hobby. In his own words, "My makeup is such that I am attracted to this form of expression. It's extremely relaxing, satisfying, and very demanding mental work to write even simple verse. It requires the most total kind of concentration, but losing yourself totally is very personally satisfying, especially if you put something together you like."[38]

On August 1, 1975 Dr. John Autian (Figure 156) was appointed permanent Dean of the University of Tennessee College of Pharmacy by Chancellor James C. Hunt. He continued in that role and managed the College well until his appointment as Dean of the Graduate School of Medical Sciences and Vice Chancellor for Research in 1982.[36]

There were three changes in the leadership within the U.T. College of Nursing during the brief period of 1977–1981. Dean Ruth Neil Murry, who since 1949 had led the College in exemplary fashion, retired in 1977 and was appointed as a Professor on the Emeritus faculty. Dr. Norma J. Long, who at the time of Dean Murry's retirement was a Professor and Assistant Dean for the University of Tennessee College of Nursing, was appointed Acting Dean from 1978–1979. Norma Long obtained her B.S.N. degree in 1958 from the University of Arkansas, and she earned an M.S.N. from Washington University in St. Louis in 1964. She completed her D.N.Sc. degree in 1975 from Catholic University in Washington, D.C. She first came to the University of Tennessee College of Nursing as an Assistant Professor in 1967, and thus she completed her postgraduate doctoral work on a part-time basis. After serving for one year as Acting Dean, she was appointed as an Associate Dean and Director of Academic Affairs. She resigned from this position on March 11, 1981, and she resigned permanently as a Professor in the Department of Basic Nursing Concepts on June 15, 1981.[15,19,36]

Marie C. Josberger, Ed.D. was appointed as permanent Dean of the U.T. College of Nursing in 1979 and resigned from that position on March 16, 1981. She had obtained her B.S. degree in Nursing from Florida State University in 1962 and an Ed.D. degree in Nursing from Indiana University in 1972. Prior to coming to the University of Tennessee, she had also been affiliated with Penn State University, the University of Florida, and Wayne State University. Dr. Josberger left the University on February 25, 1982.[36]

Roland H. Alden, Ph.D. (Figure 140), who was Dean of the Graduate School of Medical Sciences from 1961, retired from the University of Tennessee in 1979. John L. Wood, Ph.D. (Figure 163) was named as Acting Dean and served from 1979–1980 in that capacity.[36]

The concept of developing a College of Allied Health at U.T. Memphis was approved by the University of Tennessee Board of Trustees in 1969, as part of a nationwide impetus to the formation of such colleges, provided by newly available Federal funding. However, it was not until 1972 that the College of Community and Allied Health Professions was organized at the University of Tennessee, Memphis. Although it was established as the newest of the six Colleges on the health science campus, most of the programs within the College were developed prior to 1972 as part of the Colleges of Medicine, Dentistry, and Basic Medical Sciences. For example, Medical Technology is the oldest program in the United States, having been started as a part of the U.T. Department of Pathology in 1922. Dental Hygiene also is one of the oldest such programs in the nation, having originated in the U.T. College of Dentistry in 1926. Radiologic Technology, although not active as a program at the present time, was developed in 1953 as part of the U.T. Department of Radiology, and Physical Therapy had its genesis in 1965 as part of the Section of Physical Medicine in the University of Tennessee College of Medicine. Medical Record Administration began as a program based in the Baptist Memorial Hospital in Memphis in 1954, and it was transferred to the University of Tennessee in 1973. The Cytotechnology Program was developed in 1952 and Clinical Immunohematology in 1966, both in the U.T. Department of Pathology. In 1985 the name of the College was changed to the College of Allied Health Sciences to reflect more accurately the growing complexity and sophistication of the various Allied Health Professions, of which the College is comprised.[13,14]

In having a College of Allied Health Sciences, the University of Tennessee joined over 85 percent of all other land grant institutions in the nation. These distinct and separate administrative units for the Allied Health Sciences are recognized as the most appropriate and effective means for the education and training of qualified allied health professionals. Nevertheless, the College of Allied Health Sciences is unique on the U.T. Memphis campus. Unlike other Colleges, it represents several very different health disciplines, each with a distinct professional mission. Although each program is different, each shares with the others the responsibility for educating health professionals, who contribute to the quality of medical care by complementing and enhancing the efforts of primary health care providers. In addition to the undergraduate educational programs offered by the various Departments within the College, continuing educational courses for allied health practitioners in Tennessee have been a significant statewide contribution by the U.T. College of Allied Health Sciences' faculty. Annual enrollments of 400–500 individuals in a variety of programs in each professional area have been the norm for over a decade. Since the inception of the U.T. College of Allied Health Sciences in 1972, three individuals have served as its Dean (Appendix F). The first was Lee Holder, Ph.D. (1972–1982), the second was Ralph Hyde, Ed.D., Acting Dean (1982–1984), and the third was William G. Hinkle, Ph.D. (1984—present).[36]

Dr. Lee Holder was born January 19, 1932 in Upland, California. His B.S. and M.P.H. degrees were obtained in 1953 and 1958, respectively, from the University of California in Berkeley. In 1968 he received his Ph.D. degree in Public Health Administration from the University of Michigan. From 1959 through 1963 he worked in the Department of Public Health for Monterey, California and the State of Wyoming. From 1963 through 1966 he was an Associate in Public Health Administration at the Johns Hopkins

"Pathology is a demanding mistress."

George Margolis, M.D.

203

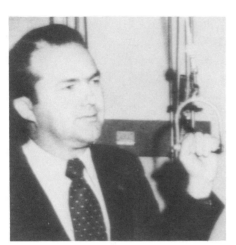

University School of Hygiene in Public Health in Baltimore. During that time he also served on the National Commission on Community Health Services in Bethesda, Maryland. From 1968–1971 he was an Associate Professor in the Department of Health Education for the School of Public Health at the University of North Carolina in Chapel Hill. In 1972 Dr. Holder was appointed as Dean of the U.T. College of Community and Allied Health Professions and also a Professor in the Department of Community Medicine of the U.T. College of Medicine (Figure 182).[36]

Dr. Holder is involved in many professional societies, including serving on the Board of Directors for the American Society of Allied Health Professions from 1972–1982; he also served as President of this organization from 1979–1981. He is a Fellow of the American Public Health Association, a Fellow of the Society for Public Health Education, a member of the Royal Society of Health, and a member of the International Union for Health Education. He was the co-author and editor of eight publications of the Governor's Committee on Aging for the State of Wyoming, published in 1960. He also served from 1972 through 1982 on the Editorial Board of the *Journal of Allied Health*. Dr. Holder saw active duty with the U.S. Army in Europe from 1953–1955, and he remained as a Lieutenant Colonel in the U.S. Army Reserve (Infantry). On September 13, 1982 Dr. Holder resigned from the University of Tennessee, Memphis and accepted an appointment as Dean of the College of Allied Health at the University of Oklahoma Medical Center.[36]

A comparison of Table 12 and Table 13 reveals that enrollment during the 1970's decade rose dramatically in the U.T. College of Medicine, 560 in 1969 to 718 in 1979, making it the largest medical school in the United States. There was also a marked rise in enrollment for the U.T. College of Dentistry from 399 in 1969 to 533 in 1979. The U.T. College of Nursing rose less dramatically from 139 in 1969 to 191 in 1979. The U.T. College of

Table 13

The University of Tennessee, Memphis—Enrollment 1970–1979

Fall Term	College of Medicine	College of Dentistry	College of Pharmacy	College of Nursing	Graduate School of Medical Sciences
1970	570	411	315	138	120
1971	575	417	314	145	112
1972	574	430	359	174	115
1973	600	446	391	187	113
1974	606	450	396	192	114
1975	611	467	406	239	114
1976	611	469	370	158	121
1977	715	545	335	159	134
1978	723	540	316	170	129
1979	718	533	325	191	113

Pharmacy enrollment figures remained in the 300 category except for 1975, when they reached 406. The Graduate School of Medical Sciences continued to show a small increase with enrollments during the 1970's fluctuating between 112 and 134 graduate students.

The 1970's were years of continued building at the University of Tennessee, Memphis. In 1972 a permanent Chancellor's residence was acquired by the University at 343 Goodwyn Street, and Chancellor Joe Johnson was the first occupant of this home. Both he and the succeeding Chancellors have been most generous in allowing the use of their lovely home for numerous important University social functions. The Physical Plant Building was completed in 1975 and serves as the headquarters of the Vice Chancellor for Facilities and Human Resources; this building is located at 201 East Street. The Doctors' Office Building is located at 66 North Pauline Street and houses the majority of the office space utilized by the University Physicians Foundation. The Dunn Dental Clinical Building was named for Governor Winfield Dunn, when it was completed in 1977 and is located at 875 Union Avenue (Figure 180).

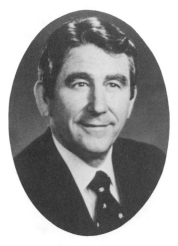

Winfield Culbertson Dunn, D.D.S. was born July 1, 1927 in Meridian, Mississippi. He earned his B.A. degree from the University of Mississippi in 1950 and graduated in the September, 1955 class of the University of Tennessee College of Dentistry with his D.D.S. degree. As a dental student, he was selected for membership in the Deans' Honorary Odontological Society and Omicron Kappa Upsilon, the dental honor society. Dr. Dunn entered the private practice of dentistry in Memphis from 1955 to 1970. During that time he served as a member of the Board of Trustees of the City of Memphis Hospitals, and as Chairman (in March of 1964) of the Republican Party of Shelby County. He was elected and served as Governor of the State of Tennessee from 1971 to 1975 (Figure 183). He attended the Advanced Management Program at Harvard University and holds an honorary Juris Doctorate degree from Rhodes College in Memphis. Dr. Winfield Dunn joined the management of Hospital Corporation of America soon after completing his term of office as Governor. He served as Vice President for Public Affairs, prior to his appointment in November of 1977 as Senior Vice President. In addition to these responsibilities, he was a Director on the Boards of Hospital Corporation of America, First American Bank, and the Tennessee-Alabama-Georgia Railroad until his gubernatorial bid again for the State of Tennessee in 1986. He is a past President of the Federation of American Hospitals and Chairman of the Executive Committee of the National Committee on Quality Health Care.[12,13]

The last building to be completed in the 1970's decade was the General Education Building, which is located at 8 South Dunlap Street; this structure was built at a cost of $21,486,400. The General Education Building was the result of intensive planning by a large number of University of Tennessee, Memphis faculty under the leadership of Chancellor Joe Johnson. Another key figure in the planning concept and execution of this building was Earle Bowen, Ph.D., who at that time was Director of Educational

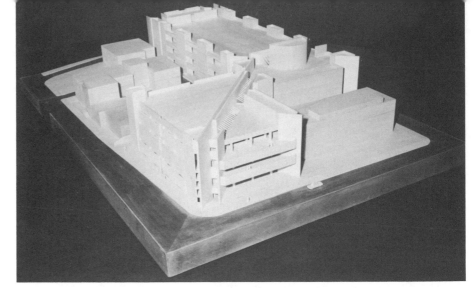

FIGURE 184. *General Education Building, Architect's Model, 1977*

Services for U.T. Memphis. The urgent need for space, due to expanding class sizes in each College, enlarging faculties within the U.T. Medical Center, and the growth of new programs, left no real alternative except to build a proper educational facility. The decision was made to consolidate the preclinical teaching spaces, which at that time were located in multiple departments, into one large, multi-use building. The teaching space that would thus be freed-up could then be recycled by the various departments to meet their own internal space needs. The purpose of the General Education Building was stated to be: a structure that would encompass all non-clinical instruction with the exception of laboratories in gross anatomy, postmortem pathology, and industrial pharmacy. Figure 184 depicts the architect's model of this massive structure, which is divided into three main components: a series of modern lecture rooms around a central core on each floor with adjacent smaller study/lecture areas, an independent study area to be utilized by students, and the high and low bench laboratories for multiple use. Both the lecture/teaching facilities, the independent study areas, and the laboratory facilities are used by students and faculty from all of the University of Tennessee, Memphis Colleges. For example, the same multi-use high bench laboratory could be used for medical biochemistry on Monday morning, dental physiology on Monday afternoon and pharmacy pharmacology on Tuesday afternoon, and so on. There are three floors of independent study spaces, each floor containing six to eight individual study rooms, three to four group study rooms, and about 130 individual study areas.[26]

The University of Tennessee, Memphis announced on February 24, 1978 that a $1,000,000 gift from Memphis philanthropist Abe Plough would be used to support new research and to recruit outstanding faculty. Reflecting a wish by Mr. Plough, the University of Tennessee Board of Trustees named the new General Education Building in honor of Dr. Cecil C. Humphreys, a University of Tennessee alumnus, who has made significant contributions to higher education in the State of Tennessee. Cecil Humphreys was a 1936 University of Tennessee (Knoxville) graduate and played end on the U.T.

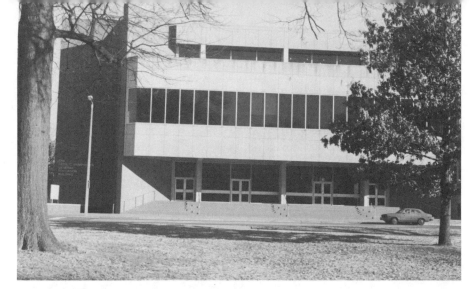

FIGURE 185. *Cecil C. Humphreys' General Education Building, front view, 1986 (courtesy of James E. Hamner, III, D.D.S., Ph.D.)*

Volunteer Football Teams of the 1933–1935 era. He taught and coached at the University of Tennessee, Martin campus for one year before joining the Memphis State University faculty in 1937. Later he earned an M.S. degree at the University of Tennessee and a Ph.D. degree at New York University. From 1960 to 1972, Dr. Humphreys was President of Memphis State University, which made tremendous strides under his Presidency and leadership. In 1972 he became the first Chancellor of the State Board of Regents. He retired in 1975. The front entrance of the Cecil C. Humphreys General Education Building is seen in Figure 185, looking across Dunlap Street from Forrest Park.[31]

Because the University of Tennessee, Memphis was on the four-quarter system with a new class admitted each three months for many years, this structure allowed certain students to attend school and then drop out for several quarters and enter again, without losing an entire year of work. Thus, many professional athletes were able to complete a health profession education, while they played their particular professional sport. The following list is a compilation of as many of these individuals as could be located: Dr. Edward C. Baker (New York Giants), Dr. Edwin M. Beatty, Jr. (Pittsburgh Steelers), Dr. Ernest J. Borghetti, Jr. (Kansas City Chiefs), Dr. Billy A. Cannon (Kansas City Chiefs), Dr. Gary S. Cuozzo (Minnesota Vikings), Dr. Walter M. Dennis (Los Angeles Rams), Dr. James R. Detwiler (Baltimore Colts), Dr. Cary G. Dischinger (Detroit Pistons), Dr. David Dowling (St. Louis Cardinals and Chicago Cubs), Dr. Bernard Erickson (Cincinnati Bengals), Dr. Clyde D. Goodnight (Green Bay Packers and Washington Redskins), Dr. White S. Graves, III (Boston Patriots), Dr. Louis B. Guy (New York Giants), Dr. Charles ("Chuck") P. Latourette (St. Louis Cardinals—football), Dr. William E. Linkaitis (San Diego Chargers), Dr. David H. Middleton (Detroit Lions), Dr. Stephen J. O'Neil (New York Jets), Dr. Edward W. Sutton (Washington Redskins), Dr. Harry E. Taylor (Kansas City Athletics), Dr. Edward J. Weiner (Philadelphia Warriors), and Dr. Kendall C. Wise (Detroit Tigers).[2,12,21]

On June 15, 1976 John F. Griffith, M.D. succeeded James G. Hughes, M.D., who served as Chairman of the U.T. Department of Pediatrics for 16 years and as Medical Director of Le Bonheur Children's Hospital. This year also featured the continuation of leadership by the U.T. Department of Pediatrics in planning the development of a Children's Medical Center, which evolved from the original Le Bonheur Children's Hospital. In order to provide better and more comprehensive medical and surgical care for the children of Memphis and the Mid-South, to improve the Department of Pediatrics' teaching programs by concentrating patients and faculty in one location, and to stimulate and further research, the headquarters for the Department was moved to a spacious suite on the third floor of Le Bonheur Children's Hospital. At that time the pediatric patients of the Frank T. Tobey Memorial Children's Hospital were transferred to Le Bonheur Hospital. The U.T. Department of Pediatrics has a special commitment to the physicians and institutions of the Mid-South who are involved with the health care of children. The High-Risk Infant Program is committed to the care of ill neonates, which has been described previously under the direction of Dr. Sheldon Korones. The High-Risk Infant Program is comprised of the Newborn Center, the Term and Premature Nurseries, the Special Care Clinic, and the Transport Service; it serves the western third of Tennessee, northern Mississippi, eastern Arkansas, and a small area in southern Missouri. The Sidney Shelton Pediatric Hemodialysis Unit, which is located in Le Bonheur Children's Medical Center, serves pediatric patients with end stage kidney disease, residing in Tennessee, Arkansas, Mississippi, southern Missouri, and northern Alabama. A Child Abuse and Neglect Program began July 1, 1977 under the direction of James G. Hughes, M.D. It is a comprehensive program for early detection, prompt reporting, rapid evaluation, and integrated treatment of abused and neglected children and their parents. The program, which began in 1977, has evolved into a Center for Children in Crisis; this facility is located in the Le Bonheur Children's Hospital Annex.[9,30]

John Francis Griffith, M.D. was born on February 14, 1934 in Humboldt, Saskatchewan, Canada. He received his B.A. degree in 1956 and his M.D. degree in 1958, both from the University of Saskatchewan. Dr. Griffith completed a rotating internship and a pediatric residency at the Montreal General Hospital, residing there from 1958 through 1963. He completed his residency in Pediatrics and Infectious Diseases in 1964 at the Cleveland Metropolitan General Hospital. From 1964–1966, he was Assistant Resident in Neurology, and from 1965 through 1966 he was also a Pediatric Neurology Resident at the Massachusetts General Hospital. His postgraduate training was also taken at the Harvard Medical School and Massachusetts General Hospital as a Neuropathology Research Fellow from 1966–1967 and an Infectious Disease (Virology) Research Fellow from 1967–1969. From Boston, Dr. Griffith went to Duke University Medical Center in Durham, North Carolina where he served as an Associate Professor in both Pediatrics and Medicine from 1969–1976. During that

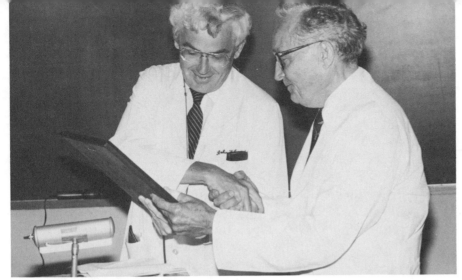

FIGURE 186. *John Francis Griffith, M.D. (1934–   ) Professor and Chairman, U.T. Department of Pediatrics, 1976–present (presenting a research award to Dr. James N. Etteldorf)*

time he received the prestigious Howard Hughes Medical Investigatorship Award from 1971–1974. Dr. Griffith came to the University of Tennessee, Memphis in 1976 to become Professor and Chairman of the Department of Pediatrics.[14,36]

Figure 186 illustrates Dr. John F. Griffith presenting Dr. James N. Etteldorf with an award plaque for pediatric research. Dr. Griffith is board certified in Pediatrics by the Royal College of Physicians and Surgeons of Canada (1965) and the American Board of Pediatrics (1966). He is a member of numerous professional societies, has served as an Examiner on the American Board of Pediatrics from 1979 through the present, has been a member of the Residency Review Committee of the Accreditation Council for Graduate Medical Education of the American Medical Association from 1982 through the present, a member of the American Pediatric Society, a member of the American Academy of Pediatrics, and a member of the Association of Medical School Pediatric Department Chairmen. Dr. Griffith has served as an Editor on the *Journal of Developmental and Behavioral Pediatrics* and the *Synopsis of Pediatrics*. He is the author of over 30 scientific publications, the recipient of 5 major grants, and is a Trustee for the Crippled Children's Hospital Foundation Forum on Child Health. He has served as the Chairman of the Scientific Program Committee for the Forum on Child Health since 1984.[6,36]

Dr. Frank P. Bowyer was born January 29, 1917 in Tampa, Florida. His predental education was taken at the University of Florida, and he graduated with honors from the University of Tennessee College of Dentistry in 1939. He took his advanced training in Orthodontics as an Associate of Dr. Oren A. Oliver in Nashville, Tennessee from August of 1939 through October of 1942. At that time, he was sent to Knoxville by the Procurement and Assignment Division of the Manpower Commission to render orthodontic service in Knoxville and Oak Ridge, Tennessee and to serve as Dental Consultant to the Manhattan Project until the end of World War II.

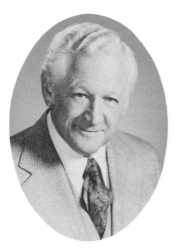

FIGURE 187. *Frank P. Bowyer, D.D.S. (1917–   ) U.T. College of Dentistry graduate, 1939 President, American Dental Association, 1977–1978*

Dr. Bowyer also served from 1952–1955 as a Major in the U.S. Air Force Dental Corps during the Korean War. He is a Diplomate of the American Board of Orthodontics. Dr. Bowyer has given generously of his time and talents, and he has served in many positions within organized Dentistry. From 1964–1965 he was President of the Tennessee Dental Association, and earlier he had served as Secretary (1948–1952) and as President (1956–1957) for the Southern Society of Orthodontists. He has served in the top leadership positions within many prominent dental organizations. Dr. Bowyer was President of the following professional groups: the American Board of Orthodontics (1963–1964), the American Association of Orthodontists (1965–1966), and the American College of Dentists (1969–1970, which was the fiftieth anniversary of the founding of the American College of Dentists).[20] Continuing on a national scale, his most important position was President of the American Dental Association from 1977–1978. Previously, he had been Chairman of the Committee on Dental Education and Hospitals for the A.D.A. in 1967. He was Chairman of the A.D.A. Council of International Relations in 1972 and was Speaker of the House of Delegates from 1972–1976 (Figure 187). Dr. Frank Bowyer has also been very much involved in international affairs, being a Fellow of the International College of Dentists since 1949. On a People to People Tour in 1976, he joined a group of Tennessee dentists, who toured Great Britain, Hungary, Russia, Poland, and Yugoslavia in order to study dental practice systems, education, and research in those countries. At the Pierre Fauchard Academy Centennial Meeting in Paris in 1978, the Lord Mayor of Paris presented Dr. Bowyer with a gold medal for "the Pursuit of Excellence in International Health." As a long-time member of the Federation Dentaire Internationale, he was elected Vice President for a three-year term at the annual International Congress in Helsinki, Finland in 1984. Governor Frank Clement appointed Dr. Frank Bowyer in 1959 for a 12-year term as a member of the University of Tennessee Board of Trustees. He was reappointed in July of 1971 by Governor Winfield Dunn for another 9-year term. Dr. Bowyer has received numerous citations during his distinguished professional career, four of which will be listed in this chapter: in 1979 he was given the "Governor's Outstanding Tennessean Award" by the State of Tennessee (this occasion marked the first time that this award was given, and it was presented to him by Governor Lamar Alexander); the University of Tennessee National Alumnus Award was given to him "in recognition of dedicated service to the University of Tennessee"; in 1982 he was given the American Dental Association's Presidential Citation "for significant contributions to the oral health of the public and to the profession of dentistry"; and in 1983 he became the first recipient of the Jack E. Wells Memorial "Dedication to Dentistry Award".[1] This distinction has been designated as the highest award presented by the Tennessee State Dental Association. On January 29, 1980 Dr. Bowyer generously endowed the Frank P. Bowyer Visiting Lectureship for the University of Tennessee College of Dentistry. The College's gratitude was expressed by Dean William F. Slagle as follows:

"The University of Tennessee expresses its sincere appreciation to Dr. Frank P. Bowyer for his unselfish gifts, which made the Bowyer Visiting Lectureship in the U.T. College of Dentistry a reality. Dr. Bowyer's dream of making available lectures by prominent individuals from the profession of Dentistry will add an important dimension to the educational environment of the College."[13]

Alvin J. Ingram obtained his M.D. degree from the University of Tennessee College of Medicine in 1939. He was born March 31, 1914 in Jackson, Tennessee and received both his B.S. and M.D. degrees from the University of Tennessee in 1939. He also earned an M.S. degree in Orthopedic Surgery in 1947 from the University of Tennessee. In 1948 he was certified as a Diplomate of the American Board of Orthopedic Surgeons, after earlier taking his residency at the Campbell Clinic. During World War II he was a Major in the U.S. Army Medical Corps. Dr. Ingram served as Professor and Chairman of the Orthopedic Department at the University of Tennessee College of Medicine from 1971 through 1979. During that time he was also Chief-of-Staff for the Campbell Clinic from 1971–1976 (Figure 188). Dr. Ingram acquired numerous honors during his distinguished career. From 1976–1977 he was President of the American Board of Orthopedic Surgery. He was also President of the American Orthopedic Association in 1973–1974, as well as serving as President for the American Academy of Cerebral Palsy from 1958–1959. He is a Fellow of the American College of Surgeons, a member of the Board of Trustees for the American Medical Association from 1964–1970, and Secretary-Treasurer of the American Medical Association from 1968–1970. He served for a decade as a member of the National Academy of Sciences' Institute of Medicine from 1971–1981. Also, he is the author of 22 scientific publications. Dr. Ingram became an Emeritus Professor of the University of Tennessee in 1979.[4,14]

Herbert C. Butts, D.D.S. was born August 24, 1924 in Dover, Tennessee. After serving in the U.S. Navy during World War II, he completed his predental education at Memphis State University in 1947. He graduated from the University of Tennessee College of Dentistry with his D.D.S. degree in June of 1950 and began general practice and part-time affiliation with the University in Memphis. From 1958 through 1960 he was a full-time faculty member at the U.T. College of Dentistry in the Operative Dentistry Department. He left Memphis in 1960 and continued until 1963 as a Dental Education Advisor with the International Cooperation Administration (I.C.A.), a branch of the United States State Department. This organization is presently called the Agency for International Development (A.I.D.). From 1963 through 1964, he remained as Chairman of the Department of Operative Dentistry and Clinical Director of the El Salvador School of Dentistry after his A.I.D. contract was completed. He returned to the United States in 1964 and obtained an M.S. degree in 1966 from the University of Iowa Graduate School in Operative Dentistry and Education.[13]

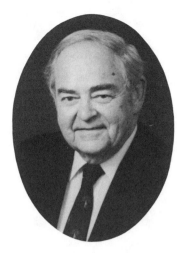

FIGURE 188. *Alvin J. Ingram, M.D. (1914–   ) Professor and Chairman, U.T. Department of Orthopedics, 1971–1979*

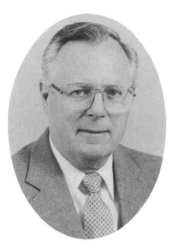

FIGURE 189. *Herbert Clell Butts, D.D.S. (1924–   ) U. T. College of Dentistry graduate, June, 1950, Editor, American Dental Association, 1974–1977, Dean, School of Dental Medicine, Southern Illinois University, 1981–present*

From 1967–1970 Dr. Butts served as Professor and Chairman of the Department of Operative Dentistry at the Medical University of South Carolina College of Dental Medicine in Charleston. In June of 1970 he became Assistant Dean for Admissions and Student Affairs within the College of Dental Medicine, and in February of 1971 due to illness of the Dean, he was named as Acting Dean of the Medical University of South Carolina College of Dental Medicine. In March of 1974 he was selected as Editor of the American Dental Association by the A.D.A. Board of Trustees and assumed this position in July of 1974. The Editor has a staff of approximately 30 editors, writers, production people, and secretaries and is responsible for the budgeting and publication of the following journals: *Journal of the American Dental Association, A.D.A. News, Journal of Oral Surgery, Dental Abstracts, Oral Research Abstracts, Journal of Endodontics,* and the *Journal of Dental Research.* He left Chicago in January of 1978 to become the Associate Dean for Academic Affairs of the University of Tennessee College of Dentistry and remained in that position until August of 1981, when he left the University of Tennessee, Memphis to become Dean of the Southern Illinois University School of Dental Medicine (Figure 189). Dr. Butts is a member of numerous professional societies, including the Dean's Honorary Odontological Society and Omicron Kappa Upsilon (while he was a student at the University of Tennessee College of Dentistry), the American College of Dentists, and the International College of Dentists. He was named as the Outstanding Alumnus of the University of Tennessee College of Dentistry in 1975.[12,36]

Bland Wilson Cannon, M.D. was born on April 4, 1920 in Brownsville, Tennessee. He obtained a B.S. degree from Southwestern College in Memphis (1941), an M.S. degree from Northwestern University Graduate School (in Neurology—1943), an M.B. degree from Northwestern University Medical School (1944), and an M.D. degree from Northwestern University Medical School (1945). During the year 1944–1945, he interned in New York Hospital in New York City. Afterwards, he served as a Captain in the U.S. Army Medical Corps from April of 1946 to February of 1948 at the 98th General Hospital in Munich, Germany. Returning to the United States, he was accepted as a Fellow at the Mayo Foundation of the Mayo Clinic, Rochester, Minnesota from 1948–1950. Previously, he had completed one year of his fellowship at the Mayo Foundation from 1945 to 1946. His training in neurosurgery was completed at the Mayo Clinic, and he was certified as a Diplomate of the American Board of Neurological Surgeons in 1952. The following year he was elected as a Fellow of the American College of Surgeons.[14,36]

From 1953 to 1980, he moved through the academic ranks from Assistant to Professor of Neurosurgery at the University of Tennessee College of Medicine. On August 22, 1980 Dr. Cannon was named as an Emeritus Clinical Professor of Neurosurgery by Chancellor Al Farmer. Dr. Bland Cannon has rendered many special services to the University of Tennessee, Memphis (Figure 190), including being Special Advisor to the Chancellor since 1972 and also serving as Vice Chancellor for Academic Affairs, *pro tem* from January through September of 1974. He has held many appointments within the American Medical Association, including the Council on Medical Education (1965–1975), the Committee on Federal Health Programs, and the Committee on Professional Standards Review Organizations (1973–1974). His service for the U.S. Department of Health, Education, and Welfare included serving on the National Advisory Council for the Regional Medical Programs Service. Dr. Cannon has been extremely active in professional societies, serving as a delegate for the American Medical Association from 1964–1972. He is the founder and first President (1955–1956) of the Congress of Neurological Surgeons. He chaired the Membership Committee for the American Association of Neurological Surgeons in 1964. His academic and scientific background led him to become one of the founding members of the Sigma Xi Chapter at the University of Tennessee, Memphis. Dr. Cannon has been President of the following professional societies: Memphis and Shelby County Medical Society (1961), Tennessee Medical Association (1963–1964), the Memphis Neurological Society (which he founded—1965), and the Tennessee Neurological Society (1972–1973). His community activities and accomplishments have been numerous. He was Vice Chairman of the Regional Medical Program Advisory Group, and he was both founder and Vice Chancellor of the Mid-South Medical Center Council for Comprehensive Health Planning. The following four awards are typical of the recognition for his community health services: the L. M. Graves Memorial Health Award (1973), the Tennessee Medical Association's Distinguished Service Award (1973), the American Medical Association House of Delegates Award for Service (1964–1972), and the Mid-South Medical Center Council Award for Leadership and Service as a Consultant to the Council (1973).[36]

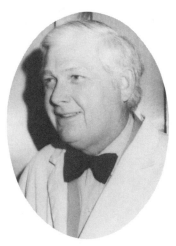

FIGURE 190. *Bland Wilson Cannon, M.D. (1920–   ) Emeritus Clinical Professor of Neurosurgery, 1980–present Special Advisor to the Chancellor, 1972–present*

A large debt of gratitude is owed to Dr. Bland W. Cannon for his continuing support and guidance since the inception of the Frank M. Norfleet Forum for the Advancement of Health in 1980, for which he was the motivating force. Bland Cannon has served as a staunch Trustee of the Norfleet Forum since 1980. He is the author of over 30 scientific publications and has produced the following three films in the clinical area of Neurosurgery: "The Nature of Paresis Following Lesion of Pyramidal Tracts", "The Lateral Position for Lumbar Disc Surgery", and "Acrylic Cranioplasty for Skull Defects." His son, Dr. John S. Cannon, received his undergraduate education at the University of the South, Sewanee and obtained his D.D.S. degree from the University of Tennessee College of Dentistry in December of 1974. Dr. John Cannon trained in oral and maxillofacial surgery at the Mayo Clinic Graduate School of Medicine from 1976-1979 and practices in Memphis.[13,36]

Other U.T.-associated medical accomplishments during the 1970's decade include the following individuals. Alexander Carter Lewis graduated from the U.T. Department of Microbiology and Immunology in 1972; currently, Dr. Lewis is an Associate Dean of Medicine at the Louisiana State

University School of Medicine in New Orleans.[33] Dr. Alton A. Register, III is a December, 1961 graduate of the University of Tennessee College of Dentistry. He was a University of Tennessee faculty member from 1972–1978. During that time he performed the first controlled study of acid demineralization of tooth root surfaces, using cats, dogs, and monkeys as experimental animals with the aim of enhancing and accelerating reattachment of periodontal tissue to diseased root surfaces. His further studies defined the type of acid, the pH, and the time of application to the tooth root for optimal clinical effects. Dr. Register performed additional studies in dogs and reported success in repairing chronic periodontal disease defects in certain sites. His research is cited regularly in the periodontal literature and is recognized both nationally and internationally. These scientific investigations created a great renewal of interest in the use of acid demineralization as an adjunct to new attachment therapy in periodontal treatment.[13]

Dr. Thoralf M. Sundt, Jr. obtained his M.D. degree from the University of Tennessee College of Medicine in 1959. During the 1970's he developed a special surgical clamp, which is used in the successful repair of carotid aneurysms. Currently, Dr. Sundt is a faculty member of the Mayo College of Medicine's Department of Neurosurgery in Rochester, Minnesota.[6]

Dr. Hubert Bell obtained his D.D.S. degree from the University of Tennessee in 1946 and earned an M.S. in postgraduate orthodontics from the University of Tennessee, Memphis in 1948. Dr. Bell served as President of the American Association of Orthodontists from 1974–1975.[12] Since a well-informed public is of prominent importance in effective health care, Dr. Andrew Lasslo (Figure 165—a faculty member of the U.T. College of Pharmacy) developed and served as both producer and moderator of the "U.T.C.H.S. Health Care Perspectives" television series, a color production carried by commercial and public service television stations throughout Tennessee. The audio portions of the 28 thirty-minute programs were re-recorded for radio broadcast and were aired by 44 radio stations from 1976–1978. Nationally prominent and internationally respected clinical specialists and research scientists, whose views had significant influence on emerging health care policies, appeared on these University of Tennessee programs, which were partially funded by a Federal grant under the Higher Education Act of 1965.[16]

Dan P. Greer, M.D., a native of Kentucky, received his premedical education at the George Washington University in Washington, D.C., and then obtained an M.D. degree from the University of Tennessee, Memphis in 1943. Dr. Greer was certified by the American Board of Surgery in 1952 and has been extremely active in the American Cancer Society for the State of Wyoming. For distinguished service in cancer control, he was awarded the St. George's Medal by the American Cancer Society in 1968.[8]

Albert W. Biggs, III, M.D. succeeded his stepfather, Dr. Samuel L. Raines, as Chairman of the U.T. Department of Urology in January of 1969. He served in that position until July of 1972. Previously, Dr. Biggs had received his undergraduate education and his M.D. degree in 1952 from the

University of Virginia in Charlottesville. He also obtained an M.S. in Urology from the University of Tennessee, Memphis in 1959. He moved from Assistant in Urology in 1959 to become Professor of Urology and Chairman of the Department in January of 1969, exhibiting rapid advancement through that decade of educational service. His Chairmanship occurred during the early 1970's, when a rapid change from part-time to full-time faculty was beginning to occur. He was shortly promoted to Director of the Clinical Education Center for the University of Tennessee's Medical Facility in Knoxville in January of 1972. In March of 1975 he was appointed as Vice Chancellor for Knoxville for the University of Tennessee Center for the Health Sciences. The responsibilities of that position encompassed the following divisions: Area Health Education Center, Clinical Education Center, Eastern Tennessee Cancer Research Center, the University of Tennessee Memorial Research Center, and the University of Tennessee Memorial Hospital.[6,14] The University of Tennessee Memorial Research Center and Hospital in Knoxville are under the aegis of the University of Tennessee, Memphis, with the Vice Chancellor for Knoxville reporting directly to the Chancellor in Memphis.

Dr. Al Biggs was succeeded as Professor and Chairman of the University of Tennessee, Memphis Department of Urology by Clair Edward Cox, II, M.D., who prior to his appointment was Professor of Urology at the Bowman Gray School of Medicine of Wake Forest University in Winston-Salem, North Carolina. Dr. Clair Cox obtained his undergraduate education at the University of Michigan and earned an M.D. degree from that institution in 1958. He is a distinguished urologist with over 75 scientific publications and is a Diplomate of the American Board of Urology (1966), a Fellow of the American College of Surgeons (1967), and the recipient of the Hugh Hampton Young Award from the American Urological Association (1976).[36]

Dr. Marvin Chris Meyer joined the University of Tennessee College of Pharmacy faculty as an Assistant Professor in January of 1969. He first obtained a B.S. degree in Pharmacy in 1963 and an M.S. degree in 1965 from Wayne State University in Detroit, Michigan. His postgraduate education was continued at the State University of New York at Buffalo, where he obtained his Ph.D. in 1969 with a major in Pharmaceutics. He was awarded financial support for this graduate training in the form of a Fellowship from the American Foundation for Pharmaceutical Education and in the form of a predoctoral Fellowship grant from the National Institutes of Health. In January of 1972 he was named as Director of the Division of Drug Metabolism and Biopharmaceutics in the U.T. Department of Medicinal Chemistry. He continues to serve as Director of this Division, becoming an Associate Professor in July of 1972 and a full Professor in July of 1976 (Figure 191). Dr. Meyer is a member of Rho Chi, the National Pharmacy Honor Society, Sigma Xi, Associate Fellow—American College of Apothecaries, and Member—Academy of Pharmaceutical Sciences. In addition to his many activities on University committees, Dr. Meyer has served as a

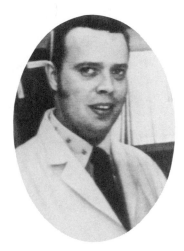

FIGURE 191. *Marvin Chris Meyer, Ph.D. (1941–   ) Professor and Director, Division of Drug Metabolism & Biopharmaceutics, U.T. Department of Medicinal Chemistry*

215

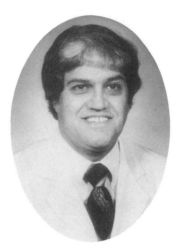

FIGURE 192. *Abbas E. Kitabchi, Ph.D., M.D. (1933–) Professor, U.T. Department of Medicine, 1973–present, Director, U.T. Clinical Research Center, 1968–present*

Member of the University of Tennessee Faculty Senate (1971–1974), a scientific review panelist for the American Pharmaceutical Association Drug Interactions Project (1972), and a consultant for Bioavailability Studies for the Veterans Administration (1972). He has been extremely active in the area of drug testing and evaluation, receiving 19 grants, which total $1,878,587. Dr. Marvin Meyer (principal investigator) and Dr. Seymour M. Sabesin, Professor of Medicine-Gastroenterology in the U.T. College of Medicine (co-principal investigator) were awarded a $558,000 research grant in 1984 by the Federal Drug Administration to investigate the manner that common prescription drugs are absorbed by the elderly. It was the first such grant awarded in the nation.[39] Dr. Meyer has also authored over 30 scientific publications and has been an invited speaker at 25 professional meetings.[16]

Abbas E. Kitabchi, Ph.D., M.D. was born August 28, 1933 in Teheran, Iran; he is now a citizen of the United Staes. Dr. Kitabchi's educational background is extensive. He received a B.S. degree from Cornell College in Mt. Vernon, Iowa in 1954. At the University of Oklahoma Medical Center he obtained an M.S. degree in 1956 and a Ph.D. degree in 1958. His postdoctoral work in Biochemistry was performed at the Oklahoma Medical Research Institute in Oklahoma City from 1958 through 1960. He entered medical school at the University of Oklahoma and obtained his M.D. degree in 1965. After a year of straight Medicine internship, he completed three years as a Senior Fellow in Endocrinology in the Department of Medicine of the University of Washington in Seattle, Washington from 1966–1968 as a National Institutes of Health Special Fellow (Figure 192). He came to the Veterans Administration Hospital in Memphis in 1968 and was soon appointed as the Director of the U.T. Clinical Research Center in the University's William F. Bowld Hospital. Dr. Kitabchi has been a Professor of Medicine in the U.T. College of Medicine since 1973, and also he has been a Professor in the U.T. Department of Biochemistry since 1972.[36]

Dr. Kitabchi has served as a member of the Editorial Board of the following three journals: *Journal of Clinical Endocrinology and Metabolism* (1976–1979), *Capsules and Comments* (1977–present), and *Diabetes* (1981–1984). He served as a member of the National Research Committee of the American Diabetes Association from 1978–1981. Also, he has served as Vice President of the Board of Directors for the National Pituitary Foundation from 1980 to the present. Dr. Kitabchi has been a member of numerous University of Tennessee, Memphis committees and holds membership in 17 professional societies, including being President (1973–1974) of the Tennessee Diabetes Association. He is a Diplomate of the American Board of Internal Medicine (1973). He has been the principal investigator/program director for six major grants in the diabetes/endocrinology area, and he is the author of over 100 scientific publications and 135 abstracts.[14] In 1975, Dr. Kitabchi simplified therapy for diabetic coma and substantially reduced mortality rates by administering small amounts of insulin every hour, instead of a single large dose, during the first day of treatment.[10]

Dr. Leonard Share (Figure 193) came to the University of Tennessee, Memphis as Professor and Chairman of the Department of Physiology and Biophysics in 1969. He continued the environment of excellence in research, which had been a hallmark of this University of Tennessee Department. Earlier, he obtained his A.B. degree from Brooklyn College (1947), his A.M. from Oberlin College (1948), and his Ph.D. in Physiology from Yale University (1951). He was awarded a U.S. Public Health Service Postdoctoral Fellowship in the training course for cardiovascular investigators; his program was directed by Dr. C. J. Wiggers, Department of Physiology, Western Reserve School of Medicine. Dr. Share remained with Western Reserve University School of Medicine as an Instructor in 1952, becoming a full Professor in 1968, and joining the University of Tennessee, Memphis in 1969. He is a member of the American Physiological Society, the Endocrine Society, and Sigma Xi. From 1966–1969 he had the honor of serving on a Study Section for the National Institutes of Health at Bethesda, Maryland. As an active member of the Association of Chairmen of Departments of Physiology, Dr. Share served as Secretary-Treasurer (1974–1976) and as President (1978–1979). Dr. Share has provided excellent administrative leadership, teaching capabilities, and excellence in research—publishing over 60 scientific articles, mainly in the cardiovascular area.[14,36]

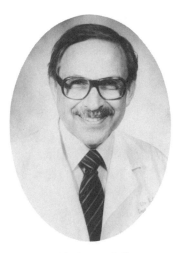

FIGURE 193. *Leonard Share, Ph.D. (1927–   ) Professor and Chairman, U.T. Department of Physiology & Biophysics, 1969–present*

On October 1, 1975 Preston V. Dilts, Jr., M.D. was named as Chairman of the U.T. Department of Obstetrics and Gynecology, moving from a similar position he had held at the University of North Dakota College of Medicine. Dr. Dilts, a native of Missouri, earned his A.B. degree in 1955 at Washington University in St. Louis. He obtained his M.D. degree from Northwestern University Medical School in 1959, as well as an M.S. degree in Gynecologic Pathology in 1961 from the same institution. Dr. Preston Dilts held the offices of President, Vice President, Secretary, and member of the Board of Directors for the Society for Obstetrical Anesthesia and Perinatology. He also served as an Examiner for the American Board of Obstetrics and Gynecology and is a member of numerous professional and academic organizations. He is the author of chapters in five different medical textbooks and the author of numerous research articles in the field of Obstetrics and Gynecology.[14]

Richard James Reynolds, D.D.S., who is a 1939 graduate of the University of Tennessee College of Dentistry, has been a tremendously devoted alumnus and has attained many medical accomplishments in his distinguished career (Figure 194). Dick Reynolds was born on April 7, 1915 in Memphis, Tennessee. He obtained his undergraduate education at the University of New Mexico and Memphis State University, before enrolling in the University of Tennessee College of Dentistry in 1935— his D.D.S. degree was obtained in June of 1939. From 1939 to 1942 he served as a full-time Instructor in the U.T. Department of Fixed and Removable Partial Denture Prosthesis. With the outbreak of World War II, he entered the United States Navy Dental Corps and ended the War as a Lieutenant

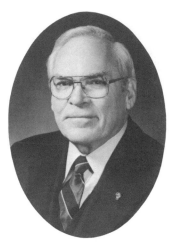

FIGURE 194. *Richard James Reynolds, D.D.S. (1915–) U.T. College of Dentistry graduate, June, 1939, President, Tennessee Dental Association, 1968 President, American College of Dentists, 1981–1982*

Commander. He continued in the U.S. Naval Reserve in Memphis and was the Commanding Officer of Dental Company 6-6 from 1950–1965. In 1945 he returned to Memphis and began the private practice of general dentistry, although he did maintain his affiliation with the University of Tennessee College of Dentistry as a part-time Instructor in the Prosthetics Department. His honors, awards, and activities in organized Dentistry have been extensive. He is a member of Omicron Kappa Upsilon, as well as the Deans' Odontological Honor Society. In 1982 he was named as the University of Tennessee College of Dentistry's Outstanding Alumnus. In addition to membership in the Memphis, Tennessee, and American Dental Association, Dr. Dick Reynolds is a member of the American Prosthodontics Society, the Federation Dentaire Internationale, and the Pierre Fauchard Academy. He has worked extensively on the Tennessee Board of Dental Examiners from 1973 to the present time, serving as President of the Tennessee Board of Dentistry in 1979. He is also a member of the American Association of Dental Examiners.[13,20]

Dr. Reynolds was elected as President of the Memphis Dental Society in 1967 and the Tennessee Dental Association in 1968. He is a Fellow of the American College of Dentists and has been Secretary-Treasurer of the Tri-State Section from 1959 through the present time. Also, he was a Regent of the American College of Dentists from 1973–1977, Vice President of the American College of Dentists 1979–1980, and President of the American College of Dentists 1981–1982. He was also elected a Fellow of the International College of Dentists in 1982. In 1982, he was appointed to the University of Tennessee Chancellor's Advisory Council and Search Committee for the Dean of the U.T. College of Dentistry. His other services to the University of Tennessee, Memphis include: member of the Advisory Committee in the search for a Dean of the College of Community and Allied Health Professions 1983–1984, commencement speaker for the University of Tennessee Center for the Health Sciences graduation exercise in June of 1983, and member of the Board of Directors of the University of Tennessee Quintard House. His civic duties have also been most commendable. From 1974–1975 he was the President of the Board of the Mid-South Regional Blood Center. In addition to his numerous professional activities, Dr. Dick Reynolds is an accomplished musician, being principal clarinetist for the Memphis Symphony Orchestra from 1935–1978. He was a member of the Board of the Memphis Orchestral Society from 1950–1980. In 1985, he received the most distinguished award given by the Memphis Rotary Club, being named as a Paul Harris Fellow with 23 years of perfect attendance. He is the 1986 President of the Memphis Wine and Food Society, is a member of Confrerie des Chevaliers du Tastevin and Chaine des Rotisseurs, and is a charter member of the newly organized Memphis Medical Historical Society in 1986. [12,20] His eldest son, Richard James Reynolds, III, M.D., is also a graduate of the University of Tennessee, Memphis' medical class of June, 1972. His son-in-law, Charles Richard Patterson, M.D., is a 1975 graduate of the U.T. College of Medicine and presently is Chief-of-Surgery at the Regional Medical Center at Memphis. [20,36]

The University of Tennessee College of Nursing was housed in the buildings of the City of Memphis Hospital until 1952. At that time a remodeled residence was converted into an office and classroom building at 817 Court Street. In 1962 the College was housed in the old Lindsley Hall, located at 879 Madison Avenue, adjacent to the Physicians and Surgeons Building of Baptist Memorial Hospital to the east and the Campbell Clinic to the west. In 1973 the College of Nursing administrative headquarters was moved to the Goodman House, situated at 777 Court Street, where it remains today in 1986. The U.T. College of Nursing has had three faculty members who have served as Chairman of the Accreditation Board of Review of the N.L.N. Council of Baccalaureate and Higher Degree Programs. These faculty members are Dean Ruth Neil Murry, Dr. Norma J. Long, and Dr. Mary Lou Shannon, the current Chairman. Dr. Shirley F. Burd was the first faculty member of the University of Tennessee College of Nursing to be inducted as a Fellow in the American Academy of Nursing in 1976. She also served as the initial Chairman of the Certification Board for the A.N.A. Division of Psychiatric and Mental Health Nursing Practice from 1966 to 1976. The mental retardation content in baccalaureate nursing programs was studied from 1967 to 1971 along with two other nursing schools under a program funded by the Mental Retardation Division, Social Rehabilitation Services of the Department of Health, Education, and Welfare. Two publications, a follow-up study of a day-care center for retarded children, and continuing conferences, workshops, and lectures resulted from this study. In 1975, at the request of the Division of Nursing of the U.S. Public Health Service, the U.T. College of Nursing, along with two other selected nursing schools, undertook the task of determining whether or not selected college graduates could follow an accelerated curriculum and obtain the skills necessary for graduation with a Bachelor of Science in Nursing and for meeting licensing requirements. The success of this program was evident by satisfactory state board grades and nursing practice as graduates. In 1954, the new four-year curriculum program was begun in the U.T. College of Nursing so that the B.S.N. degree could be awarded in Memphis. The M.S.N. degree program was initiated in 1973 and graduates approximately 28-30 candidates annually.[15] Ruth Neil Murry was the first nurse to be appointed to a regional association of colleges and schools. From 1970 to 1974, Dean Murry was a member of the Southern Association of Colleges and Schools and was on the Commission on Colleges and on the Committee on Standards and Reports for Institutions.

J. T. Jabbour, M.D., who was a University of Tennessee College of Medicine graduate in 1951, received prominence nationally in reporting studies that related viral infections (measles and infectious mononucleosis) to the etiology of subacute sclerosing pan encephalitis. He contributed to the classification and pathological description of this disease, and he initiated and maintains a registry, which currently is international in scope. Another member of the U.T. Department of Pediatrics, Professor Ellen S.

"Love cures people— both the ones who give it, and the ones who receive it."

Karl Menninger, M.D.

219

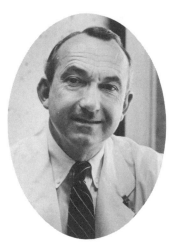

FIGURE 195. *Hershel Patrick Wall, M.D. (1935–)*
Associate Dean for Admissions
U.T. College of Medicine,
1978–present

Kang, M.D., designed an animal model system to study Reye's syndrome which will help to establish the etiology and evaluate treatment of this particular condition. Dr. Ellen Kang has also reported extensive research in regard to the role of lipids in brain growth and differentiation.[6]

The individual, who so well manages one of the most demanding positions on the campus of the University of Tennessee, Memphis, is Hershel Patrick Wall, M.D., the Associate Dean for Admissions for the U.T. College of Medicine (Figure 195). He was appointed Assistant Dean for Admissions for the College in 1974 when it organized a separate Office of Admissions and served in this administrative capacity until January of 1977, when he left the Dean's office, while retaining his Chairmanship of the Committee on Admissions. In 1978 his title was changed to Associate Dean for Admissions. Dr. Pat Wall is a Tennessee product, being born in Murfreesboro, Tennessee on November 10, 1935. He obtained his B.S. degree from Middle Tennessee State University in 1957 and his M.D. degree in 1960 from the University of Tennessee College of Medicine, in Memphis. His rotating internship was taken at the University of Tennessee Memorial Hospital and Research Center in Knoxville; then he completed his residency in Pediatrics through the University of Tennessee, Memphis and the City of Memphis Hospitals, with a two-year interlude from 1963 to 1965 when he served on active duty with the U.S. Army Medical Corps as Chief of Pediatrics for the 60th Station Hospital and Chief of Pediatrics for the 130th General Hospital. He has maintained an active role in the U.S. Army Reserve and is a Colonel and Commanding Officer for the 330th General Hospital Reserve Group located in Tennessee. In addition to his administrative duties within the U.T. College of Medicine, Dr. Wall has served on the medical faculty since 1965 and is a Diplomate of the American Board of Pediatrics. He is the recipient of the following awards: Student American Medical Association Golden Apple Award (1968), William Furgang Memorial Faculty Award (1968), the University of Tennessee Alumni Association "Outstanding Teacher Award" (1974), and the Medical Staff of the City of Memphis Hospital Distinguished Service Award (1977). Dr. Wall is quite concerned with maintaining and building an even stronger rapport with the medical students, the undergraduate pre-professional counselors, and friends and parents of the students. His feelings are best summed up in his own words: "The rapport which we have established and maintain with the students and faculty on undergraduate college campuses relates to the understanding which we have with own own faculty, which is excellent. I think that this is extraordinarily important. We look forward to increasing the caliber and quality of the applicant pool, both majority and minority. This you do in large part by maintaining a high level of communication between this campus and the undergraduate campuses. The Committee on Admissions is the front door to the College of Medicine. The caliber and quality of the students that we attract will have a significant bearing on performance in our educational programs and on the end product of our school, who largely will constitute the physicians of the future for the State of Tennessee."[32]

Alan L. Bisno, M.D., Professor of Medicine and Chief of the Division of Infectious Diseases in the U.T. Department of Medicine, was appointed as the Associate Dean for Academic Affairs on July 1, 1981 in the College of Medicine. A native of Memphis, Dr. Bisno has been on the University of Tennessee, Memphis faculty since 1969. After earning his A.B. degree from Princeton University in 1958 and being elected to Phi Beta Kappa, he obtained his M.D. degree from Washington University in St. Louis in 1962. Working with Dr. Gene Stollerman in the U.T. Department of Medicine as a Fellow in Infectious Diseases, he was a member of the research team that worked to develop a safe, effective vaccine for the streptococcal bacteria which causes rheumatic fever. He was certified as a Diplomate of the American Board of Internal Medicine in 1970 and has lectured and published widely in the area of cardiology and rheumatic fever.[14]

Solomon S. Solomon, M.D. is the Chief of the Endocrinology-Metabolism Section, Medical Service, of the V.A. Hospital in Memphis, Tennessee. He is also a Professor of Medicine for the University of Tennessee College of Medicine and serves as the Associate Dean for Research. He won a four-year scholarship to Harvard College, made the Dean's List for four years, and obtained his B.A. degree from that institution in 1958. At the University of Rochester Medical School in New York, he was a recipient of the prestigious Whipple Scholarship for three years and received his M.D. degree in 1962. Dr. Solomon has been associated with the University of Tennessee College of Medicine since 1969, is a member of the Society of Sigma Xi, served as President of the Tennessee Diabetes Association in 1975, trained eight Fellows in Medicine, and has numerous research publications in the field of endocrinology and metabolism.[14]

Malcolm Alexander Lynch, D.D.S. graduated in the September, 1955 class of the University of Tennessee College of Dentistry. After four years of service in the U.S. Navy Dental Corps, he returned to medical school and obtained his M.D. degree from Washington University in St. Louis in 1963. After a straight internship in Medicine at Grady Hospital in Atlanta, Georgia, he joined the faculty of the University of Pennsylvania School of Dental Medicine in 1964. Dr. Lynch is Professor and Chairman of the Department of Oral Medicine, and he also serves administratively as the Associate Dean for Hospital and Extramural Affairs for the University of Pennsylvania School of Dental Medicine. One of his most significant medical accomplishments was the total revision and editorship of Dr. Lester Burket's famous textbook—*Oral Medicine: Diagnosis and Treatment.* [11,13]

Eugene W. Fowinkle, M.D. was the Tennessee Commissioner of Public Health from 1969 to 1983. He was born in Memphis, graduated from Southwestern College in Memphis, and obtained his M.D. degree from the University of Tennessee College of Medicine in 1958; he also earned a Master of Public Health degree at the University of Michigan School of Public Health. After joining the Memphis-Shelby County Health Department in 1961, he became Director in 1966; in July of 1969 he was appointed as Commissioner of the Tennessee Department of Public Health. Dr.

Fowinkle is certified by the American Board of Preventive Medicine, is a Fellow and member of the Governing Council of the American Public Health Association, and is a Fellow of the American College of Preventive Medicine. Currently, he is a Clinical Professor of Community Medicine at the University of Tennessee College of Medicine in Memphis.[22,36]

John Adrian Shively, M.D. assumed the duties as Professor and Chairman of the Department of Pathology at the University of Tennessee, Memphis in 1971, succeeding Cyrus C. Erickson, M.D., who returned to full-time teaching and research. Dr. Shively is a Diplomate of the American Board of Pathology with subspecialty boards in Clinical Pathology, Anatomic Pathology, Hematology, and Blood Banking. From 1967–1968 he was President of the American Association of Blood Banks and Chairman of that Association's Scientific Advisory Committee. He earned his M.D. degree at Indiana University, where he also received an A.B. degree with highest honors. He is a member of Phi Beta Kappa, Alpha Omega Alpha, American Men of Science, and Sigma Xi. Dr. John Shively served as a member of the Editorial Board for the *American Journal of Clinical Pathology* (1965–1976) and a member of the Editorial Board for *Annals of Clinical Laboratory Science* (1971–1982). He is a Fellow of the American Society of Clinical Pathologists, the American College of Physicians, the American Association of Blood Banks, and the International Academy of Pathology. In July of 1976 he was named by Chancellor Al Farmer to be the U.T. Memphis Vice Chancellor for Academic Affairs. He managed the academic affairs of the University in a smooth, exemplary fashion, well-respected by his professional colleagues. In December of 1982, Dr. Shively retired from the University of Tennessee, Memphis to accept the position of Director for Smith Kline Clinical Laboratories in Tampa, Florida.[25]

John A. Shively, M.D. was succeeded in 1983 as Vice Chancellor for Academic Affairs by Bob A. Freeman, Ph.D., who had been Chairman of the U.T. Department of Microbiology and Immunology since 1972. A native of Texas, Dr. Freeman obtained his B.A., M.A., and Ph.D. degrees from the University of Texas in 1949, 1950, and 1954, respectively. Bob Freeman's professional memberships include: the American Society of Microbiology, the Society of Sigma Xi, the Society for Experimental Biology and Medicine, and the American Association of Dental Schools. In the summer of 1968 he was a Consultant in Immunology for the World Health Organization, assigned to the Cholera Research Centre in Calcutta, India. From 1980–1983 he was a member of the Editorial Board of the *Journal of Dental Education*. Dr. Freeman is the author of numerous scientific articles, but perhaps his greatest medical accomplishment has been the authorship of *Burrows Textbook of Microbiology*, which is considered one of the major textbooks in this discipline.[36]

After earning his B.S. and M.A. degrees in Physiology and Chemistry from Southern Illinois University, Edsel T. Bucovaz obtained his Ph.D. degree in Biochemistry in 1962 from St. Louis University under the direction of Dr. Edward A. Doisy. That same year he accepted a postdoctoral position in the laboratory of Dr. John L. Wood, Chairman of the University of Tennessee Department of Biochemistry. He continued in that position until 1964, at which time he accepted a faculty appointment in the Biochemistry Department. Dr. Ed Bucovaz has led the way in many of his research accomplishments. His laboratory at the University of Tennessee, Memphis was the first to purify the Glutamyl-RNA Synthetase and Cysteinyl-RNA Synthetase. He was a pioneer in the use of Sephadex filtration in the purification of enzymes involved in protein biosynthesis. He was the first investigator to purify the cysteine specific tRNA by a unique procedure, employing an organomercurial polysaccharide column. This procedure was one of the early affinity chromatography columns used in biological research. In collaboration with Dr. John L. Wood, he proposed a pathway for carcinogenesis by polycyclic hydrocarbons. He was also involved in the development of the L/S Assay procedure which is presently used for determining fetal lung maturity. He elucidated the cause for fetal respiratory depression in newborn babies, whenever Demerol was used during delivery. Ed Bucovaz discovered and named the Coenzyme A-Synthesizing Protein Complex (CoA-SPC) of bakers' yeast. He also developed and named the low molecular weight material T-factor, which is responsible for the release of CoA-SPC from its binding site on the membranes of the yeast cell.[14,32]

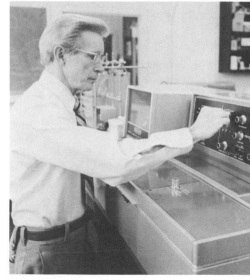

FIGURE 196. *Edsel T. Bucovaz, Ph.D. (1928–) Professor, U.T. Department of Biochemistry, 1975–present*

Dr. Ed Bucovaz discovered a protein which is present in the serum of patients with cancer, which he named B-Protein and developed an assay procedure for the detection of B-Protein. This simple diagnostic blood test is potentially useful for routine screening purposes and has shown an accuracy rate of about 90% in tests on more than 5,000 patients. The cancer test is based on a reaction that occurs between a protein fraction of ordinary bakers' yeast and proteins found in the blood of cancer victims, called the B (or Bucovaz) protein. The University of Tennessee, Memphis has been awarded a patent from the U.S. Office of Patents and Trademarks for this cancer test. Currently, Dr. Ed Bucovaz (Figure 196) is a Professor in the U. T. Department of Biochemistry, was a member of the Editorial Board of *Chemico-Biological Interactions* (1969–1974), a member of the Board of Directors for the Southeastern Cancer Research Association, a member of the American Association for Cancer Research, a member of the American Society of Biological Chemists, a member of the American Chemical Society, and a member of Sigma Xi.[14,32,36]

One of the classic textbooks developed at the University of Tennessee, Memphis has been *Campbell's Operative Orthopaedics*. It was first published in 1939 by Willis C. Campbell, M.D. The Second Edition in 1949 was edited by J. Spencer Speed, M.D. and Hugh Smith, M.D. Dr. Speed had served as President of the American Orthopaedic Association, and Dr. Hugh Smith had served as President of the American Academy of Orthopaedic Surgeons and as President of the American Board of Orthopaedic Surgery. The Third Edition in 1956 was edited by J. Spencer Speed, M.D. and Robert A. Knight, M.D. The Fourth Edition (1963), the Fifth

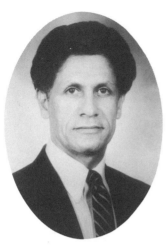

FIGURE 197. *Mustafa K. Dabbous, Ph.D. (1939–) Professor, U.T. Department of Biochemistry, 1977–present, Assistant, Dean for Research U.T. College of Dentistry, 1984–present*

Edition (1971), and the Sixth Edition (1980) were edited by A. Hoyt Crenshaw, M.D. The Sixth Edition was compiled in conjunction with Alan S. Edmundson, M.D., who has made significant surgical contributions in the treatment of scoliosis.[14] Dr. Crenshaw is currently also editing the seventh revision. Many of the University of Tennessee and Campbell's Clinic orthopedic surgeons have contributed chapters to this book which continues to remain the standard reference for orthopedic surgery. It has been translated into many languages, including French, Spanish, Portuguese, and Japanese. One of the chapter contributors, Marcus J. Stewart, M.D., was named as the Outstanding Alumnus by the University of Tennessee College of Medicine in 1976. His daughter, Jeanne Stewart Jemison, M.D., is a 1981 U.T. College of Medicine graduate, who completed her pediatric residency in 1985 and is a staff physician in Ambulatory Care at Le Bonheur Hospital and an Instructor in Pediatrics.[21, 22]

James T. Robertson, M.D. became Professor and Chairman of the University of Tennessee College of Medicine Department of Neurosurgery in 1973 and continues in that position. He is a 1954 graduate of the University of Tennessee, Memphis and obtained his surgical and neurosurgical training at the John Gaston Hospital (1956), the Baptist Memorial Hospital and City of Memphis Hospitals (1956–1959), and the Peter Bent Brigham Hospital in Boston (1959–1960). He served in the Medical Corps of the U.S. Air Force from 1960 through 1964, attaining his certification by the American Board of Neurological Surgery in 1962. Dr. Jim Robertson is a member of the Harvey Cushing Society, a Fellow of the American College of Surgeons, Treasurer (1981) of the American Academy of Neurological Surgery, and President (1977) of the Memphis Neurological Society. He joined the U.T. Department of Neurosurgery in 1964 and became Chairman in 1973. He is a member of Alpha Omega Alpha, was an Associate Examiner of the American Board of Neurological Surgery, was a member of the American Board of Neurological Surgery from 1977 through 1983, has participated in national studies on neurological tumors conducted by the National Cancer Institute, and has published 74 scientific publications.[36]

In June of 1984 Mustafa K. Dabbous, Ph.D. was appointed to the newly created position of Assistant Dean for Research for the U.T. College of Dentistry. He is among the few individuals who hold unique joint appointments in both the University of Tennessee College of Medicine and College of Dentistry, a Professor of Biochemistry since 1977 in the former, and a Professor of Periodontics since 1980 in the latter (Figure 197). This dynamic individual was born January 25, 1939 in Egypt and obtained his B.S. degree in Chemistry from the University of Cairo in 1958. He earned an M.S. in Leather Chemistry in 1962 at the Lowell Technological Institute in Massachusetts and another M.S. degree in Biochemistrty in 1965 at the Massachusetts Institute of Technology in Cambridge, Massachusetts. After obtaining his American citizenship, he followed his M.I.T. professor, the late Dr. Maurice Drake, to the University of Tennessee, Memphis and obtained a Ph.D. degree in Biochemistry in 1967.[5,36]

His dental-related research began in 1967, when he was an Assistant Professor of Biochemistry at the University of Pittsburgh School of Dental Medicine. While there, he investigated the role of components of saliva in calculus formation and periodontal disease. After a year at the University of Pittsburgh, he spent two years as a research Fellow at the National Research Center and Faculty of Medicine for Cairo University in Egypt. Dr. Dabbous returned to the United States to become an Assistant Professor of Biochemistry at the University of Tennessee, Memphis in 1970, and within the short time span of seven years he became a full Professor. Dr. Mustafa Dabbous has an unquenchable appetite and enthusiasm for his research and teaching activities. He is well-respected by both his faculty colleagues and students within the Colleges of Dentistry and Medicine. He has been the recipient of four major N.I.H. grants, both from the National Cancer Institute and the National Institute for Dental Research, and he has published over 85 scientific articles. He holds membership in the following scientific societies: the American Society of Biological Chemists, the American Association for Cancer Research, the International Association for Dental Research, the Southeastern Regional Cancer Association, the Southern Connective Tissue Society, and the Society of Sigma Xi. He is an active participant in the newly created University of Tennessee Comprehensive Cancer Center, organized by Dr. Alvin Mauer. In addition to these responsibilities, Dr. Dabbous also served for two years as the Acting Chairman of the U.T. College of Medicine's Department of Biochemistry. He has been a vigorous participant in the University of Tennessee, Memphis— Tanta University in Egypt P.L. 480 Project. This faculty/student exchange program will be discussed further in Chapter 9. Dr Dabbous serves as the catalyst for the cooperative spirit that has been created within the U.T. College of Dentistry in the area of research as typified by his own words, "Research is what makes any school a leading institution. You cannot disassociate good academics from good research. A classroom teacher must always be a good researcher, a good reader, and a creative person to function well in the classroom. To be a successful academician, you must do research."[5]

Many significant medical contributions have been made by University of Tennessee College of Medicine graduates and departmental faculty within the U.T. Department of Ophthalmology. Dr. David Meyer, who received his M.D. degree from the U.T. College of Medicine in 1962, has become an internationally renowned ophthalmological surgeon, limiting his practice to the retina. Dr. Steven Charles, a Clinical Assistant Professor within the U.T. Department of Ophthalmology, has pioneered a number of operations in vitreal/retinal surgery, including operations for retinal fibroplasia. Dr. Audrey W. Tuberville, who obtained her M.D. degree from the University of Tennessee in 1975 and is an Assistant Professor in the U.T. Department of Ophthalmology, has produced notable research in inflammatory conditions, which are associated with intraocular lens and has received national recognition for her research.[18]

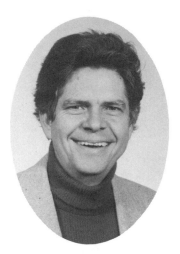

FIGURE 198. *Jerre Minor Freeman, M.D. (1933–) Clinical Associate Professor U.T. Department of Ophthalmology*

Dr. Jerre Freeman, who obtained his M.D. degree from the U.T. College of Medicine in 1963 and serves as a Clinical Associate Professor in the U.T. Department of Ophthalmology, has pioneered phacoemulsification and intraocular lens implantation, extracapsular cataract surgery, and aphacia treatment. Jerre Freeman was born in Memphis, Tennessee on April 7, 1933 and obtained his B.S. degree in Mechanical Engineering from Auburn University in 1955. He served with the U.S. Navy from 1956–1959, qualifying as a Naval aviator. He returned to Memphis to attend the University of Tennessee College of Medicine and graduated in 1963. He was selected for an N.I.H. Fellowship at Harvard Medical School with the Massachusetts Eye and Ear Infirmary, Howe Laboratory, in 1964. Two years were spent in an Ophthalmology residency at the University of Tennessee; then his final year was taken as a Heed Fellow at the Harvard Medical School, Massachusetts Eye and Ear Infirmary in 1968. He was certified by the American Board of Ophthalmology in 1970 and is also a Fellow of the American Academy of Ophthalmology. Dr. Jerre Freeman has been in private practice since 1968, specializing in cataract surgery, microsurgery of the anterior segment of the eye, and intraocular lens implants (Figure 198). From 1968–1973 he was Director of Training for Ophthalmology at the Methodist Hospital, Memphis, Tennessee. His efforts as a medical emissary to underdeveloped nations of the world have been tremendous. He has done outreach medical work at Hospital de La Amistad, a 35-bed hospital located in southwest Mexico; he is the Chairman of a project to secure funds for this hospital under the organization entitled "Ometepec Friends." As an active member of the Memphis Council of International Friendship, he visited the People's Republic of China in 1977 and was the first individual to introduce intraocular lenses and punctum plugs for dry eyes. Again in 1979, he led a group of 47 members of the International Intraocular Implant Congress from five nations to Peking and Shanghai to teach Ophthalmology. He serves as Chairman of the World Lens Project, whose goal is to develop a high-quality lens implant for developing countries at a cost of $10 or less. Dr. Freeman has been involved in fund raising efforts for Good Shepherd Hospital in Kananga, Zaire in Africa and has traveled to Egypt on numerous occasions to demonstrate ophthalmological surgical techniques to the Egyptian medical schools' faculties. For these and other medical missionary efforts, he received the National Medal of Honor for Humanitarian Services from the Daughters of the American Revolution in 1981, being the third Tennessean in the nation ever to receive this award.[14,18,36]

On July 1, 1970 Sam Houston Sanders, M.D. retired from the Chairmanship of the U.T. Department of Otolaryngology and Maxillofacial Surgery; he had headed this Department for 16 years and continues to teach in the Department with the title of Clinical Professor Emeritus. He was succeeded by Charles W. Gross, M.D., who came to the University of Tennessee, Memphis in September of 1968, after teaching assignments at the Harvard Medical School and the University of Cincinnati Medical School. He earned his M.D. degree from the University of Virginia Medical

School in Charlottesville and completed his internship and residency in ENT both at the University of Virginia Hospital and at Massachusetts Eye and Ear Infirmary. Previously, Dr. Gross' appointment at the University of Tennessee involved responsibilities for the residency training program and teaching assignments in the Department of Otolaryngology and Maxillofacial Surgery.[36]

E. Eric Muirhead, M.D. was born September 13, 1916 in Recife, Pernambuco, Brazil where his parents from Texas were medical missionaries. He obtained both his B.A. undergraduate degree and his M.D. degree from Baylor University in 1939. His residency in Pathology was taken at the Baylor University Hospital in Dallas, Texas. During World War II, he served as a Lieutenant (MC) U.S. Naval Reserve, seeing service in Australia, New Guinea, and the Philippines. He returned to Dallas and joined the faculty of the Pathology Department of Southwestern Medical School, becoming Professor and Chairman of the Department from 1950-1956. He was Director of Laboratories and the Blood Bank for the Women's Hospital in Detroit, Michigan from 1959 through 1965. At that time, Dr. Muirhead had become Director of the Department of Pathology and Blood Bank for the Baptist Memorial Hospital in Memphis, Tennessee. Also, he joined the University of Tennessee College of Medicine as a Clinical Professor of Pathology and Medicine.[17,36]

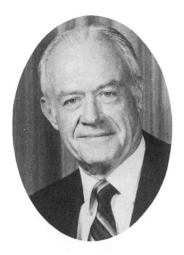

FIGURE 199. E. Eric Muirhead, M.D. (1916–   ) Professor and Chairman, U.T. Department of Pathology, 1980–January 31, 1986

Over his outstanding career, Dr. Eric Muirhead has been prominent nationally in many scientific societies (Figure 199). In addition to the usual medical societies, he has held active membership in the following: the American Physiological Society, the American Association of Pathologists, the Society of Experimental Biology and Medicine, the American Society of Clinical Pathologists (Chairman of the Council on Immunohematology, 1965–1967), the American Society of Nephrology, the Sigma Xi Society, Alpha Omega Alpha, and the International Society of Hypertension. From 1956–1957 he was President of the American Association of Blood Banks. Dr. Muirhead is a Fellow of the College of American Pathologists, the American College of Physicians, and the International Society of Hematology. His research activities have led him to be an active participant in the American Heart Association, especially as a member of its Council for High Blood Pressure Research. In 1982 he was President of the Tennessee Affiliate of the American Heart Association and has served on its Board of Directors since 1968. Earlier in 1978 he was President of the Memphis Chapter of the American Heart Association. Eric Muirhead is a Diplomate of the American Board of Pathology with subspecialties of Anatomic and Clinical Pathology, Blood Banking, and Hematology. He has served as a member of the Editorial Boards for the following three professional journals: *American Journal of Clinical Pathology* (1959–1973), *Transfusion* (1963–1969), and *Hypertension* (1981–present). Dr. Muirhead has also been the recipient of the following prestigious honors and awards: the Emily Cooley Lectureship for the American Association of Blood Banks (1963), the Arthur C. Corcoran Lecture for the Council for High Blood Pressure

Research (1979), the Arthur Grollman Lecture for the University of Texas, Southwestern Medical School, Dallas, Texas (1981), the Distinguished Service Award of the American Association of Blood Banks (1982), and the Merck, Sharpe, and Dohme Award of the International Society of Hypertension (1982).[14,36]

In December of 1985 a University of Tennessee Chair of Excellence in Pathology was established as the E. Eric Muirhead Professorship in Pathology, honoring the distinguished career of Dr. Muirhead, who has served since 1965 as the Director of Baptist Memorial Hospital's Department of Pathology and Blood Bank. He has been a member of the University of Tennessee College of Medicine faculty since 1965 and led the U.T. Department of Pathology as Chairman from 1980 through January 31, 1986. In announcing the Chair of Excellence, Mr. Joseph Powell, President of Baptist Memorial Hospital, stated, "Baptist Memorial Hospital has fulfilled a vital role in the provision of health care in this community, this State, and this region since 1912. While patient care is a primary function of the hospital, in order to excel, we must be involved in other endeavors—especially education and research. Today, the missions of the University of Tennessee, Memphis and Baptist Memorial Hospital are being enhanced by these two entities entering into an agreement for the establishment of the E. Eric Muirhead Professorship in Pathology. This agreement expresses the deep interest of Baptist Memorial Hospital and its Department of Pathology in the future of pathology research at the University of Tennessee, Memphis."[40] This Chair of Excellence was possible because of a $500,000 gift from Baptist Memorial Hosptial and members of its Department of Pathology, which matched $500,000 provided by the State of Tennessee through its Better Schools Program. In receiving this generous gift, James C. Hunt, M.D., Chancellor of U.T. Memphis, said, "Eric Muirhead is a leader of men. He has created one of the outstanding Departments of Pathology in more than 20 years at Baptist Hospital. We are honored and privileged that his colleagues in Pathology and the leadership of Baptist Memorial Hospital have come forth to honor him for his contributions with the establishment of a Chair of Excellence."[40]

With over 250 scientific publications, numerous abstracts, and contributions to book chapters, it is impossible to detail all of the research contributions made by Dr. Eric Muirhead, so only a few of these medical accomplishments will be highlighted. Along with Dr. Kossmann and others at the University of Tennessee, Dr. Muirhead obtained in 1971 the first specialized Center of Research in Hypertension. Many of his early papers in research contributions dealt with peripheral circulatory failure (shock) both in humans and induced experimentally in animals. Dr. Muirhead developed a standarized method for producing an irreversible shock with hemoconcentration in the dog. In 1947, he reported the first case of acute renal failure (due to an incompatible transfusion) treated by peritoneal irrigation successfully, outside of hospital institutions in Boston. His description of the first resin artificial kidney and its application to the dog was published in

1948. Dr. Muirhead's interest in experimental hypertension commenced with his association with Dr. Arthur Grollman, which began with their description of the application of the Kolff artificial kidney to the nephrectomized dog in 1949. Some of their succeeding papers were concerned with vascular disease of renoprival hypertension, which pointed out that the disease of small arteries in arterioles resembles that which is seen in humans having severe or accelerated hypertension. The 1950 JAMA publication by Muirhead, Vanatta, and Grollman first described capillary necrosis of the kidney in an experimental animal (the dog), due to complete urethral obstruction, plus some diuresis, and they described this phenomenon as being due to ischemia of the renal papilla. Receiving more than $1,000,000 in funding from the National Institutes of Health over the last ten years, Dr. Eric Muirhead has conducted and directed research with his professional associates on the cardiovascular system for more than 45 years. This research has resulted in the identification of a unique endocrine system, informally called a "gland of internal secretion" within the kidney. This extensive research has resulted in an "equilibrium" concept of blood pressure control and the elaboration of a naturally-occurring antihypertensive hormone, the antihypertensive neutral renomedullary lipid (AHRL), which is secreted by the renal interstitial cells. The research is best described in Dr. Muirhead's own words, "This system of cells in the innermost portion of the kidney secretes a hormone which modulates major factors elevating blood pressure. Left to themselves, these factors cause hypertension. Blood pressure elevating factors include the effects of salt, certain aspects of the sympathetic nervous system, and the actions of the potent vasoconstrictor agent, angiotensin. This hormone is partly characterized, and its final characterization appears quite promising. The importance of such a molecule results from the fact that it is produced by body cells for the body's own biologic economy. Thus, the body not only uses it for its own purposes, but at the same time, the body has means of controlling it. This combination favors its use over the foreign molecules available with current therapeutic treatments, which often have unwanted side effects."[14,17]

James Edward Hamner, III, D.D.S, Ph.D. (Figure 200) was born July 29, 1932 in Memphis, Tennessee. He was educated at the following institutions: B.S. degree in 1954 from the University of Tennessee, Knoxville; D.D.S. degree in 1955 from the University of Tennessee, Memphis; M.S. Degree in 1964 (in experimental pathology) from the Medical College of Virginia; Ph.D. degree in 1970 (in general pathology) from Georgetown University; M.B.A. in 1981 (in executive health care management) from Loyola College in Baltimore. After four years of service in the U.S. Navy Dental Corps with the 3rd Marine Division in Asia and at the U.S. Naval Air Station, Norfolk, Virginia, he made a direct military transfer to the U.S. Public Health Service and was assigned to the U.S.P.H.S. Hospital in Baltimore, Maryland in Oral Surgery. From 1961–1965 his residency in General Pathology and Oral Pathology was taken at the Medical College of Virginia, the National Institute of Dental Research at N.I.H., and at the Armed

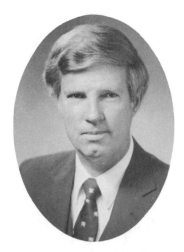

FIGURE 200. *James Edward Hamner, III, D.D.S., Ph.D. (1932–) U.T. College of Dentistry graduate, September, 1955, Associate Director, National Cancer Institute, N.I.H., 1975–1978*

Forces Institute of Pathology in Washington, D.C. In 1973 he left the National Institute of Dental Research to join the National Cancer Institute, also at the National Institutes of Health in Bethesda, Maryland, in a number of leadership positions, culminating in being named Associate Director for the National Cancer Institute in 1975. He served in this capacity until 1979, when he joined the Immediate Office of Secretary Joseph Califano in the Department of Health, Education, and Welfare, as a special consultant from the National Institutes of Health. His last two years at the National Cancer Institute were devoted to duties as Special Assistant to the Director.[36]

From 1969–1972 Dr. Hamner's laboratory at the National Institutes of Health was a Collaborating Center for the World Health Organization's International Reference Center for Oral Precancerous Conditions in Copenhagen, Denmark. He was a member of the Editorial Board of the *Journal of Medical Primatology* from 1972–1977, a member of the National Cancer Institute's Breast Cancer Task Force from 1975–1982, and a member of the American Joint Committee for Cancer Staging and End-Results Reporting from 1975-1982. This latter group was responsible for the consensus publication for all cancer staging in the United States. He is a Diplomate of the American Board of Oral Pathology and a Fellow of the American Academy of Oral Pathology, the American Society of Clinical Pathologists, and the American College of Dentists. He is also a member of the Deans' Society (the University of Tennessee), Omicron Kappa Upsilon Honor Society (the University of Tennessee), and the Society of Sigma Xi. The three most important research projects, in which he has had direct leadership involvement, include the following: (1) P.L. 480 Project between the National Cancer Institute in Bethesda, Maryland and the Tata Institute for Fundamental Research in Bombay, India—the longest continuously supported cancer project (1966–present) by the N.I.H. Fogarty International Center. This project ("Oral Cancer and Precancerous Conditions Among Rural Indian Villagers") has resulted in 41 scientific publications, one book on cancer and tobacco habits in India, and two award-winning scientific films; (2) the joint U.S.A.-U.S.S.R. Oncology Program Agreement between the National Cancer Institute and the Petrov Cancer Institute in Leningrad, Russia ("The Search For Effective Methods of Early Detection of Breast Cancer") from 1976–1978; and (3) the editing of the N.C.I. *Management Guidelines for Head and Neck Cancer* in 1979—this publication was used nationally in medical schools and residency programs in surgery, head and neck surgery, and radiation therapy, and because of its popularity and the number of reprint requests, it was reprinted twice. During the time frame of the late 1960's and early 1970's there were four significant medical research contributions made by Dr. Hamner. The first was the definitive histopathological description and extensive A.F.I.P. study of benign fibro-osseous jaw lesions, which was published in *Cancer* in 1968. Second was the demonstration of perivascular cuffing of collagen by histochemical staining, which is currently used as a definitive marker in the histopathological diagnosis of cherubism (1969). Third was the extensive analysis of the treatment of cherubism, published jointly in 1969 with Alfred S. Ketcham, M.D., who was Chief of Surgery at the National Institutes of Health Clinical Center. Fourth was the demonstration in 1973, after three years of research, that carcinoma could be produced experimentally in the buccal mucosa of subhuman primate (baboons) by the use of betel quid, which contained tobacco. This was an important discovery in the indictment of tobacco as a carcinogen.[36] For these medical contributions, while he was a member of the National Cancer Institute, Dr. Jim Hamner was awarded the Commendation Medal by the U.S. Public Health Service. His son, H. Wentzell Hamner, is completing his freshman year (Class of 1989) at the U.T. College of Medicine.

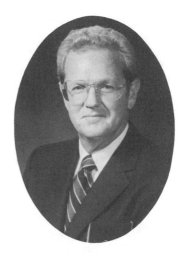

FIGURE 201. *Louis G. Britt, M.D. (1931–   ) Professor, U.T. Department of Surgery, 1973–present, Deputy Chairman, U.T. Department of Surgery, 1974 present*

Louis G. Britt, M.D. was born May 30, 1931 in Akron, Ohio. Early in his life, his family moved to Memphis, Tennessee, and he was reared in this city. His premedical education was obtained at the University of Tennessee, Knoxville, and he received his M.D. degree from the University of Tennessee, Memphis in March of 1955. After a year of rotating internship at the Cook County Hospital in Chicago, Dr. Britt served as a Major in the U.S. Air Force Medical Corps from 1957–1959. He served his residency in General Surgery at the University of Tennessee and City of Memphis Hospitals from July of 1959 through June of 1963 under the tutorship of Dr. Harwell Wilson.[36]

He joined the faculty of the University of Tennessee Department of Surgery in July of 1963 as an Instructor and in one decade moved rapidly to full Professorship in July of 1973. Dr. Louis Britt's sound sense of principle and integrity, his driving leadership, and his commitment to excellence in surgery have made him respected and admired by his patients, U.T. faculty colleagues, and University students (Figure 201). He has been the recipient of numerous honors, including: Alpha Omega Alpha, the Society of Sigma Xi, the Golden Apple Award, the Distinguished Alumni Award of the U.T. College of Medicine, the L.M. Graves Award, and the U.T. Alumni Distinguished Service Professor Award. Dr. Britt is a Fellow of the Southeastern Surgical Congress, the American College of Surgeons, and the American Surgical Association. Among his many other professional affiliations are the Harwell Wilson Surgical Society, the American Society for Transplant Surgeons, the American Association for the Surgery of Trauma, and the International Society of Surgery. He has served on numerous University of Tennessee committees and other faculty assignments, including being Vice President for the U.T. College of Medicine faculty from 1968–1969. He is widely known as an excellent teacher and a stimulating Director of the Surgical Residency Program. Since 1974, Dr. Britt has been the Deputy Chairman of the U.T. Department of Surgery.[14,23]

Beginning with the significant, original medical contributions in kidney research made in 1952 by C. Riley Houck, Ph.D. in the U.T. Department of Physiology, the University of Tennessee steadily developed an excellent Renal Dialysis Program and a superior Nephrology Section in the Depart-

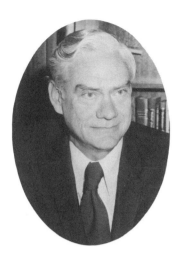

FIGURE 202. *James W. Pate,
M.D. (1928–   ) Professor
and Chairman, U.T.
Department of Surgery,
1974–present*

ment of Medicine, under the direction of Fred E. Hatch, M.D. The development of a full range of diagnostic and therapeutic techniques began around 1960 at the University of Tennessee and expanded to encompass long-term patient care through hemodialysis. With an expanding pool of patients suffering nephrotic failure, the preliminary clinical and basic research work on a complimentary Renal Transplantation Program was commenced by members within the U.T. Department of Surgery. These efforts culminated in the first human kidney transplant at the University of Tennessee, Memphis on April 9, 1970 on a 39 year old male recipient. The second human kidney transplant occurred 12 days later, both operations being performed successfully by Louis G. Britt, M.D. Since this beginning, 499 kidney transplants have been performed at U.T. Memphis with a 95% patient survival rate, which is higher than the national average. His leadership in developing the kidney transplant program and his active involvement as a member of the liver transplant group at the University of Tennessee, Memphis have been two of Dr. Britt's many medical accomplishments and contributions.[23]

On June 1, 1974 a momentous change, which boded a dynamic, positive future for the University of Tennessee Department of Surgery, occurred. Following the unanimous recommendation of a search committee composed of U.T. faculty members, representatives from the practicing medical community, and national leaders in surgery, Dr. T. Albert Farmer, Dean of the U.T. College of Medicine, named James W. Pate, M.D. (Figure 202) to succeed Dr. Harwell Wilson as Chairman of the U.T. Department of Surgery. Dr. Harwell Wilson, who had served as Chairman of the U.T. Department of Surgery since 1948 (a record tenure of 26 years), retired to devote his time to private practice and some teaching within the Department.[28]

James W. Pate, M.D. was born in Wedowee, Alabama on August 28, 1928. He took his premedical education at Emory University in Atlanta, and in 1950 he received his M.D. degree from the Medical College of Georgia. While in medical school he was a member of Alpha Omega Alpha and the Society of Sigma Xi. He entered the U.S. Navy and took his rotating internship at the National Naval Medical Center in Bethesda, Maryland from June 1950 through July 1951, at which time he began a General Surgery residency at the same institution. While serving the first two years of his General Surgery residency, he also headed the Division of Experimental Surgery at the National Naval Medical Center from July 1952 through July 1953. While there, he helped develop the freeze-dried process for preserving arteries to use as grafts and proved the practicality of this process with combat-wounded casualties during the Korean War. He also was a co-discoverer of the bioelectrical causes of blood clots in arteries and veins. He took two additional years of residency in General Surgery from 1953–1955 at the Medical College of Alabama and completed two further years (1955–1957) of residency in Thoracic Surgery at the Veterans Administration Medical Teaching Group in Memphis, Tennessee. Dr. Pate (Figure

202) is a Diplomate of both the American Board of Surgery and the American Board of Thoracic Surgery. He joined the University of Tennessee, Memphis faculty in 1955 as an Assistant Professor of Surgery and rapidly rose to become Professor of Surgery July 1, 1965. Dr. Pate established the open-heart surgery program at the City of Memphis Hospital and the Veterans Administration Hospital, and he was instrumental also in establishing the open-heart surgery program at Baptist Memorial Hospital in Memphis. Jim Pate is a Fellow of the American College of Surgeons, the American College of Chest Physicians, and the American College of Cardiology. He also holds membership in the American Association for Thoracic Surgery, the Society for Vascular Surgery, was a founding member of the Society of Thoracic Surgeons, and has served on the Board of Directors for the Tennessee Heart Association, as well as being President of the Memphis Heart Association, President of the Memphis Thoracic Society, and was the founder and first President of Directors of Training in Thoracic Surgery. In addition to these affiliations, he is a past President of the Southern Thoracic Surgical Association and President of the University of Tennessee College of Medicine faculty (1963–1964).[14,28,36]

Dr. Jim Pate has been a national leader in developing several new techniques for open-heart surgery. He was the first surgeon in this country to replace a heart valve with an artificial valve in pediatric surgery, and also he was the first surgeon to replace a heart valve and implant a pacemaker for emergency surgery, following a gunshot wound of the heart. He has authored over 125 papers for scientific journals, primarily dealing with cardiovascular surgery and the physiology related to surgery and transplantation. His work in cardiac transplantation will be described in Chapter 9. Dr Pate is the co-author of *Science of Surgery*, and he has contributed chapters in several widely-used surgery textbooks.[14]

On November 17, 1982 both Dr. Louis G. Britt and Dr. James W. Pate were honored for outstanding and distinguished public service and received awards from the medical staff at the City of Memphis Hospital. Dr. Britt was honored for his efforts in training general surgery residents, his leadership in emergency surgical services, his development of renal transplantation in the Mid-South, and his work in the field of endocrinological surgery. Dr. Pate was given his award in recognition of his efforts in training general and thoracic surgical residents, his leadership in establishing surgical intensive care for this region, his guidance in establishing the Trauma Center, and his development of cardiovascular surgery and training.[37]

The 1970's decade began on a sad note with the death of Dr. Thomas Palmer Nash, Emeritus Dean of the School of Biological Sciences and Emeritus Professor of Biochemistry, on October 21, 1970 at the age of 80. In collaboration with the late Dr. O. W. Hyman, he played a leading role in the early development of the University of Tennessee, Memphis. The 1970's decade ended on an upswing note, which would witness tremendous leadership changes in a positive direction going into the 1980's.

REFERENCES

1. Bowyer, Frank P. : "Tributes to Two Deans", *J. Tenn. Dent. Assoc.* 61:8-9, 1981.
2. Bruesch, Simon R.: Personal Communication, 1985.
3. *Commercial Appeal*: April 10, 1984 (Dr. Farmer).
4. Crenshaw, Andrew Hoyt: Personal Communication, 1986.
5. *Dental Alumni News*: Fall, 1985 (Dr. Dabbous).
6. Etteldorf, James N: Personal Communication, 1984.
7. Seldon D. Feurt Building—Dedication Program.
8. Greer, Dan B.: Personal Communication, 1985.
9. Hughes, James G.: *Department of Pediatrics—UTCHS: 1910–1985*, 1985.
10. Lollar, Michael: *Commercial Appeal* Mid-South Magazine, May, 1984.
11. Lynch, Malcolm A.: Personal Communication, 1986.
12. McKnight, James P.: Personal Communication, 1985.
13. Medical Accomplishments: U.T. College of Dentistry.
14. Medical Accomplishments: U.T. College of Medicine.
15. Medical Accomplishments: U.T. College of Nursing.
16. Medical Accomplishments: U.T. College of Pharmacy.
17. Muirhead, E. Eric: Personal Communication, 1985.
18. Murrah, William F.: Personal Communication, 1985.
19. Murry, Ruth N.: Personal Communication, 1985.
20. Reynolds, Richard J.: Personal Communication, 1985.
21. Stewart, Marcus J.: Personal Communication, 1985.
22. Stewart, Marcus J. and Black, William T., Jr.: *History of Medicine in Memphis*, (McCowat-Mercer Press, Inc: Jackson, TN.), 1971.
23. *Tennessee Medical Alumnus*: Fall, 1970 (Dr. Britt; Dr. Overman; Dr. Gross; Dr. Nash).
24. *Tennessee Medical Alumnus*: Spring, 1971 (Dr. Johnson).
25. *Tennessee Medical Alumnus*: Fall, 1971 (Dr. Shively).
26. *Tennessee Medical Alumnus*: Spring, 1973 (GEB Building).
27. *Tennessee Medical Alumnus*: Fall, 1973 (Dr. Pellegrino; Dr. Johnson).
28. *Tennessee Medical Alumnus*: Fall, 1974 (Dr. Farmer; Dr. Pellegrino; Dr. Pate).
29. *Tennessee Medical Alumnus*: Spring, 1975 (Dr. McCall; Dr. Rosenberg).
30. *Tennessee Medical Alumnus*: Spring, 1977 (Pediatrics).
31. *Tennessee Medical Alumnus*: Summer, 1978 (Dr. Hunt; Dr. Humphreys—Building).
32. *Tennessee Medical Alumnus*: Fall, 1979 (Dr. Bucovaz; Dr. Wall).
33. Todd, William M.: Personal Communication, 1985.
34. *University of Tennessee College of Medicine Alumni Directory*, 1985.
35. *University of Tennessee Medical Units Newsletter*, February 1, 1970 (Dr. Farmer and Dr. Williams).
36. University of Tennessee, Memphis: Personnel Records.
37. U.T.C.H.S. News Release: November 18, 1982 (Dr. Pate; Dr. Britt).
38. *U.T.C.H.S. Record*: March 16, 1981 (Dr. Martin Hamner).
39. *U.T.C.H.S. Record*: July 18, 1984 (Dr. Meyer; Dr. Sabesin).
40. *U.T.C.H.S. Record*: December 11, 1985 (Muirhead Chair of Excellence).

CHAPTER NINE

1980–1986

A historical perspective of the 1980's decade reveals new leaders for a new era, dynamic stimulating events, and a surge of growth and optimism for the University of Tennessee, Memphis. The first four years witnessed a complete turnover of the Chancellorship and all of the College Deans, and a new covenant developed between the University of Tennessee, Memphis and its statewide affiliates, its fellow schools in Memphis, St. Jude Children's Research Hospital and the other Memphis hospitals, the City of Memphis, and the State of Tennessee. Its motto became—"Our business today is the quality of life tomorrow."

The first and most significant change in leadership, as was mentioned in Chapter Eight, was the appointment of James C. Hunt, M.D., Dean of the U.T. College of Medicine since July of 1978, to the Chancellorship of the University of Tennessee, Memphis. Dr. Jim Hunt, who was approved unanimously by the University of Tennessee Board of Trustees in November of 1980, succeeded T. Albert Farmer, Jr., M.D., who accepted the position as Chancellor of the University of Maryland Medical Units in Baltimore on January 1, 1980.[33]

At the time, Dr. Hunt stated that one of his major areas of concentration in the future would be the development and expansion of manpower and teachers for the University of Tennessee, Memphis, and he emphasized that the University must have accomplished researchers to move ahead in the future. His aim was to increase the number of the teaching faculty who had expertise in research and/or patient care—across the board in Medicine, Dentistry, Nursing, Pharmacy, and all fields that are encompassed in Memphis in the health sciences. The new Chancellor also underlined the need for improvement in the faculty-student ratio, as emphasized by his following remarks: "The teaching load is so great that our scientists and clinicians spend too little time in research and patient care—and either or both are essential for good teachers."[33]

A summation of Dr. Hunt's biography and certain of his medical accomplishments were described in Chapter Eight; however, there are six additional significant contributions which should be mentioned. In 1983, the Mayo Alumni Association established the James C. Hunt Lecture in Nephrology as part of the annual meetings of the Alumni Association. This recognition noted his responsibilities as the organizing Chairman of the Division of Nephrology and the Nephrology Chapter of the Mayo Alumni Association. Dr. Hunt was responsible for the development of the Nephrology Research Training Program and the subspecialty discipline of

> *"My Grace is sufficient for thee; for my strength is made perfect in weakness."*
>
> St. Paul's Second Epistle to the Corinthians 12:9

235

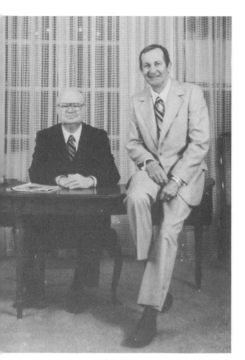

FIGURE 203. *James C. Hunt, M.D. (right) Chancellor, U.T. Memphis, 1981–present; Robert L. Summitt, M.D. (left) Dean, U.T. College of Medicine, 1981–present*

Nephrology at the Mayo Clinic. From 1974 to 1979 he served as a member of the National Heart, Lung, and Blood Advisory Council, on which he chaired the Publications Committee of the Advisory Council for two years and had a major responsibility for research training programs. He helped to establish the Preventive Cardiology Award Program, and S. Edwards Dismuke, M.D., of the University of Tennessee, Memphis was one of the seven original appointees in Preventive Cardiology. Dr. Jim Hunt was President of the National Kidney Foundation from 1973 to 1976, a time when it became a nationwide entity. He was also involved in the leadership role of developing such programs as the National High Blood Pressure Education Program. In this work he collaborated with Dr. Theodore Cooper and Secretary of Health, Education, and Welfare, Caspar Weinberger, the President-Elect of the American Heart Association, and the President-Elect of the American College of Cardiology. When he was Chairman of the Division of Nephrology at the Mayo Clinic, he worked with Dr. George Hollenbeck to establish the Mayo End-Stage Renal Disease Program, which included chronic dialysis and renal transplantation. This program, which was established in 1960, is one of the nationally recognized Organ Transplant Programs in the United States. Both his undergraduate school, Catawba College, and the Bowman Gray School of Medicine of Wake Forest University awarded Dr. Jim Hunt their Distinguished Alumnus Award. In addition, he was elected to Honorary Fellowship in the American College of Clinical Pharmacology.[10,56]

After launching an intensive search for a new Dean of the U.T. College of Medicine, on April 1, 1981 Dr. Hunt appointed Robert L. Summitt, M.D., who had been Associate Dean for Academic Affairs in the U.T. College of Medicine since January of 1979, as the new Dean for the University of Tennessee College of Medicine. Chancellor Hunt and Dean Summitt are depicted in Figure 203.

Robert Layman Summitt, M.D. joined the U.T. College of Medicine faculty in 1964 as an Instructor in Pediatrics and Anatomy; he now is a Professor of both. During his tenure with the University of Tennessee, Memphis, he was Chief of the Genetics Department of the Child Development Center and Chief of the Genetics Section, Department of Pediatrics, U.T. Memphis from July 1, 1964 to March 31, 1981. Also, he was Director of the National Foundation Medical Service Program for Birth Defects within the U.T. Department of Pediatrics from July 1, 1970 to December 31, 1978.[16]

Dr. Bob Summitt was born December 23, 1932 in Knoxville, Tennessee; he was reared in LaFollette in nearby Campbell County, Tennessee. His undergraduate education was taken at Davidson College in North Carolina, and he received his M.D. degree from the University of Tennessee College of Medicine in December of 1955. After a year of rotating internship at the University of Tennessee Memorial Research Center and Hospital in Knoxville, he entered the Medical Corps of the U.S. Navy in January of 1957 and served until June of 1959. During his active duty service, he was designated

Naval Flight Surgeon on September 13, 1957. On December 16, 1985 Dr. Bob Summitt was promoted to Rear Admiral (Medical Corps) U.S. Naval Reserve (Figure 204). Admiral Summitt was instrumental in developing the Naval Medical Reserve's PRIMUS (Physician Reservists In Medical Universities and Schools) Program nationwide. The University of Tennessee PRIMUS Detachment has been the nation's prototype for this program and is, by far, the nation's largest and most active. For his accomplishments in the PRIMUS Program, Admiral Summitt was awarded the Navy Commendation Medal in September of 1985.[24,28]

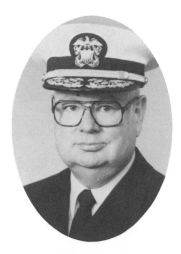

FIGURE 204. *Robert Layman Summitt, M.D. (1932–) Rear Admiral (MC) U.S. Naval Reserve*

Dean Bob Summitt served his residency in Pediatrics at the University of Tennessee College of Medicine and City of Memphis Hospital from 1959 to 1961. He was a U.S. Public Health Service Postdoctoral Trainee in Pediatric Endocrine and Metabolic Diseases at the University of Tennessee College of Medicine from July 1, 1961 to December 16, 1962. At that time, he received an M.S. degree in Pediatrics under the Pediatric Postgraduate Training Program administered by Dr. James N. Etteldorf, as mentioned earlier. During the year of 1963 he worked as a Postdoctoral Fellow in Medical Genetics at the University of Wisconsin, completing his pediatric training. He is Board certified by the American Board of Pediatrics (1962) and the American Board of Medical Genetics (1982). Dr. Summitt was President in 1970 of the Memphis and Mid-South Pediatric Society, and he is a member of the following professional societies: the Southern Society for Pediatric Research, the American Society of Human Genetics (Board of Directors 1980–1982), the American Pediatric Society, the Association of Military Surgeons of the United States, and the Association of American Medical Colleges and its Council of Deans. He was appointed as an official Oral Examiner for the American Board of Pediatrics from 1977 to the present time; he was Chairman of the Written Examination Committee from 1984–1985 and continues to serve on that Committee, and is Co-Chairman of the 1989 Recertification Task Force and has served in that capacity since 1986. Dr. Summitt was elected to a four-year term on the Board of Directors of the American Board of Medical Genetics in October of 1985. His many honors include membership in Alpha Omega Alpha Honor Medical Society, Sigma Xi (President of the University of Tennessee, Memphis Chapter 1973–1974), membership in the Society for Pediatric Research (1970), the University of Tennessee Alumni Public Service Award (1980–1981), the U.T. College of Medicine, Medical Student Executive Council Distinguished Teaching Award (1981–1982, 1982–1983, 1983–1984), and the Outstanding Alumnus Award of the University of Tennessee College of Medicine (1984). His editorial appointments include the following: *Birth Defects Atlas and Compendium; Cancer and Genetics; Syndrome Identification; American Journal of Medical Genetics; Birth Defects Atlas and Compendium, Second Edition; Cell Surface Factors, Immune Deficiencies, and Twin Studies; Recent Advances and New Syndromes; Sex Differentiation and Chromosomal Abnormalities;* and the *Journal of Clinical Dysmorphology.* In addition to these many administrative, teaching, and research accomplishments, Dr. Sum-

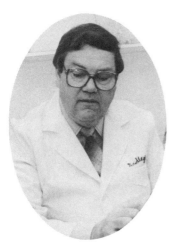

mitt has trained 11 graduate students, postdoctoral trainees, and fellows. He has read 68 papers before professional society meetings, contributed 72 articles in scientific books, has written 66 scientific papers, and has published 15 abstracts.[16,56]

On March 14, 1981 with the sudden death of Dean Jack Wells, the U.T. College of Dentistry was again thrown into a leadership quandary. William F. Slagle, D.D.S. (Figure 205), who was Professor, Executive Associate Dean, and Director of Clinical Programs in the U.T. College of Dentistry since 1979, was named Acting Dean from March, 1981 to March, 1982, when he was selected as permanent Dean. Dr. Slagle had first joined the U.T. College of Dentistry faculty in 1972 as a protege of Dean Wells, who had known him since their days together at the University of Missouri at Kansas City. Bill Slagle was born February 3, 1929 in Alpina, Arkansas. He received his B.S. degree in Chemistry from Central State University in 1950 and taught high school chemistry in Edmond, Oklahoma until he entered the University of Missouri at Kansas City School of Dentistry. He obtained his D.D.S. degree from that institution in 1957, and later while in Memphis as a faculty member at the University of Tennessee, he obtained a Master of Education degree from Memphis State University in 1975.[15,34]

After serving two years as an Instructor in the Department of Operative Dentistry for the University of Missouri at Kansas City, Dr. Slagle entered the full-time private practice of Dentistry from 1959–1972. He joined the University of Tennessee, Memphis faculty as an Assistant Professor and Administrative Assistant to the Dean in 1972. He became an Associate Professor in 1973 and was the Director for the Division of Restorative Dentistry until 1975. Dr. Slagle was the founder and Director of the Temporomandibular Joint Facial Pain-Oral Rehabilitation Clinic at the University of Tennessee, Memphis. He became a Professor and Associate Dean for Clinical Affairs in 1977 and the Executive Associate Dean in 1979 for the U.T. College of Dentistry. In announcing Dr. Slagle as the new Dean, Chancellor James Hunt stated, "The College of Dentistry has a proud tradition. It is first in the nation in terms of its stature in the clinical field. In fact, for many years it was the only dental school in the South. It trained dentists in Texas, Mississippi, Georgia, Alabama, Arkansas, and other states, producing one of the largest dental alumni bodies in the nation. It possesses a stature that all dental colleges have tried to emulate. But, the College of Dentistry, as are all other Colleges on this campus, is funded only for instruction. It has become apparent, especially since the explosion of new knowledge in the 1980's, that instruction cannot be accomplished without excellence in patient care and very active biomedical research by the faculty. Consequently, it is the imperative for the College of Dentistry and the challenge for Dr. Slagle and the Alumni of the College to upgrade this College in the research field."[34]

Among his awards and honors, Dr. Slagle was named as "Man of the Year" in Dentistry for the State of Oklahoma (1968), President of the Board of Governors of Registered Dentists in Oklahoma (1970–1971), Fellow of the American College of Dentists, a member of Omicron Kappa Upsilon, and a member of the Pierre Fauchard Academy. Dr. Slagle has written seven scientific papers and has presented 26 continuing education courses.[56]

With the retirement of Dr. Roland Alden on June 30, 1979, there was a vacancy created in the Deanship of the Graduate School of Medical Sciences. From July 1, 1979 through June 30, 1982, the Graduate School was led under the Acting Dean aegis of Dr. John L. Wood, Dr. John A. Shively, Dr. Robert E. Taylor, and Dr. James Calvin Hunt. After a nationwide search, John Autian, Ph.D., Dean of the U.T. College of Pharmacy and a nationally recognized clinical investigator in industrial poisons and toxicology, was named to be Dean of the U.T. Graduate School of Medical Sciences, effective July 1, 1982 by Chancellor James C. Hunt. As part of a new concept at the University of Tennessee, Memphis of coordinating biomedical research and research training in the Colleges, Dr. Autian was also appointed as Vice Chancellor for Research. In naming this appointment Dr. Hunt stated, "Dr. Autian will be an outstanding leader in these new roles, because of his excellent research credentials and his knowledge of this campus and this University. His excellent relationships with the other Deans and our faculty will provide needed continuity to our programs. Dr. Autian was the unanimous choice of the Advisory Committee."[36]

Dr. Autian was appointed by the Chancellor with four major challenges, each a major component of the new concept of graduate education at U.T. Memphis:

(1) Establishment of a new Division of Biostatistics to help health care professionals with biostatistical support and epidemiology.
(2) Development of a program in Computer Science with the eventual formation of a formal Computer Science Department for the training of students. This program was stressed to have a high priority with our academic community and the production of health science student graduates as computer-competent individuals.
(3) Further development of a Bioengineering Program at U.T. Memphis, an effort which was begun earlier in 1982 when the Rehabilitation Engineering Program received a large gift from the Crippled Children's Hospital Foundation and was moved to the U.T. Child Development Center. This program was one of only 15 in the United States and one of only two, which designs and fabricates special wheelchairs and other devices for handicapped children.
(4) Development of a Program in Comparative Medicine, which would include U.T. Memphis' current Animal Resources Programs and would open pathways of cooperation between the University of Tennessee, Memphis and the U.T. College of Veterinary Medicine in Knoxville and other University of Tennessee institutions.

Dr. Autian's medical achievements have been depicted earlier in Chapter Seven.[18,36,56]

With Dr. John Autian's decision to return to teaching and laboratory

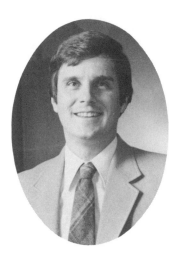

FIGURE 206. *Michael Allen Carter, D.N.Sc. (1947–) Dean, U.T. College of Nursing, 1983–present*

research in 1985, the leadership responsibility for the Graduate School of Medical Sciences was placed under the direction of Bob A. Freeman, Ph.D., Vice Chancellor for Academic Affairs.[56]

After the long, distinguished Deanship of Ruth Neil Murry and her subsequent retirement in 1977, the U.T. College of Nursing witnessed a rapid turnover in its leadership. Norma J. Long, D.N.Sc. was Acting Dean from 1978–1979. Marie C. Josberger, Ed.D. was Dean from 1979–1981. From 1981 through October of 1982 E. Dianne Greenhill, Ed.D. served as Interim Dean, and she did an excellent job of holding the College of Nursing together. Effective November 1, 1982, Michael Allen Carter, D.N.Sc., the former Chairman of the Medical-Surgical Nursing Department at the University of Colorado School of Nursing, was appointed by Chancellor James C. Hunt to be the permanent Dean of the U.T. College of Nursing. Dr. Carter, who holds a master's degree as a Nurse Clinician and a doctorate degree in Nursing Science, became in 1982 the youngest nurse ever to be admitted to Fellowship in the prestigious 130-member American Academy of Nursing. Dr. Carter (Figure 206) received his B.S.N. degree in Nursing from the University of Arkansas College of Nursing in 1969. He received an M.N.Sc. degree in Family Nursing from the same institution in 1973, and in 1979 he completed his D.N.Sc. degree in Nursing Science from the Boston University School of Nursing.[17]

Mike Carter served as a 1st Lieutenant in the U.S. Army Nurse Corps from 1969–1971. He was an Assistant Professor at the Boston University School of Nursing from 1975–1976. He joined the faculty of the University of Colorado School of Nursing in 1976 and remained there until 1982 as Chairman of the Medical-Surgical Nursing Department. He was named as the Volunteer of the Year for the Salvation Army Western U.S. Region in 1978, and in 1985 he was listed as a Distinguished Practitioner by the National Academies of Practice. He has been President of Sigma Theta Tau, the nursing honor society, both at the University of Colorado and the University of Tennessee. He is a charter member of the Society for the Advancement of Nursing, and he is also a member of the American Association for the Advancement of Science and the American Academy of Nursing. He has been the recipient of five research grants. In naming Dr. Carter to the Deanship of the U.T. College of Nursing, Chancellor Hunt stated, "Dr. Carter's experience as a Departmental Chairman will be invaluable to him as a Dean. He has already been deeply involved in nursing and biomedical research as part of a multi-discipline arthritis center, and he has demonstrated his ability to work with people from other departments and colleges in interdisciplinary efforts." With Dr. Michael Carter's arrival at U.T. Memphis, the University gained the added benefit and expertise of a husband-wife team. His wife, Sarah Carter, M.D., served as Assistant Chief of the Ambulatory Care Section of the Veterans Administration Hospital in Denver, and she also joined the University of Tennessee Department of Medicine with an appointment to the staff of the Memphis VA Medical Center.[17,56]

After a distinguished 27-year career in the U.S. Navy and the National Cancer Institute, James E. Hamner, III, D.D.S., Ph.D. (Figure 207) returned to his original Alma Mater, the University of Tennessee, Memphis in December of 1982, being appointed as Executive Assistant to the Chancellor by James C. Hunt, M.D. In addition to these administrative duties, he assumed line responsibilities as the Director of the Norfleet Forum and the University's International Programs, with the retirement of James R. Gay, M.D. in June of 1983. Dr. Jim Hamner also serves as a Trustee for the Health Resources Development Corporation (the federally funded Health Service Agency for Shelby, Tipton, Fayette, and Lauderdale Counties), the Memphis Health Care Coalition, and the Biomedical Research Zone. He is Director of the Special Programs, which are briefly described below.[38]

The Frank M. Norfleet Forum for the Advancement of Health is an annual invitational forum on selected issues or topics related to health care. It was created by the University of Tennessee, Memphis to focus on the improvement of the health status of the community, the state, the nation, and the world, through timely emphasis on effective health policies and organization. This Forum was initiated in 1980 as the result of a continuing generous gift from prominent Memphis businessman, Dunbar Abston, Sr., and it is named in honor of his adopted stepson, Frank M. Norfleet (Figure 208). Current Trustees for the Norfleet Forum are: Bland W. Cannon, M.D., Maurice W. Elliott, Mrs. Harry J. Phillips, John W. Runyan, M.D., and James D. Witherington, Jr.[16]

In September of 1983, the Trustees of the Crippled Children's Hospital Foundation in collaboration with the Chancellor of the University of Tennessee, Memphis, James C. Hunt, M.D., agreed to establish a Forum on Child Health to be supported with revenues from a generous $200,000 gift from the Foundation and administered by a senior administrative officer of the University, appointed by the Chancellor and approved by the Trustees. Figure 209 depicts James C. Hunt, M.D., Chancellor of the University of Tennessee, Memphis, and Mrs. Michael F. Sheahan, President of the Crippled Children's Hospital Foundation, signing the official agreement. The purpose of this Forum is to concentrate on improving health care for children at the national level, through concern for major, pertinent issues and promotion of research findings related to child health. The first Crippled Children's Hospital Foundation Forum on Child Health, "The Biology of Transplantation", was held September 24-25, 1984 in the auditorium of the Le Bonheur Children's Medical Center in Memphis. Its Board of Trustees include as members: Miss Margaret Hyde (Chairman); Mrs. Albert M. Austin, III; John F. Griffith, M.D. (Professor and Chairman, U.T. Department of Pediatrics and Medical Director, Le Bonheur Children's Medical Center); Mrs. G. Blair Macdonald; Joseph V. Simone, M.D. (Director, St. Jude Children's Research Hospital); Robert L. Summitt, M.D. (Professor of Pediatrics and Anatomy, and Dean, U.T. College of Medicine); and Mrs. Russel L. Wiener. Dr. Hamner is ably assisted in the management of these two Forums and the publishing of their *Proceedings* and *Abstracts*, respec-

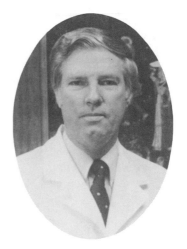

FIGURE 207. *James E. Hamner, III, D.D.S., Ph.D., M.B.A. (1932–) Assistant to the Chancellor, 1982–present; Professor, U.T. Department of Pathology, 1982–present*

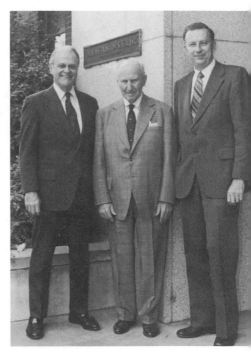

FIGURE 208. *Frank M. Norfleet, Dunbar Abston, Sr., T. Albert Farmer, Jr., M.D., (left to right)*

tively, by Barbara S. Jacobs, J.D., who is the Associate Director of each Forum and also is the University's Affirmative Action Officer and Assistant Vice Chancellor, Academic Affairs. [40,56]

Through the efforts of Chancellor Hunt, an annual Forum on Cancer Research was established in March of 1986 via a significant five-year, $250,000 grant from the Dorothy Snider Foundation. The first Forum on Cancer Research is scheduled to be held April 10, 1987 at the University of Tennessee, Memphis. The Trustees for this Forum are: Costan W. Berard, M.D. (Chairman); Terrance G. Cooper, Ph.D.; Irvin D. Fleming, M.D.; James E. Hamner, III, D.D.S., Ph.D; W. Neely Mallory; Alvin M. Mauer, M.D.; John D. "Jack" Pigott, M.D.; and Michael E. Wilson. [55]

A generous $140,000 gift from the Memphis Cancer Society established the Ralph R. Braund Distinguished Visiting Professorship and the Ralph R. Braund Young Investigator Award to be presented annually to a student or recent postdoctoral graduate for achievements in cancer research. This Visiting Professorship and Award were also funded in March of 1986. Jack Pigott, M.D., a surgical oncologist and Assistant Professor in the U.T. Department of Surgery, stated: "Dr. Braund was the first Medical Director of the first cancer treatment center established in Tennessee in the 1940's as the West Tennessee Cancer Clinic. Dr. Braund brought modern cancer treatment to Memphis. He was immediately comforting to patients and quickly recognized as a remarkable teacher by students, interns, and residents. Thousands of physicians, who have trained in Memphis over the years, are better for his having been here."[21] Funds from this gift will provide travel to a scientific meeting for the Braund Young Investigator.

It would be appropriate at this point to discuss the other four original Distinguished Visiting Professorship Lectures, which were inaugurated in July of 1979 at the University of Tennessee, Memphis with the endowment of the Phineas J. Sparer, M.D. Distinguished Visiting Professorship. The Harwell Wilson, M.D. and the Charles C. and Mary Elizabeth Lovely Verstandig Distinguished Visiting Professorships were endowed in August of 1980 and November of 1981, respectively. In November of 1981, Mrs. Mildred A. Reeves made the initial endowment, which resulted in the first Reeves Distinguished Visiting Professorship in Nutrition, commencing in the Spring of 1984. Chancellor Hunt decided in 1983 that these University of Tennessee, Memphis Distinguished Visiting Professorship Lectures would provide greater benefit for a much larger audience by having them published on an annual basis and distributed nationally to other health science centers and appropriate libraries. Dr. Hamner has edited the 1983, 1984, and 1985 series of these Lectures.[16]

The University of Tennessee, Memphis is involved in five formal International Programs, which are directed through the Chancellor's Office. Three of these programs involve a faculty and/or student exchange with Tanta University in Egypt, Hirosaki University in Japan, and Hadassah University in Israel. The fourth program is a P.L. 480 grant involving epidemiological and cancer control research in oral cancer and oral precancerous condi-

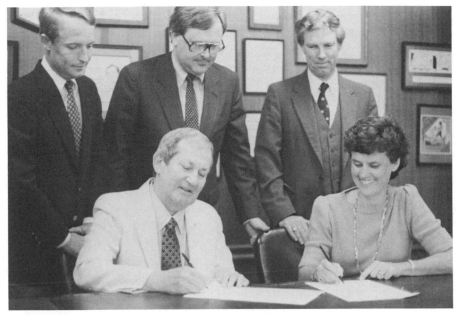

FIGURE 209. *Chancellor James C. Hunt and Mrs. Michael F. Sheahan signing the agreement for the Crippled Children's Hospital Foundation Forum on Child Health, 1983*

tions; this project with the Tata Institute of Fundamental Research in Bombay, India has been funded by the National Cancer Institute since 1966. The fifth program is another scientific collaborative program in neuroscience with the Curie Institute in Paris, France; this program is also funded through Dr. Steve Kitai by N.I.H. grants.[8,37]

With Dr. John Autian's movement in July of 1982 from Dean of the U.T. College of Pharmacy to Dean of the U.T. Graduate School of Medical Sciences, Michael R. Ryan, Ph.D. (Figure 210) was named as the Executive Associate Dean for the U.T. College of Pharmacy. He served in that capacity until March 1, 1983 when Chancellor James C. Hunt appointed him to be the permanent Dean. He first joined the University of Tennessee faculty as an Assistant Professor in the Division of Pharmacy Administration in July of 1972. Prior to that time, Dr. Mike Ryan had served as a hospital pharmacist in the United States Army and had attended graduate school at the University of Mississippi. He obtained his B.S. degree from the St. Louis College of Pharmacy in 1967, his M.S. degree from the Department of Pharmacy Administration, University of Mississippi in 1969, and his Ph.D. degree from the Department of Health Care Administration at the University of Mississippi in 1973.[39]

Dr. Mike Ryan was Associate Director of the American College of Apothecaries (1972–1978), Associate Editor for the *Voice of the Pharmacist* (January–December 1973), Managing Editor for the *Voice of the Pharmacist* (1974–1977), and Editor for the *American College of Apothecaries Newsletter* (1975–1977). He rose to become a Professor in the Department of Phar-

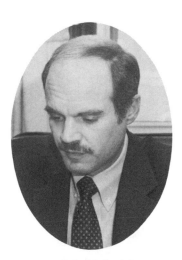

FIGURE 210. *Michael R. Ryan, Ph.D. (1944–   ) Dean, U.T. College of Pharmacy, 1983–present*

243

maceutics in the U.T. College of Pharmacy in 1977; he also was appointed as Assistant Dean in 1977. Administratively, he became Associate Dean for Academic Affairs in 1979, then Executive Associate Dean in 1982, and finally Dean in 1983. Dr. Ryan is a member of the American Association of Colleges of Pharmacy, the American Pharmaceutical Association, Rho Chi Honor Society, and the American Society of Hospital Pharmacists. He has been the recipient of 12 grants, has trained 7 graduate students, has presented 62 continuing education courses, and has authored 44 scientific papers.[18,39]

With the departure of Dean Lee Holder to become Dean of the College of Allied Health for the University of Oklahoma Medical Center in September of 1982, Ralph A. Hyde, Ed.D. became Acting Dean. Dr. Hyde first joined the University of Tennessee, Memphis in October of 1954 as an Administrative Assistant to the Director of the U.T. Extension Center in Memphis. From August 1, 1973 he had been Associate Dean for the U.T. College of Allied Health Sciences. He served commendably as Acting Dean until October 1, 1984 when William G. Hinkle, Ph.D., a speech pathologist and educator, was named by Chancellor James C. Hunt to be the permanent Dean of the University of Tennessee College of Allied Health Sciences. Dr. Hinkle came to the University of Tennessee, Memphis from Indiana University Northwest in Gary, Indiana, where he headed the Division of Allied Health Sciences. His Ph.D. degree is in special education and learning disabilities, and his expertise resides in educating students with hearing and speech disorders. Dr. Hinkle is the author of numerous articles about this subject. In addition to his responsibilities as Dean of the multi-disciplined College of Allied Health Sciences (which has been described earlier), Dr. Hinkle has maintained his professional ties as a speech pathologist with the VA Hospital, Memphis State University, and the University of Tennessee Child Development Center. He also holds a joint appointment in the U.T. Department of Otolaryngology. His major medical accomplishment has been as a recognized authority in voice and language disorders. With the filling of this last Deanship vacancy, the total changeover of the Deans of the five Colleges and the Graduate School of Medical Sciences was completed within three years.[42,56]

Table 14 illustrates the administrative organizational chart for the Chancellor, the Deans of the Colleges, and the Vice Chancellors for the University of Tennessee, Memphis. William R. Rice, J.D. was appointed Executive Vice Chancellor for U.T. Memphis in 1979 and served in that capacity until October of 1983. From November of 1983 to the present he has served as Associate Vice President, Health Affairs of the University of Tennessee based in Knoxville, where he is responsible for the University-wide management of the University's hospitals and related facilities. Robert L. Blackwell was appointed Vice Chancellor, Business and Finance in August of 1981. Bob A. Freeman, Ph.D. was named Vice Chancellor, Academic and Student Affairs in December of 1982 with the retirement of John A. Shively, M.D. Howard S. Carman, who was Director of Facilities Management since

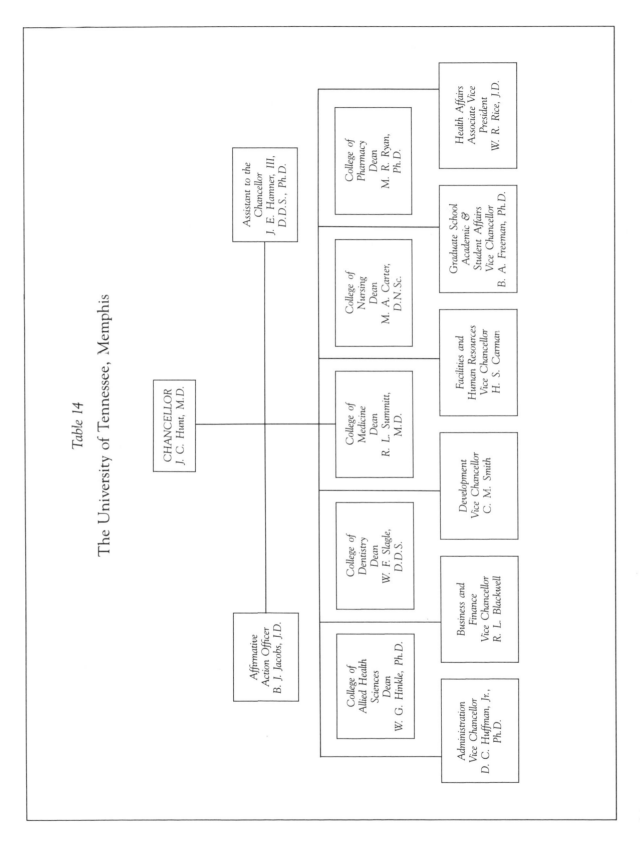

Table 14

The University of Tennessee, Memphis

CHANCELLOR
J. C. Hunt, M.D.

Assistant to the Chancellor
J. E. Hamner, III, D.D.S., Ph.D.

Affirmative Action Officer
B. J. Jacobs, J.D.

College of Allied Health Sciences Dean
W. G. Hinkle, Ph.D.

College of Dentistry Dean
W. F. Slagle, D.D.S.

College of Medicine Dean
R. L. Summitt, M.D.

College of Nursing Dean
M. A. Carter, D.N.Sc.

College of Pharmacy Dean
M. R. Ryan, Ph.D.

Administration Vice Chancellor
D. C. Huffman, Jr., Ph.D.

Business and Finance Vice Chancellor
R. L. Blackwell

Development Vice Chancellor
C. M. Smith

Facilities and Human Resources Vice Chancellor
H. S. Carman

Graduate School Academic & Student Affairs Vice Chancellor
B. A. Freeman, Ph.D.

Health Affairs Associate Vice President
W. R. Rice, J.D.

1981, was promoted to Vice Chancellor, Facilities and Human Resources on July 1, 1984. D.C. Huffman, Jr., Ph.D. was also appointed on July 1, 1984 to the newly created position of Vice Chancellor, Administration. Curtis M. Smith, who had previously worked in the U.T. Memphis Office of Development, was named as Vice Chancellor, Development on November 1, 1984, following the decision by Carley E. "Mickey" Bilbrey, III to accept an executive position in the private business sector in September of 1984.[41,56]

For the 1980's decade, Table 15 exhibits an overall reduction in the number of total students during the time span 1980 to 1985 in the College of Medicine (759 to 703), the College of Dentistry (570 to 366), and the College of Pharmacy (316 to 214). The College of Nursing showed an increase from 215 to 252 total students, and the Graduate School of Medical Sciences remained fairly constant in its total enrollment. The national health manpower statistical situation and the glut of health care providers, predicted by economists for the 1990's, provided the impetus for the decision to reduce overall student enrollment, beginning in the 1980's, in the U.T. Memphis Colleges, as shown in Table 16. The College of Medicine had accepted 204 matriculating students in 1981; this figure was reduced to 180 in 1982, and it was further reduced to 150 in 1986. The U.T. College of Dentistry reduced its entering class size from 128 in 1982 to 90 in

Table 15

The University of Tennessee, Memphis—Enrollment 1980–1985

Fall Term	College of Medicine	College of Dentistry	College of Pharmacy	College of Nursing	Graduate School of Medical Sciences
1980	759	570	316	215	76
1981	769	555	301	188	63
1982	770	492	272	227	59
1983	762	410	264	285	52
1984	742	390	218	273	64
1985	703	366	214	252	70

Table 16

Reduction in Student Enrollment—U.T. Memphis *

College	1982	1983	1984	1985	1986
Medicine	180				150
Dentistry	128	90			
Pharmacy	95	85			65**
Nursing	85				

* = size of each entering annual class in the fall
** = the Pharm.D. degree program began in 1984

246

1983 and has continued at that level. The U.T. College of Pharmacy admitted 95 new students in 1982 and reduced this number to 85 in 1983. In 1984 the U.T. Memphis Executive Council approved the decision to change the College of Pharmacy's B.S. degree program to a Pharm.D. degree program only. Thus, in 1986 the newly enrolling class size was reduced to 65. The U.T. College of Nursing has maintained a consistent entering class size of 85 students since 1982.[15,16,17,18]

The dedication of the E. P. and Kate Coleman College of Medicine Building (Figure 211) on May 1, 1980, marked not only the beginning of a

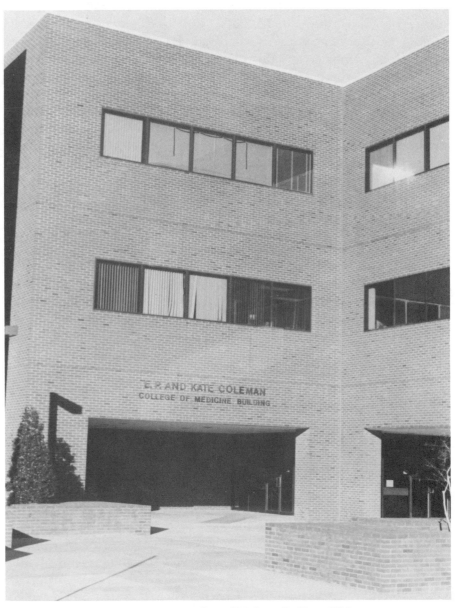

FIGURE 211. *E. P. and Kate Coleman College of Medicine Building, 1980*

new decade for the U.T. College of Medicine, but it also symbolized a new era of excellence in medical education and research. This new building brought together the majority of the College of Medicine's offices and research laboratories in a modern, 158,000 square-foot facility. The $12 million Coleman Building at 956 Court Avenue houses approximately 350 individuals in 110 offices and more than 100 research laboratories. Two auditoriums, several conference rooms, an exhibit area, a dining area, and the Animal Division are located on the first floor. Occupying the second floor are the U.T. Departments of Surgery, Neurology, Neurosurgery, Urology, and Ophthalmology, including both their administrative offices and research laboratories. The third floor contains the administrative unit of the U.T. Department of Medicine and the Divisions of Connective Tissue, Medical Oncology, Hematology, Infectious Diseases, Allergy/Immunology, Dermatology, and Physical Medicine. The research facilities for Obstetrics/Gynecology, Pediatrics, and Orthopedic Surgery are located there, also. Before her death, Mrs. Kate Coleman made one of the largest, single gifts in the history of the University of Tennessee, Memphis in memory of her husband, E. P. Coleman, a prominent Southeast Missouri farmer, landowner, and philanthropist. The building, which was under construction at the time this gift was announced, was named for the Colemans in appreciation of their generosity.[25] The off-campus Animal Care Facility was completed in 1981.

The new University of Tennessee, Memphis Library Building (Figure 212) was completed in 1985 at a cost of $7,264,600. In moving the Library from the old C. P. J. Mooney facilities to its new address at 877 Madison Avenue, it was in a literary sense "coming home". The first Library at the University of Tennessee, Memphis was housed in old Lindsley Hall, which once stood on this same site, facing Madison Avenue. The new Library opened for business on July 15, 1985 under the guidance of Jess A. Martin, Library Director and Professor. It will eventually consume the first five floors of the building, with the sixth floor devoted to the University of Tennessee College of Nursing Administrative Offices; the Division of Biometry will occupy the seventh floor. The first floor houses the acquisition, binding, and serials sections, plus a shipping and receiving area. The second floor contains the current journals and basic reference books and a special Medical History Room, which emphasizes medical history in the Mid-South. This room also features the Wallace Collection (see Appendix J), a collection of books authored by University of Tennessee, Memphis faculty and alumni. The Library staff offices occupy the third floor, which also contains a large conference room and temporary offices for the Division of Biometry. When the Division of Biometry moves to the seventh floor, this space will revert to its original purpose—study areas designed for student groups of four to six students, plus typewriter rooms. The fourth floor houses the new reserved-locked carrels, designed to meet the needs of graduate students working on dissertations and faculty members writing papers or books. The Library is equipped for eight computer terminals and an on-line

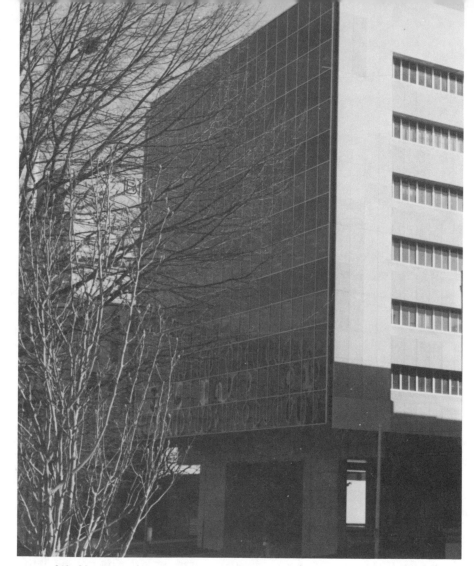

FIGURE 212. *University of Tennessee, Memphis Library, 1985 (courtesy of James E. Hamner, III, D.D.S., Ph.D.)*

catalog data base. Presently, the Library collection is housed in both the old and new facilities with approximately 24,000 books remaining in the old Library, awaiting completion of the fifth floor. Of the 110,000 journal volumes, 66,000 have been moved to the new quarters with the balance scheduled to be transferred with completion of all construction. In 1913 the U.T. Memphis Library was opened with 400 volumes; today, the collection contains 147,000 volumes.[13]

The Elvis Presley Memorial Trauma Center, the only Level I Trauma Center in the Mid-South, is a combination emergency room, operating room, and intensive care unit that treats victims of gunshot wounds, stabs, motor vehicle and industrial accidents, and other victims of severe trauma. It was opened as part of the Regional Medical Center at Memphis (the MED) in November of 1983 (Figure 213). All necessary life-support services are clustered around the patient. The Trauma Center has the capacity to stabilize five shock/trauma victims in the admitting area with a critical care

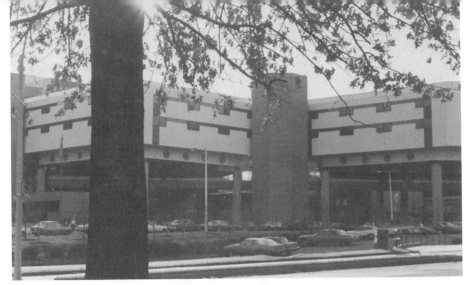

FIGURE 213. *Elvis Presley Memorial Trauma Center, Regional Medical Center, 1983 (courtesy of James E. Hamner, III, D.D.S., Ph.D.)*

assessment area for overflow. It contains four operating rooms, twelve Trauma Intensive Care beds, and a nine-bed recovery room. It is staffed by three trauma teams that work 24-hour shifts. Each team consists of physicians who are specially trained in traumatology, orthopedic surgery, neurosurgery, and anesthesiology, as well as oral surgeons, nurses, technicians, and other necessary skilled personnel.

Pertinent events, which affected and involved the University of Tennessee, Memphis during the first-half decade of the 1980's, moved at such a fast and furious pace that another Domesday Book would be required to chronicle them adequately. Thus, only the salient features will be sketched in this narrative.

In July of 1981 the University of Tennessee, Memphis was awarded a three-year Health Careers Opportunity Program grant, which was administered in a noteworthy fashion by the husband-wife team composed of Robert E. Taylor, Jr., Ph.D. and Billye S. Fogleman, Ph.D. The success of this program, which was directed toward high school and college students, was directly related to the deep personal commitment and dedication of these two Directors to introduce minorities and disadvantaged students to health science careers. Dr. Bob Taylor has been a Professor in the U.T. Department of Physiology and Biophysics since 1973; Dr. Billye Fogleman is an Associate Professor in the U.T. Department of Psychiatry and also is an Assistant Dean for Student Affairs in the University of Tennessee College of Medicine. The federal funding for this program ended in July of 1984. Robert M. Netherland, who formerly was associated with the University of Tennessee College of Engineering in Knoxville, was appointed as Executive Director of the U.T. Memphis Minority Health Careers Program on April 1, 1984. Since 1984, U.T. Memphis has supported, in collaboration with the Coalition of Memphis Colleges and Universities, the Tennessee Minority Health Careers Program, which is a summer academic enrichment program for black high school students. This program receives funding from the City of Memphis, Shelby County, and the University of Tennessee, Memphis.[47]

The first liver transplantation carried out by the University of Tennessee Medical Center was performed in May of 1982 under the direction of James W. Williams, M.D., who headed the University's Liver Transplant Team, prior to his leaving for Rush-St. Luke's-Presbyterian School of Medicine in Chicago in 1985. This program began after extensive preliminary preparations and research before clinical liver transplants were conducted. This preparation, coupled with the immuno-suppressive success of the drug, Cyclosporine, has led to a very successful survival rate. The U.T. Liver Transplant Team, composed of Drs. Louis G. Britt, Thomas G. Peters, Santiago Vera, Steven Van Voorst, James W. Williams, and Mr. Gary Hall (the Coordinator), received the Memphis Rotary Club's Community Service Award as a team effort in their pioneer medical accomplishments in liver transplantation for 1984. In September of 1984 the Inaugural Session of the Crippled Children's Hospital Foundation Forum on Child Health chose the theme, "The Biology of Transplantation", which was attended by over 300 physicians, health professionals, and students. It brought together in Memphis the leading specialists in the field of transplantation for the session held at the Le Bonheur Children's Medical Center, and the keynote address was given by Senator Albert Gore, Jr.[29,30]

On June 12, 1982 Chancellor Hunt informed graduates and faculty at the commencement excercises that the Simon Rulin Bruesch Alumni Professorship in Anatomy was established with gifts totaling more than $1,000,000 from his former students. More than 6,000 graduates of the U.T. College of Medicine passed through the portals of anatomy under the tutelage of Dr. Bruesch during his four decades as a distinguished faculty member of the University. This professorship was not only an honor for Dr. Bruesch, but it was a milestone for University of Tennessee, Memphis, since it was the first endowed Alumni Professorship. It made possible the attraction of a national caliber anatomist to lead the Department, as will be described later under the medical accomplishments of Steve Kitai, Ph.D., who currently holds this chair as Professor and Chairman of the U.T. Department of Anatomy and Neurobiology.[35]

Robert G. Jordan, M.D., who served as Director of the University of Tennessee Child Development Center since 1957, was named as the first Herbert Shainberg Professor in Developmental Pediatrics in October of 1982. This professorship is named for the late Herbert Shainberg, Memphis philanthropist and former President of the company which operated Shainberg's and Kent's stores in the Mid-South area. Gerald S. Golden, M.D., a nationally known pediatrician, succeeded Dr. Jordan on November 1, 1984 as the Director of the U.T. Child Development Center and as the second Shainberg Professor.[9,56]

One of the most dynamic ideas to germinate in the 1980's in Memphis was the concept of a Biomedical Research Zone (BRZ). The father of this concept was Dr. John Autian, who was Vice Chancellor for Research and Dean of the Graduate School of Medical Sciences at the University of

Tennessee, Memphis. The first suggestion that Memphis should consider a high technology center appeared in the December, 1982 issue of the Mid-South Business newspaper under the title, "U.T. Scientist Suggests Memphis as High-Tech Corridor", based on an interview with Dr. Autian. Mr. John Dudas, Executive Director of the Center City Commission, invited Dr. Autian to speak at a meeting of the Commission which took place in January of 1983. Mr. Dudas realized this idea to be an opportunity for the City of Memphis, Memphis State University, the University of Tennessee, Memphis, and the Memphis business community. He suggested that the land area between the Medical Center and the downtown portion of Memphis would be an ideal site for revitalization through the development of a high-tech corridor. His enthusiasm became contagious, and in the summer of 1983 the City Mayor Dick Hackett and County Mayor Bill Morris announced a joint plan to develop a Biomedical Research Zone. It was guided initially under the Jobs Conference Health Committee, headed by County Commissioner Jim Rout, with the supporting Co-Chairman, John Dudas and Dr. John Autian. The City Council and the Board of Commissioners of Shelby County granted seed money ($190,000) to help support the initial funding for activities of the BRZ. June 7, 1985 proved to be a memorable day for the Memphis community and the BRZ, because at a press conference Mayor Hackett, Mayor Morris, and Chancellor Hunt announced that a California firm would build a $65 million, 18-story building, in which the first five floors would become a medical mart, and the remaining floors would be used for offices, research laboratories, and other functions relating to biomedical activities; construction would be initiated in April of 1986. It was proposed to be followed by a 1,500-room hotel to house visitors for the BRZ. A third project would be concerned with the building of a facility to become an incubator for research and developmental activities, related to biomedical research. The Biomedical Research Zone would be planned to become an attractive campus-like business/industrial/academic area, linking the University of Tennessee, Memphis and the Medical Center to the downtown business area. The boundaries of the BRZ have been extended to encompass an area bordered by Third Street, Poplar Avenue, Cleveland Avenue, and Beale Street in a large rectangle, which thus would also include the Baptist Hospital, the VA Hospital, Le Bonheur Hospital, and the Methodist Hospital, as well as the U.T. Bowld Hospital and the MED. The smaller segment of the BRZ would be bordered by Second Street, Auction Avenue, Danny Thomas Boulevard, and Interstate 40; thus, this portion of it would include St. Jude Children's Research Hospital and St. Joseph Hospital.[3,5]

In 1984 the University of Tennessee, Memphis became the first health sciences center in the United States to establish a Department of Education, a development which reflected the University's ultimate commitment to education in the health sciences for professionals, scientists, patients, and the general public. The new Department functions within the U.T. Graduate School of Medical Sciences. The courses offered by the Department are designed to enhance the quality of teaching in all the Colleges and to prepare health care professionals and biomedical scientists to be more effective teachers and communicators. The Department of Education is headed by Raoul A. Arreola, Ph.D., Associate Professor and Chairman. He has initiated research programs in the development of new techniques, procedures, and products designed to give the faculty more effective means of teaching and assessing student learning.[43]

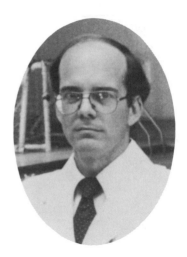

FIGURE 214. *S. Edwards Dismuke, M.D. (1946–   ) Associate Professor, U.T. Department of Medicine and Community Medicine, 1978–present*

Alumni of the U.T. College of Dentistry raised $235,000 for the Weber Orthodontics Research Fellowship in 1983. This Fellowship was established to honor Faustin Neff Weber, D.D.S., former Chairman of the Department of Orthodontics from 1951–1978 (Figure 127). Dr. Weber's medical contributions have already been described in Chapter Six. The Fellowship was formally announced at a dinner at the Memphis Country Club, and in his response remarks Dr. Weber stated, "Establishment of an Orthodontics Research Fellowship would make our dream of an internationally known center for Orthodontics' teaching and research at the University of Tennessee, Memphis more real than chimerical."[15]

The W. K. Kellogg Foundation awarded the University of Tennessee, Memphis a record $1,845,000 grant to begin the first comprehensive program in the nation to teach its students to be health role models and health promoters, as well as traditional health care providers. It marked the first time that a Health Promotion and Disease Prevention Program of such depth and breadth has been developed and undertaken by an American health science university. This program involves collaboration among all of the U.T. Memphis Colleges, and is under the overall direction of S. Edwards Dismuke, M.D., who developed the grant proposal (Figure 214). It is designed to lead the way in promoting wellness as an intrinsic part of curbing health care costs, as described by Dr. Dismuke, who is an Associate Professor of Medicine and Community Medicine in the University of Tennessee College of Medicine. As another important component of the program, U.T. students in Memphis will undergo a complete health appraisal when they enter one of the professional Colleges. At the end of four years, the same students will again be evaluated, health-wise. The results will be compared to the appraisals of students at other health science centers as a means of measuring the effectiveness of the Health Promotion and Disease Prevention Program. The concept of wellness, as well as illness, will be emphasized in the first quarter classes of entering medical students.[31,42]

On September 28–29, 1984, the University of Tennessee College of Dentistry held a two-day seminar for the dental faculty entitled, "Dental Professional Ethics Workshop." This workshop was funded by a special grant from the Tri-State Section of the American College of Dentists to promote ethics within the dental curriculum. Currently, there are two courses within the U.T. College of Dentistry on professional ethics, and a third course will be added for seniors in 1986.[15]

A year-long campaign to make the U.T. College of Dentistry a front-

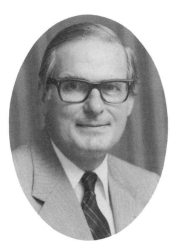

FIGURE 215. *Alvin M.
Mauer, M.D. (1928–   )
Professor, U.T. Department of
Medicine, and Director, U.T.
Comprehensive Cancer
Center, 1984–present*

runner in dental research exceeded its $1,000,000 goal. This announcement was made by Rear Admiral Frank H. Anderson (DC) U.S. Naval Reserve of Johnson City, Tennessee and Dr. Kirby P. Walker, Jr. of Jackson, Mississippi, the two alumni leaders who were national campaign co-chairmen of the Renewal Campaign. This good news was announced on March 1, 1985. Kirby P. Walker, Jr., D.D.S. was named recipient of the U.T. College of Dentistry's Outstanding Alumnus Award for 1985. Principal from the established permanent endowment fund will remain intact, but the annual interest income will be used for alumni clinical research fellowships for exceptional postdoctoral students to pursue teaching or research, alumni clinical research grants to purchase equipment and support dental research, alumni professional development grants to establish special educational opportunities for selected faculty, alumni dental scientist awards, and alumni academic enrichment grants.[14,15]

Alvin M. Mauer, M.D. (Figure 215), former Medical Director of St. Jude Children's Research Hospital, joined the U.T. College of Medicine full-time faculty in January of 1984. Dr. Mauer is an internationally recognized specialist in children's blood dyscrasias and serves as both Professor of Medicine and Chief of the Division of Oncology and Hematology within the U.T. Department of Medicine. The most arduous task commissioned to Dr. Mauer is that of being Chairman of the U.T. Cancer Center Advisory Committee to identify the resources, needs, and planning which will lead to the formation of a Comprehensive Cancer Center, following successful grant application to the National Cancer Institute for a core center grant. Because of the need to coordinate education and research activities, the Comprehensive Cancer Center will essentially be University-based, but it will involve all of the major health provider groups in Memphis. This Center will combine the facets of education, research, patient care, and public education into a comprehensive program of detection, diagnosis, treatment, and prevention of cancer in adults; it will also have a strong component of health professional education, in which all of the U.T. Colleges will be involved. St. Jude Children's Research Hospital has long been a leader in terms of treating and conducting research of cancer in children, and, consequently, Memphis is recognized as a national center for Pediatric Oncology. From 1962–1964 treatment protocols developed at St. Jude's helped increase the survival rate of children with acute lymphocytic leukemia (which is the most common form of childhood cancer) from 4% in 1962 to 17% by 1965. Currently, more than 50% of these patients now have cancer-free remissions for five years or longer. During the 1970's decade a 64% remission rate among patients with neuroblastoma, the most common solid tumor in children, doubled the previously reported positive results. St. Jude has been a pioneer in the field of out-patient cancer treatment and research investigation regarding influenza virus.[12,16,45]

Dr. Al Mauer was born January 10, 1928 in Le Mars, Iowa and received both of his academic degrees from the State University of Iowa: a B.A. in 1950 and an M.D. in 1953. During his educational years, he was a member of Phi Beta Kappa, Alpha Omega Alpha, and Sigma Xi. He is a member of numerous scientific societies and has been President of the American Society of Hematology (1979–1981), Executive Vice President of the International Society for Hematology (1980), and President of the Association of American Cancer Institutes (1981). He has chaired and served as a member of numerous national committees, involving the American Academy of Pediatrics, the United States Department of Agriculture, the United States Department of Health, Education, and Welfare, and the National Institutes of Health. He has published over 160 professional papers in scientific journals and has served as a member of the Editorial Boards for: the *Journal of Blood, Journal of Cancer, Cancer Research, Leukemia Research,* and *Medical and Pediatric Onology.* He is a Diplomate of the American Board of Pediatrics with a subspecialty board certification in Pediatric Hematology-Oncology. His awards include the Distinguished Research Award for Outstanding Medical Research from St. Boniface General Hospital and Research Foundation, and the Award of Excellence from the University of Cincinnati. He was Director of the St. Jude Children's Research Hospital from 1973 to 1983 and was associated with the University of Tennessee, Memphis during that time as a Professor of Pediatrics.[16,45,56]

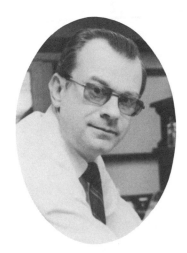

FIGURE 216. *Terrance G. Cooper, Ph.D. (1942–   ) Professor and Chairman, U.T. Department of Microbiology and Immunology, 1985 present; Harriet S. Van Vleet Professor in Microbiology and Immunology, 1985*

In November of 1984, the Van Vleet Foundation of Memphis awarded the University of Tennessee, Memphis a gift of $3,000,000 to support research and education in Pharmacy and in the Biomedical Sciences related to cancer, representing the largest, single outright bequest in the history of the University of Tennessee. These funds became available, pursuant to the wishes in her will, following the death of Mrs. Harriet Smith Van Vleet earlier in 1984. Mrs. Van Vleet was the widow of McKay Van Vleet, who in conjunction with his father—Peter P. Van Vleet—established the major pharmaceutical manufacturing firm known today as McKesson Drug Company. The Van Vleet family had previously been generous donors to the University of Tennessee, Memphis (see Figure 106), especially in the area of cancer research.[44]

The first two Van Vleet Chairs of Excellence were announced on January 7, 1985 by Governor Lamar Alexander and U.T. Memphis Chancellor James C. Hunt. The chairs, one to be endowed in the Department of Microbiology and Immunology and the other endowed in the Department of Pharmacology in the University of Tennessee College of Medicine, would be held by distinguished biomedical scientists, who were primarily involved in cancer-related research. On April 18, 1985, an internationally recognized leader in genetic research related to cancer, Terrance G. Cooper, Ph.D., Professor and Chairman of the U.T. Department of Microbiology and Immunology since January 1, 1985, was formally appointed to the Harriet Van Vleet Chair of Excellence in Microbiology and Immunology (Figure 216). Dr. Cooper's primary focuses will be on biomedical research and education, as they relate to cancer. His widely recognized medical accomplishments have been involved in the structural analysis of genes, especially the genes in yeast. His research group has identified the approximately 12 genes involved with the breakdown and regulation of allantoin, a major nitrogen source for yeast in its natural environment. After determining the primary structure of these genes, they identified what occurs when a gene is "switched on" or expressed. His current work involves understanding what exactly occurs biochemically in the gene's environment to induce how a gene is turned on and off. If the order of the genetic sequences changes by even a single nucleotide, the switch becomes inoperative. It is essential to understand how genes are switched on and off as a critical component to understanding cancer. Dr. Terry Cooper was born August 14, 1942 in Wyandotte, Michigan. He obtained his B.S. degree (1965) and his M.S. degree (1967) from Wayne State University; his Ph.D. degree was earned in 1969 from Purdue University. His postdoctoral fellowship was taken under Professor Boris Magasanik from 1969–1971 at the Massachusetts Institute of Technology's Department of Biology. Dr. Cooper was Professor of Biochemistry and Genetics at the University of Pittsburgh from 1981 until December 1984, when he joined the faculty in January of 1985 at the University of Tennessee, Memphis. Dr. Cooper is a member of numerous scientific societies and has been the recipient of many honors and awards. He has been a member and chairman of several National Institutes of Health Study Sections, chiefly in the areas of biochemistry and physiology. He has also been a very active member of the American Cancer Society. He serves on the Editorial Boards for the *Journal of Bacteriology* and the *Journal of Molecular and Cellular Biology*. His numerous research programs have been funded chiefly by the National Institutes of Health and by Gulf Research and Development Corporation. Dr. Cooper is the author of the widely-used textbook, *The Tools of Biochemistry,* which serves as the primary source of information concerning the use and limitations of most biochemical methodologies. He is the author of over 80 scientific publications, has contributed ten chapters to scientific textbooks, and has written abstracts for 68 presentations given at national scientific meetings. In naming Dr. Cooper as the holder of the Harriet Van Vleet Chair of Excellence in Microbiology and Immunology, Chancellor James C. Hunt stated, "We are proud to name a scientist of such distinction to this important Professorship. His great experience and his national reputation as a teacher and a scientist will enrich the work of this University and provide many benefits for all of us in the future. This is another step by this University to serve the people of Memphis and the entire Mid-South with leaders committed to excellence in teaching and biomedical research."[48,52,56]

The Chairs of Excellence Program requires an endowment of $1,000,000 each; half of this amount is awarded by the State of Tennessee as part of the Better Schools Program, and half of it is funded by the University from private gifts, such as the Van Vleet monies. On September 11, 1985 two additional Chairs of Excellence were announced by Tennessee Governor Lamar Alexander and James C. Hunt, M.D., U.T. Memphis Chancellor. The Van Vleet Foundation provided $1,000,000 for the endowment of the Harriet S. Van Vleet Professorship in Virology and the Harriet S. Van Vleet

Professorship in Biochemistry, bringing the total number of Chairs of Excellence to four at the University of Tennessee, Memphis. On November 8, 1985 John Nicholas Fain, Ph.D. (Figure 217) was named by Chancellor Hunt for the Harriet S. Van Vleet Chair of Excellence in Biochemistry. John Fain joined the University of Tennessee, Memphis faculty in July of 1985 as Professor and Chairman of the U.T. Department of Biochemistry, bringing with him 20 years of experience from Brown University, plus a distinguished reputation as a biomedical scientist. This move was more than a career change, since it also marked the homecoming of a native East Tennessean, who was born August 18, 1934 in Jefferson City, Tennessee. Both his parents and his brother received their undergraduate degrees from the University of Tennessee, Knoxville, and his father obtained his M.D. degree in 1929 from U.T. Memphis. Taking a different course, Dr. Fain received his B.S. degree from Carson-Newman College in Jefferson City in 1956 and was awarded his Ph.D. degree from Emory University in 1960.[54]

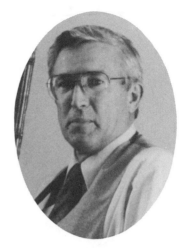

FIGURE 217. *John Nicholas Fain, Ph.D. (1934–   ) Professor and Chairman, U.T. Department of Biochemistry, 1985–present; Harriet S. Van Vleet Professor in Biochemistry, 1985*

Dr. John Fain was awarded a National Science Foundation Fellowship from 1961–1962 at the National Institutes of Health in Bethesda, Maryland. The following year he was also awarded a U.S. Public Health Service postdoctoral fellowship at the N.I.H. Afterwards, he was appointed as a biochemist in the Section on Endocrinology, National Institute of Arthritis and Metabolic Diseases at N.I.H. until June of 1965, when he joined Brown University. He was also a Josiah Macy, Jr. Foundation Faculty Scholar from September of 1977 to August of 1978 at Cambridge University in Great Britain. He was also extremely fortunate to receive a Senior International Fellowship from the Fogarty International Center of the National Institutes of Health, and he spent the year 1984–1985 in the Department of Biochemistry at the University of Nottingham, England. He served as Chairman of the Section on Biochemistry at Brown University in Providence, Rhode Island from 1975–1985. Dr. Fain has authored 178 scientific papers, and his research accomplishments have been in the area of basic hormonal processes, including diabetes mellitus and its hormonal relationships; more recently his research activities have concentrated on regulatory hormones affecting growth and metabolism.[54,56]

The fifth Chair of Excellence was established on November 8, 1985 as the E. Eric Muirhead Professorship in Pathology, honoring the distinguished career of Dr. Eric Muirhead (Figure 199), whose medical accomplishments have already been described in Chapter Eight. A $500,000 gift from the Baptist Memorial Hospital and members of its Pathology Department matched the $500,000 provided by the State of Tennessee through its Better Schools Program.[54]

On July 1, 1985 the Tennessee Higher Education Commission (THEC) approved the State funding for two Centers of Excellence at the University of Tennessee, Memphis. The first Center was the Molecular Resource Center, which is located within the U.T. Department of Microbiology and Immunology. This Center is under the coordination of Terrance G. Cooper, Ph.D., Chairman of that Department. Its main current purposes are to

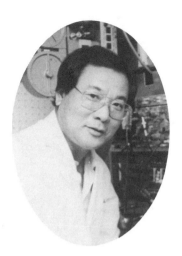

FIGURE 218. *Stephen T. Kitai, Ph.D. (1933–) Professor and Chairman, U.T. Department of Anatomy and Neurobiology, 1983–present; Director, Neuroscience Center of Excellence, 1985*

advance cancer research and to place the most advanced recombinant DNA technologies in the hands of U.T. Memphis scientists.[11]

The second funded Center, the Center of Excellence for Neuroscience, under the leadership of Stephen T. Kitai, Ph.D., Professor and Chairman of the U.T. Department of Anatomy and Neurobiology, will house a prominent and broadly interdisciplinary neuroscience research effort aimed at a better understanding of the structure and function of the nervous system to combat neurological disease and produce better health care. Stephen T. Kitai, Ph.D. (Figure 218) was born on May 14, 1933 in Osaka, Japan. His American education consisted of a B.S. degree (1959) from the University of Michigan, an M.A. degree (1962) from Wayne State University, and a Ph.D. degree (1964) from Wayne State University. After leaving the faculty of Wayne State University in 1967, Dr. Kitai was a Visiting Scientist for the American Medical Association Institute for Biomedical Research in the laboratory of Sir John Eccles in Chicago, Illinois; he was appointed a Visiting Professor in the Department of Physiology of Tokyo University, Japan in 1970. He served as the Director for the Morin Memorial Laboratory for Neurophysiology at Wayne State University from 1971 through 1978. During that time he was also a Visiting Scientist at the Max-Plank-Institut fur Hirnforschung in West Germany from 1973–1974. After serving as Professor in the Department of Anatomy of Wayne State University from 1972–1978, he became Chairman of the Department of Anatomy for Michigan State University in 1978 until he was appointed as Professor and Chairman of the U.T. Department of Anatomy on July 1, 1983. Dr. Kitai is a member of numerous scientific organizations including the American Association of Anatomists, the Sigma Xi Society, the American Physiological Association, the Society for Neuroscience, and the American Association for the Advancement of Science. In his career he has been responsible for many important administrative duties including the following: grant reviewer for the National Science Foundation (1968), field editor for *Experimental Brain Research* (1970), field editor for *Brain Research* (1970), research fellowship review Ad Hoc Committee for the National Institute of Neurological and Communicative Disorders and Stroke (1975), field editor of the *Journal of Neuroscience* (1976), President of the Society for Neuroscience—Michigan Chapter (1977–1979), editor of *Brain Research Bulletin* (1977), member of the N.I.H. Neurology Study Section A (1978), and editor of the *Journal of Comparative Neurology* (1980). His most prestigious award, given in November of 1984, was the Jacob Javits Neuroscience Investigator Award, a seven-year award made in honor of the former Senator from New York. Dr. Kitai received this $1,000,000 award from the National Institute of Neurological and Communicative Disorders and Stroke of the National Institutes of Health. He is an internationally recognized researcher on the basal ganglia, which are structures located in the interior of the brain. His research involves learning more about nerve cells and how they communicate with one another. His medical contributions include the development of a method of marking neurons in such a way that renders them visible under light and electron microscopy. By injecting these cells with certain enzymes, scientific researchers can see the structures of the cell in great detail. Dr. Kitai stated, "Scientists do not understand how neurotransmitters, which are chemicals that allow neurons to communicate, are operating in the basal ganglia. An understanding of how the neurological circuitry works in the basal ganglia might help researchers understand neurological diseases, such as Huntington's chorea and Alzheimer's disease." In commenting on this significant honor received by Dr. Steve Kitai, Chancellor Hunt reiterated, "Dr. Kitai is being recognized as one of the outstanding scientists in this research field. This is the first time we have had one of these truly prestigious awards conferred on one of our faculty. It is a great honor to have an internationally recognized neuroscientist on our faculty."[10,11,56]

The Methodist Hospitals Foundation pledged $1,000,000 to the University of Tennessee, Memphis for the funding of an endowed Professorship in Neuroscience on August 26, 1985. This agreement marked the first time a Memphis health care institution had provided endowed funds for a professorship at U.T. Memphis; with the agreement, Methodist Hospitals Foundation pledged $1,000,000 over the five-year time span of 1985–1990 to establish the Methodist Hospitals Foundation Professorship in Neuroscience. U.T. Memphis will have the responsibility of identifying an appropriate researcher and educator of international reputation to fill this position, which will be structured in the U.T. Department of Anatomy and Neurobiology. At the same ceremony, Methodist Hospitals Foundation announced that it would also establish a Memphis Neurosciences Center at Methodist Central Hospital. "The endowment to the University of Tennessee, Memphis will provide the new Methodist facility with a research arm," said Joseph Miller, M.D., who is Vice Chairman of the U.T. Neurosurgery Department and Director of the Memphis Neurosciences Center. Dr. Steve Kitai, Professor and Chairman of the U.T. Department of Anatomy and Neurobiology, as well as Director of the U.T. Neuroscience Center of Excellence, will lead the search to fill this Professorship.[51]

Chancellor James C. Hunt announced on August 8, 1985 that the University of Tennessee, Memphis had awarded a $1,670,000 contract to Digital Equipment Corporation, which marked the University's initial step in its commitment to become a national leader in information transfer and understanding. Dr. Hunt stated, "It is our intention to become the nation's model information-intensive health science university. We are trying to jump a generation—not to follow, but to lead."[50] Dr. Frank Clark, Chairman of the newly established U.T. Department of Computer Sciences, informed the audience that the new system's capabilities included support for biomedical researchers, health science educators, administrators, and hospital and patient health care providers. Installation of the system began in September of 1985 and is scheduled for completion after two years. The equipment includes VAX 8600 mainframes with some 250 work stations to be distributed throughout the campus. Interactive video display terminals and software for educational, research, patient care, and administrative needs are also included. The VAX 8600 will provide 32 megabytes of memory that can be accessed at the rate of 4.5 million instructions per second. The system will be complemented by a Local Area Network, which will link the University of Tennessee, Memphis campus with scientists across the United States. This system will form important links between huge data base computers throughout the United States, including the National Library of Medicine in Bethesda, Maryland.[50]

February 10, 1986 proved to be an important day in the history of the University of Tennessee. The U.T. Memphis Department of Obstetrics/Gynecology and the Crippled Children's Hospital Foundation both announced $500,000 challenge gifts, which, when they are matched in the future by the State of Tennessee, will create endowed professorships (Chairs of Excellence). In her comments on behalf of the Crippled Children's Hospital Foundation, Mrs. Sarah Humphreys, CCHF president, stated, "It gives me great pleasure to announce this pledge of $500,000 as a challenge gift intended to assist U.T. Memphis and Memphis State University in the development of biomedical engineering programs."[55] Dr. Hunt stressed the importance and essentiality of biomedical engineering expansion to U.T. Memphis, Memphis State University, and the Memphis Medical Center. In his response, Thomas Carpenter, Ph.D., President of Memphis State University, expressed his appreciation as follows, "The potential of our two institutions working together is absolutely unlimited. At Memphis State, we want to cast our lot with our sister institution and express our great pleasure for the arrangements now in process."[55] The $500,000 challenge gift from the U.T. Department of Obstetrics/Gynecology was announced by George M. Ryan, Jr., M.D., Acting Chairman for that Department which exhibited dynamic evidence of the strong belief by the donors in the future of the University, the College of Medicine, and their Department. In recognizing this generous gift, Chancellor Hunt said, "To the best of my knowledge this is the first time that in any University a single Department's faculty have taken their own money and come forth with the commitment to help get that one special person who will lead them into the future, recognizing that distinguished professors occupying Chairs of Excellence will move us in that direction."[55] At the same ceremony Robert L. Summitt, M.D., Dean of the U.T. College of Medicine, also announced the appointment of Joe Leigh Simpson, M.D. to the Chairmanship of the U.T. Memphis Department of OB-GYN. Once it is established by matching funds, Dr. Simpson will occupy the endowed Chair of Excellence. Dr. Simpson is a nationally recognized gynecologist who previously was Professor of OB-GYN and Head of the Section on Human Genetics at the Northwestern University Medical School in Chicago.[16,55]

After years of preliminary preparation, the first heart transplant in Memphis was performed at the Baptist Memorial Hospital by James W. Pate, M.D., Professor and Chairman of the U.T. Department of Surgery and Director of the Heart Transplant Team (Figure 219). The surgery began at approximately 10:30 p.m., but unfortunately a hyper-acute rejection of the donor organ occurred, and the first heart transplant patient died at 4:45 a.m. the following day. This hyper-acute rejection is an uncommon phenomenon, occurs very rapidly, and is caused by antibodies that are already circulating in the bloodstream at the time of the transplant operation. Cyclosporine, which is used routinely to suppress immuno-rejection of the donor organ, has little effect on these circulating antibodies. The chance of hyper-acute rejection occurs probably in 2% of all heart transplants. Dr. Pate's many medical achievements have been previously listed in Chapter Eight; however, those accomplishments relating to heart transplantation will be mentioned at this time. He played an active role in early research efforts to develop an artificial heart and prototypes for modern space suits. He helped to establish the world's first tissue bank, an endeavor which brought him into direct contact with some of the most innovative surgeons of this era. Dr. Pate was among the first surgeons to replace defective heart valves in children, and he was the first surgeon to implant a pacemaker during emergency surgery on a gun-shot victim. He established the open-heart surgery programs at the Regional Medical Center at Memphis and at the Veterans Administration Medical Center, as well as playing a pivotal role in establishing a similar program at the Baptist Memorial Hospital.[30,53] An estimated 20,000 individuals could benefit from either kidney, liver, or heart transplants annually, yet organs become available from only 2,500 donors in a typical year. Within the United States, there were 160 heart transplants performed in 1983, 130 liver transplants, and 5,400 kidney transplants, according to the American Council on Transplantation. Through April of 1986, the University of Tennessee, Memphis performed four heart transplants, three of which were successful. The U.T. Heart Transplant Team is headed by Dr. James Pate; other members of the team include: F. Hammond Cole, Jr., M.D.; V. Glenn Crosby, M.D.; Tommy Fudge, M.D.; Alim Khandekar, M.D.; and Donald C. Watson, M.D. Dr. Lewis G. Britt and Dr. Thomas Peters are involved with the procurement and retrieval of donor organs, assisted by Mr. Gary Hall, the transplant coordinator. The University's transplant program has been aided by 14 Memphis-based firms whose company jets provide free air transportation to facilitate organ retrieval. In 1984 this cooperation with private industry was expanded by an agreement with a consortium of petroleum-industry corporations that are based in Houston. This group agreed to provide air transportation on an emergency basis for surgeons, transplant patients, and other activities related to the organ transplantation program.[6,20,53]

April 25, 1986 marked the beginning of a new era for the treatment of kidney stones, with the opening of the Memphis Center for Stone Disease. This Center, which is located in the U.T. Medical Center's William F. Bowld Hospital, is a collaborative medical service of Baptist Memorial Hospital, Le Bonhur Children's Medical Center, Methodist Hospitals of Memphis, St. Francis Hospital, St. Joseph Hospital, the University of

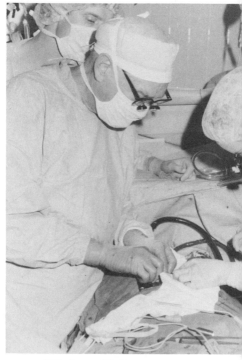

FIGURE 219. *James W. Pate, M.D. (1928–   ) Professor and Chairman, U.T. Department of Surgery, 1974–present; Director, U.T. Heart Transplant Team, 1985*

Tennessee Medical Center, and the Lithotripter Physicians' Association. This joint venture between private practicing urologists, the major hospitals of Memphis, and the University of Tennessee, Memphis represents the most comprehensive cooperative effort in Mid-South medical history.

Extracorporeal shock wave lithotripsy (ESWL) is a new technology, developed in 1980 by Dornier Systems, a West German aerospace company. Lithotripsy is derived from the Greek words which mean "stone crusher", and it is the only non-invasive procedure for the removal of kidney stones. With an estimated 5,000,000 Americans suffering from the pain and discomfort of kidney stones (in the Mid-South Region, the incidence of stone disease is twice the national average), it was indeed fortunate that this procedure was approved by the United States Food and Drug Administration in December of 1984. In this simple and virtually painless procedure, the patient is given spinal anesthesia before being partially emerged in a specially constructed tank of warm water. The high energy, short duration shock waves, which are generated by a large spark plug, travel through the water that has the same density as body tissue and harmlessly penetrate the body. However, when the shock waves hit a solid kidney stone with its higher density, the waves scatter and pulvarize the stone into sand-like particles, which are afterwards passed by the patient through normal elimination.[19]

A computerized x-ray system pinpoints the kidney stone, utilizing two fluoroscopic tubes which cross the patient's flanks. An electrocardiogram synchronizes the firing sequence to avoid any interference with the heart's conduction system. The entire procedure usually takes approximately one hour. Its many advantages include: the pain of surgery is avoided, the risk of complication and infection are drastically reduced, there is a shorter recovery time (patients are usually discharged in two or three days), and the cost reduction is evidenced both in comparison with the cost of surgery and the cost of surgery hospitalization by approximately 30%.[19]

The U.T. Department of Otolaryngology has had a stimulating history. The original Chairman, Richmond McKinney, M.D., was an outstanding surgeon who oversaw the dramatic growth of the Department until his retirement in 1938. He was followed by W. Likely Simpson, M.D. who had trained under Drs. Politzer and Hajek in Vienna; he brought to the Department a classic approach to teaching and patient management. Two of the other outstanding past chairmen include Sam H. Sanders, M.D. and Charles W. Gross, M.D. Dr. Sanders, who currently is Professor Emeritus (see Figure 69), has been a national leader in the management of diseases of the upper respiratory tract and nasal and sinus surgery. He is a founding member of the American College of Allergy and was a past President of the American Academy of Otolaryngolic Allergy. He maintained close ties to collegiate football, being an All-American halfback at Texas A & M as a student, and later served as an official for the Southern Conference and at the Rose, Orange, and Cotton Bowls. In 1985, he was inducted into the Tennessee Sports' Hall of Fame in recognition of his outstanding achievements in sports and his distinguished professional career as a physician. Dr. Charles Gross has a national reputation in general, pediatric otolaryngology, as well as facial, plastic, and reconstructive surgery. He is the immediate past President of the American Academy of Otolaryngology-Head and Neck Surgery.[2,56]

In the summer of 1983, Richard W. Babin, M.D. assumed the Chairmanship of the Department. He came to U.T. Memphis from the University of Iowa where he gained a national reputation in vestibular physiology and temporal bone histopathology. The faculty for this Department includes many notable individuals, such as John Shea, M.D. (see Figure 129), whose medical accomplishments have been previously described in Chapter Six, and John McIver Hodges, M.D. (a 1963 graduate of the U.T. College of Medicine), whose expertise in rhinoplasty is recognized nationally.[2,16]

In 1985 Henrietta S. Bada, M.D. (Figure 220) was the recipient of a $1.2 million grant to investigate why high-risk newborn infants share an often fatal event which is more commonly associated with elderly patients and other adults—stroke or brain hemorrhage. Such hemorrhage occurs unaccountably in 40% to 90% of all premature infants. Dr. Bada is the principal investigator on the multi-departmental U.T. Memphis research team to conduct this investigation, funded by the National Institutes of Health. Co-principal investigator for this prestigious grant is Sheldon B. Korones, M.D., Professor of Pediatrics and Obstetrics and Director of the U.T. Newborn Center. Figure 221 shows Governor Lamar Alexander and Dr. Korones touring the facilities of the Newborn Center in Memphis.[16] Dr. Henrietta Bada was born in 1945 in the Philippines and received both her

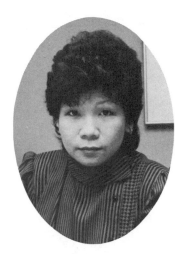

FIGURE 220. *Henrietta S. Bada, M.D. (1945–   ) Professor, U.T. Department of Pediatrics and OB-GYN, 1984–present*

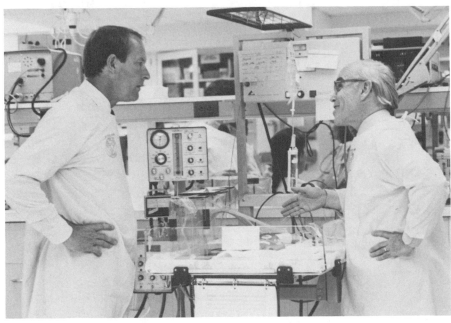

FIGURE 221. *Governor Lamar Alexander (left) Sheldon B. Korones, M.D. (right)*

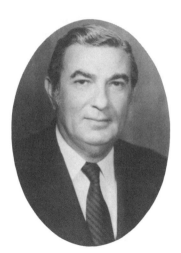

B.S. degree and M.D. degree in 1969 from the University of Santo Tomas in Manila. Her residency in Pediatrics was taken at the University of Louisville, Kentucky Hospitals, and she was certified by the American Board of Pediatrics in 1976 with a subspecialty of Neonatal-Perinatal Medicine in 1979. Dr. Bada joined the U.T. Department of Pediatrics in 1980 and currently is a Professor of Pediatrics and OB-GYN. Her research accomplishments have been in the field of postnatal brain injury.[16,56]

In addition to Drs. Willis Campbell, Harold Boyd, and Hugh Smith, Rocco A. Calandruccio, M.D. also served as President of the American Academy of Orthopaedic Surgeons (1977–1978). Dr. Calandruccio was born on February 27, 1923 in White Plains, New York. He entered Union College in Schenectady, New York in 1941 and obtained his M.D. degree from the Yale University Medical School in 1947. After a year of surgery residency at the Imogene Bassett Hospital in Cooperstown, New York (1948–1949), he entered the orthopedic residency program at the Campbell Clinic in Memphis July of 1949. He completed this program and received his M.S. in Orthopedic Surgery in 1954, after an interruption of military service in the U.S. Air Force Medical Corps from 1951–1953.[56]

Dr. Calandruccio was certified by the American Board of Orthopaedic Surgery in 1957, and he is a member of numerous professional societies, including: the American Academy of Orthopaedic Surgeons, the Orthopaedic Research Society, the American Orthopaedic Association, and the International Society of Orthopaedic Surgeons. In addition, he is a Fellow of the American College of Surgeons. He has been on the University of Tennessee, Memphis faculty since beginning as a Clinical Assistant in 1956. He was Clinical Professor and Acting Chairman of the U.T. Department of Orthopedics from April of 1979 until January of 1981, at which time he became Professor and Chairman of the Department. From 1976 until 1983, Dr. Calandruccio was the Chief-of-Staff of the Campbell Clinic (Figure 222). He has served both as Secretary-Treasurer (1964–1967) and President (1967) for the Orthopaedic Research Society. Dr. Calandruccio is the author of numerous scientific publications, and he has presented the findings of his clinical research in many professional meetings. These research accomplishments include expertise in total hip replacement, the invention of the Calandruccio nail, and the design for a patented metallic hip joint, in conjunction with the Dow Corning-Wright Company. He has been an extremely popular Visiting Professor at six American medical schools and has been the invited speaker for over 30 American and international lectures.[16,56] The current Chief-of-Staff for the Campbell Clinic is Lee Milford, M.D., an expert in hand surgery.[56]

Robert L. Summitt, M.D., Dean of the U.T. College of Medicine and a 1955 graduate, received the 1984 Outstanding Alumnus Award from the U.T. College of Medicine Alumni Association. In the awards ceremony, he was joined by Charles C. Verstandig, M.D. (Class of 1939) and John K. Duckworth, M.D. (Class of 1956), who received Distinguished Alumni Awards.[31]

Robert E. Tooms, M.D. (U.T. Medical Class of 1956) was also honored by the Variety Club for his work with handicapped children. Dr. Tooms, an orthopedic surgeon, is the national President of Children's Prosthetics and Orthotics Clinics; he has been heavily involved in research with the Spinal Cord Injury Center, the Child Amputee Clinic, and the Variety Club's electrolimb bank. Also, he is the Medical Director for the Rehabilitation Engineering Program and Professor of Orthopedics at the U.T. College of Medicine.[31]

John M. Faust, D.D.S., a 1944 graduate of the U.T. College of Dentistry and a 1951 graduate (M.S.) of the U.T. postgraduate Orthodontics Program, served as President of the American Association of Orthodontists from 1980–1981.[14]

Heber Simmons, Jr., D.D.S. is a 1957 graduate of the U.T. College of Dentistry and a 1962 graduate of the U.T. postgraduate Pedodontics Program (M.S.). Dr. Simmons is in the private practice of Pediatric Dentistry in Jackson, Mississippi and has been a guest clinician at numerous dental society meetings around the United States. In March of 1986 he became President of the American Academy of Dental Practice Administration; in May of 1986 he became President of the American Academy of Pediatric Dentistry; and in February of 1987 he will become President of the Pierre Fauchard Academy.[23]

The first pediatric hemodialysis unit in the Mid-South region was opened at Le Bonheur Children's Hospital in 1973 under the co-direction of Billy S. Arant, Jr., M.D. and Shane Roy, III, M.D. Dr. Shane Roy, III, a 1959 graduate of the U.T. College of Medicine and currently Professor, U.T. Department of Pediatrics, was selected for the 21st Annual Headliners Award by the Memphis Gridiron Show in 1980. Dr. Roy was honored for his actions in linking the chloride deficient formula, Neomullsoy, to the cause of metallic alkalosis and poor weight gain in infants. This discovery led to a nationwide recall of over $11,000,000 worth of this infant formula from retail outlets throughout the United States. This finding placed Dr. Roy, the University of Tennessee, Memphis, and Le Bonheur Children's Medical Center in the national spotlight, including personal appearances on ABC's documentary program, "20/20," and other national newscasts.[9]

During U.T. Employee Recognition Day ceremonies in December of 1985, Chancellor Hunt presented Mr. O. D. Larry with a special plaque, commemorating his 45 years of service to the University. He serves as Manager of Operations for the Student Alumni Center. Also during 1985, Greater Memphis State, Inc., a community-wide academic support organization of Memphis State University, honored James C. Hunt, M.D., Chancellor of U.T. Memphis, at its annual dinner on February 6, 1985 as the recipient of its Educator of the Year Award. Dr. Hunt's many medical contributions have been outlined in Chapters Eight and Nine.[16]

In March of 1953, W. Eugene Mayberry, M.D.—a native of Cookeville, Tennessee—graduated from the University of Tennessee College of Medicine. Two years later, he joined the faculty at the Mayo Clinic in Rochester,

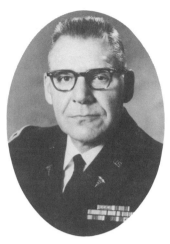

FIGURE 223. *Major General Colin F. Vorder Bruegge (MC) U.S. Army; Commanding General, Walter Reed Army Medical Center, 1970 (U.T. medical graduate, 1939)*

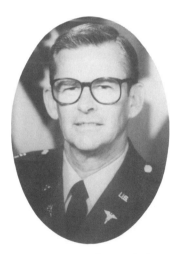

FIGURE 224. *Robert Malcolm Overbey, D.D.S. (1930–) Brigadier General (DC) U.S. Army Reserve; 1984 Trustee, American Dental Association, 1982–1988*

Minnesota and has been affiliated with that institution ever since. In 1980 Dr. Mayberry was Chairman of the Board of Governors of the Mayo Clinic, Vice Chairman of the Board of Trustees of the Mayo Foundation, and Professor of Laboratory Medicine at the Mayo Medical School.[26]

The University of Tennessee, Memphis alumni or faculty who have reached flag rank in the U.S. Armed Forces are listed in Appendix H. A sampling of that group will be mentioned at this point. Marinus Flux, M.D., U.T. medical graduate Class of 1960 and Brigadier General (MC) U.S. Air Force, retired in 1984. At the present time, Dr. Flux is Professor of Clinical Pediatrics and Director of the Cystic Fibrosis Center at the Oklahoma Children's Memorial Hospital in Oklahoma City.[16] Murphy A. Chesney, M.D., a 1950 graduate of the U.T. College of Medicine, was appointed in 1986 by President Ronald Reagan as the U.S. Air Force Surgeon General. Dr. Chesney was promoted to Lieutenant General effective August of 1985, and he is rated as a Chief Flight Surgeon.[16]

Major General Colin F. Vorder Bruegge (MC) U.S. Army is a native Memphian and a graduate in the U.T. medical class of 1939; his career in military medicine spanned more than 30 years. Following service in World War II, in 1946 he became staff pathologist and curator of the Army Medical Museum of the Armed Forces Institute of Pathology in Washington, D.C. In 1955, he received the Certificate of Achievement for service in planning the architecturally innovative construction for the Armed Forces Institute of Pathology building, which is located on the Walter Reed Army Medical Center campus in Washington. As Commanding General of the U.S. Army Medical Research and Development Command, he directed and coordinated studies in Army Medical Research Laboratories and collaborating University Medical Centers nationwide. After commanding the 9th Hospital Center comprised of 11 hospitals and supporting clinics in West Germany for three years, he returned in 1970 as Commanding General of the Walter Reed Medical Center (Figure 223). Dr. Vorder Bruegge is an outstanding pathologist, now retired from the U.S. Army. His early pathology training was taken with Dr. Lemuel Diggs and Dr. Israel Michelson at the University of Tennessee, Memphis, as well as with Dr. George Whipple (a Nobel Prize Laureate in 1934) at Rochester, New York.[27]

Robert Malcolm "Mike" Overbey, D.D.S. was selected for flag rank as a Brigadier General in the U.S. Army Reserve Dental Corps on February 29, 1984 (Figure 224). Dr. Overbey is a native Memphian, took his undergraduate education at the University of Tennessee, Knoxville, and obtained his D.D.S. degree from the U.T. College of Dentistry in Memphis in 1955. In addition to his 29 years of active duty and reserve duty in the U.S. Army, Dr. Mike Overbey has maintained a private dental practice. Also, he is on the part-time faculty of the U.T. College of Dentistry as an Associate Professor in the Department of General Dentistry. He was a member of the Deans' Odontological Honorary Dental Society and Omicron Kappa Upsilon while in dental school; he is a member of numerous professional organizations and is a Fellow of the American College of Dentists. Dr. Overbey has served as President of the Memphis Dental Society, President of the Tennessee Dental Association, and President of the Tennessee Academy of General Dentistry. He and Dr. E. Jeff Justis, Sr. are the two University of Tennessee, Memphis graduates who have served as Trustees of the American Dental Association. From 1982–1988 Dr. Overbey is the Trustee for the Sixth District which represents Tennessee, Missouri, Kentucky, and West Virginia.[1,15,22]

Murray Heimberg, Ph.D., M.D. (Figure 225) has made extensive contributions to the medical literature regarding lipid research, especially hepatic lipid transport and the area of triglyceride synthesis and its effect on atherosclerosis and hypertension. He received his B.S. degree (1948) and his M.S. degree (1949) from Cornell University in New York, then obtained a Ph.D. degree (1952) in Biochemistry from Duke University, and his M.D. degree (1959) from Vanderbilt University. From 1952–1954 he served as a postdoctoral fellow of the National Institutes of Health in the Department of Biological Chemistry at Washington University in St. Louis. From 1967–1974 he was a Professor of Pharmacology at the Vanderbilt University School of Medicine, then became Professor and Chairman of Pharmacology in 1974 at the University of Missouri School of Medicine. Dr. Heimberg joined the University of Tennessee, Memphis faculty as Professor and Chairman of Pharmacology in 1981; he is also a Professor of Medicine. He is a member of Sigma Xi, the American Society for Pharmacology and Experimental Therapeutics, the American Society of Biological Chemists, a Fellow on the Council for Arteriosclerosis of the American Heart Association, and the American Society for Study of Liver Diseases. He received the Established Investigator Award from the American Heart Association for 1962–1967. Earlier, he had been the recipient of the Lederle Medical Faculty Award (1959–1962). He has been a member of the Editorial Board for the *Journal of Lipid Research* since 1977. Dr. Heimberg is the author of over 100 scientific publications and has been an invited speaker for over 50 lectures.[16,56]

One of the most dedicated educators and productive researchers at the U.T. College of Dentistry is James E. Turner, D.D.S. Dr. Jim Turner was born in Memphis, Tennessee, on July 23, 1934, obtained his B.A. degree from Southwestern at Memphis in 1956, and earned his D.D.S. degree from the University of Tennessee, Memphis in 1960. He completed a Rotating Internship in the U.S. Air Force from 1960–1961, then served on active duty through 1963. From October of 1963 through December of 1966, he was a U.S. Public Health Service Fellow in Pathology at the U.T. Institute of Pathology in Memphis. He joined the U.T. College of Dentistry faculty in January of 1967, becoming Chairman of the Department of Oral Pathology in July of 1969. He was a member of the Deans' Odontological Honorary Society and Omicron Kappa Upsilon at the University of Tennessee, Memphis. He is a Fellow of the American Academy of Oral Pathology, a member of the American Association for Dental Research, and

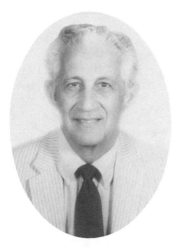

FIGURE 225. *Murray Heimberg, Ph.D., M.D. (1925–) Professor and Chairman, U.T. Department of Pharmacology, 1981–present*

267

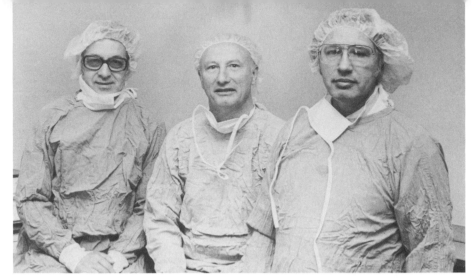

FIGURE 226. *Loys J. Nunez, Ph.D., Charles J. Shannon, D.D.S., James E. Turner, D.D.S., (left to right)*

a Diplomate of the American Board of Oral Pathology. He has been the recipient of many awards for his teaching activities, both from the University of Tennessee student body and the Memphis and Tennessee Dental Societies. His research activities have centered in the fields of: toxicity evaluation for biomaterials, carcinogenesis, epidemiology of dental caries, and oral microbiology. He has been joined in many of these teaching and research activities by Harry H. Mincer, D.D.S., Ph.D., who is also a Professor in the U.T. Department of Oral Pathology and the Chief Consultant in Forensic Odontology to the State Medical Examiner. Dr. Turner has authored over 40 scientific publications and has made 17 presentations before professional meetings. His most recent investigative work has been in the area of high intensity surgical lamps and their effect on wound healing and surgeons and dentists. He has been assisted in this project by Loys J. Nunez, Ph.D. (Professor, Biomaterials) and Charles J. Shannon, D.D.S. (Associate Professor, Oral Surgery)—(Figure 226). Their work on light and its effects was funded by a surgical lamp company which was interested in having its newest product tested for possible undesirable side effects. The results demonstrated that this surgical lamp was a proper one with a minimal amount of harmful rays. It was also noted that the warmth of light apparently had some beneficial effect on wound healing, while a wound exposed to no light at all exhibited detrimental effects. These studies were carried out in controlled conditions designed to mimic an actual surgical setting. [7,14,15]

The first nurse-sponsored ambulatory elderly clinic was developed in September of 1980 by the U.T. College of Nursing. It was co-sponsored by the U.T. Department of Community Medicine and is conducted throughout the year for 262 residents of Camilla Towers in Memphis. [17]

Patrick Tso, Ph.D. was born January 4, 1950 in the British Crown Colony of Hong Kong. His undergraduate education was taken at the University of Western Australia where he received his B.S. degree with First Class Honors in Physiology (1974); his Ph.D. degree was also obtained from the

University of Western Australia in 1978 with honors. During his time in Australia he was granted a University Research Studentship from 1975–1977. Also, he was awarded the Mary Hodgkin's Prize in 1977 and was a Raine Medical Foundation Research Fellow in 1978. After completing the year of 1978 as a Research Fellow in Physiology at the University of Western Australia, he moved to the United States and joined the faculty at the Albany Medical College in New York in 1979, serving as a research Assistant Professor until 1980. At that time, this highly sought-after young scientist joined the University of Tennessee, Memphis faculty as an Assistant Professor in the Department of Physiology and Biophysics; in 1986 he was promoted to Associate Professor within the same Department (Figure 227). He holds membership in the Australian Biochemical Society, the Australian Society for Medical Research, and the American Gastroenterology Association. Dr. Tso has been the recipient of three highly competitive National Institutes of Health grants, and his medical research accomplishments have been chiefly in the field of lipoproteins. Dr. Pat Tso has contributed chapters to four scientific books, has authored over 30 publications in professional journals, and is a member of the Editorial Board of the *American Journal of Physiology* (1985). In addition to his teaching and research duties at the University of Tennessee, Memphis, he has served as a member of an N.I.H. Site Visit Team on three occasions. He has been a special invited lecturer at seven American universities. The most recent accomplishment of Dr. Tso was being named recipient of a Visiting Scientist Fellowship from the Swedish Medical Research Council to work with Professor Bengt Borgstrom, Chairman of the Department of Physiological Chemistry at the University of Lund in Sweden from November 30, 1985 to March 29, 1986.[16,56]

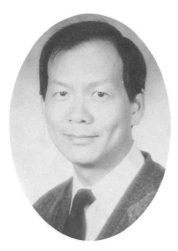

FIGURE 227. *Patrick Tso, Ph.D. (1950–   ) Associate Professor , U.T. Department of Physiology and Biophysics, 1986–present*

Preston H. Dorsett, Ph.D. devised and patented a successful, very widely-used commercial diagnostic test for rubella in 1983. His major research accomplishments have been in the area of rubella virus: host cell interactions, persistent rubella virus infections, and detection of anti-rubella virus globulins (Figure 228). He has published widely in the scientific literature in this field, in addition to his teaching responsibilities at U.T. Memphis. Dr. Preston Dorsett received his B.S. degree from Wake Forest College in 1964, then his M.S. degree in 1967 and his Ph.D. degree in 1970, both from the Bowman Gray School of Medicine of Wake Forest University. His postdoctoral fellowship was taken with Dr. Hal S. Ginsberg at the University of Pennsylvania's Department of Microbiology. He joined the University of Tennessee Department of Microbiology as an Assistant Professor in 1972 and became a tenured Associate Professor in 1976. During the year 1977, he was on special leave with the Infectious Diseases Branch of the National Institute of Neurological and Communicative Disorders and Stroke at the National Institutes of Health in Bethesda, Maryland. In his quiet, competent manner, he led the U.T. Department of Microbiology and Immunology as Acting Chairman from January of 1984 through January of 1985, in preparation for the arrival of Dr. Terrance Cooper.[16,56]

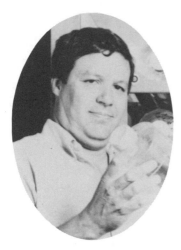

FIGURE 228. *Preston Hackney Dorsett, Ph.D. (1942–   ) Associate Professor, U.T. Department of Microbiology and Immunology, 1975–present*

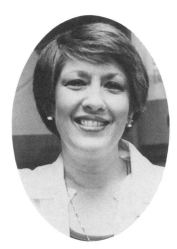

FIGURE 229. *Linda Williford Pifer, Ph.D. (1942–) Assistant Professor, U.T. Department of Pediatrics, 1978–present*

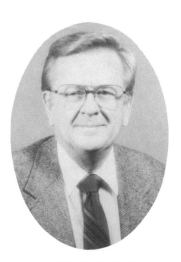

FIGURE 230. *Joe Hall Morris, D.D.S. (1922–) Professor and Chairman, U.T. Department of Oral Surgery, 1968–present*

After extensive preliminary research, Dr. Linda Pifer developed a test for the antigen of *Pneumocystis carnii* in clinical subjects and tests for the antibody. Because of their important commercial potential, her discoveries were patented and have been a major contribution to clinical laboratory medicine. Linda Williford Pifer, Ph.D. (Figure 229) was born January 1, 1942 in Greenwood, Mississippi. Both her B.A. degree (1963) and her Ph.D. degree (1972) were obtained from the University of Mississippi with a major in Microbiology. She first joined the University of Tennessee, Memphis in 1965–1966 as a Research Assistant in the Department of Medicinal Chemistry. After receiving her doctoral degree, she joined the St. Jude Children's Research Hospital in Memphis as a Research Assistant in the Infectious Disease Service. After conducting research at St. Jude from 1973–1978, Dr. Linda Pifer accepted the position as Assistant Professor of Pediatrics at the University of Tennessee, Memphis in November of 1978. She was the recipient of the McClesky Award from the American Society for Microbiology (for original research); she has been a very active member of the Society of Sigma Xi and was President of the University of Tennessee, Memphis Chapter in 1985. She is also a member of the American Society for Microbiology and the National Foundation for Infectious Diseases. Dr. Pifer has received extensive grant support from the American Cancer Society and private foundations/companies for her research activities. Her major contributions have been in the area of basic microbiology research: infections in the immunosuppressed host, new techniques in cell culture, virology, and rapid immunodiagnosis of pediatric infectious diseases.[16,56]

Following in the steeped tradition of such distinguished Chairmen of the U.T. Department of Oral Surgery as Drs. John J. Ogden, J. Roy Bourgoyne, and Lloyd C. Templeton, Joe Hall Morris, D.D.S. (Figure 230) has continued their standards of excellence in teaching and clinical practice since his appointment as Chairman in 1968. Dr. Morris was born June 23, 1922 in Cincinnati, Ohio, took his predental education at Vanderbilt University, and graduated from the University of Tennessee College of Dentistry in 1945. He was a member of the Deans' Odontological Honorary Society, Omicron Kappa Upsilon, and is a Diplomate of the American Board of Oral Surgery. He was elected a Fellow of the American College of Dentists in 1956, received the Tennessee State Dental Association Fellowship Award in 1963, and was given the Memphis Dental Society's Humanitarian Award in 1974. His internship and residency in Oral Surgery were taken at the University of Tennessee, Memphis and the City of Memphis Hospital. He joined the University staff in 1952 as an Assistant Professor in the Department of Anatomy. He was in the private practice of Oral Surgery for ten years, then rejoined the U.T. College of Dentistry faculty, becoming Professor and Chairman of the U.T. Department of Oral Surgery in 1968. His major clinical research interests have been oral surgery, radiology, and maxillofacial trauma. His greatest clinical research accomplishments have been the design of the U.T. head frame and the bi-phase external skeletal splint for mandibular fractures (see Figure 124). Dr. Joe Hall Morris has also been an inspirational teacher and an excellent Director of the Graduate Oral Surgery Program in the U.T. College of Dentistry.[14,15]

Another outstanding teacher in the specialty of Pedodontics at the University of Tennessee College of Dentistry is James P. McKnight, D.D.S. He was born September 19, 1921 in Arlington, Tennessee, obtained his B.S. degree from Memphis State University in 1948, his D.D.S. degree from the University of Tennessee, Memphis in 1951, a Certificate in Pedodontics from U.T. Memphis in 1952, and his M.S.D. degree in Pedodontics from Indiana University in 1964. Except for five years of private practice and graduate training at Indiana University, Dr. McKnight has been affiliated with the U.T. College of Dentistry. He rose through the academic ranks to become Professor and Chairman of the U.T. Department of Pedodontics in 1969, and he also serves as Director of the Graduate Program in Pedodontics. This latter Program recently moved in 1986 from the Dunn Dental Building to Le Bonheur Children's Medical Center. He has held hospital staff appointments at the John Gaston Hospital (now the MED), St. Joseph Hospital, Le Bonheur Children's Hospital, and Memphis Crippled Children's Hospital. Dr. Jim McKnight also is a consultant for the U.T. Child Development Center and a member of the Medical Advisory Board for the United Cerebral Palsy Association of Memphis and Shelby County. In addition to the usual professional organizations, he is a member of the American Society of Dentistry for Children and the Tennessee Society of Dentistry for Children, as well as the Deans' Honorary Odontological Honorary Society and Omicron Kappa Upsilon. He was certified by the American Board of Pedodontics in 1964. His main dental professional accomplishments have been in the area of formulation of an outstanding program in Graduate Pedodontics and teaching of the courses in children's dentistry. In addition to these medical accomplishments, Dr. Jim McKnight has served his community well in the unique position of another vocation. He was ordained to the Diaconate on December 18, 1974, then was ordained to the Episcopal Priesthood on December 19, 1976 (Figure 231).[14,15]

Barry E. Gerald received his M.D. degree from the University of Mississippi School of Medicine in 1958. His rotating internship and residency in Radiology were taken at the Hermann Hospital in Houston, Texas from 1958–1962. For two additional years he was a Fellow in Pediatric Radiology at the Children's Hospital in Cincinnati and was certified a Diplomate of the American Board of Radiology in July of 1963. He also spent one year at the Tufts-New England Medical Center in Boston as a Fellow in Neuroradiology from July 1971 to June 1972. He served on the faculty of medical schools in Arkansas and California prior to joining the faculty of the U.T. College of Medicine on January 1, 1969 as an Associate Professor of Radiology. He became a full Professor six months later and headed the Diagnostic Radiation Section from 1969–1972; he also served as Acting Chairman of the U.T. Department of Radiology from 1970 to 1971. In November of 1979 he was appointed as Professor and Chairman of the U.T.

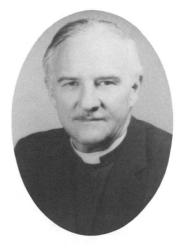

FIGURE 231. *James Pope McKnight, D.D.S. (1921–   ) Professor and Chairman, U.T. Department of Pedodontics, 1969–present*

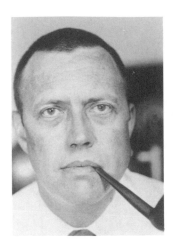

FIGURE 232. *Robert A. Crocker, M.D. (1926–1984) Associate Professor, U.T. Department of Pathology, 1966–1984*

Department of Radiology by Dr. James C. Hunt, Dean of the U.T. College of Medicine. At that time he was commissioned to develop a program in Radiation Oncology and Nuclear Medicine, which he accomplished in fine fashion.[16]

In 1985 Dominic M. Desiderio, Ph.D., Professor of Neurology and Director of the Charles B. Stout Neuroscience Mass Spectrometry Laboratory, was appointed a member of the Metallobiochemistry Study Section, Division of Research Grants of the National Institutes of Health. This honor was well deserved, since Dr. Desiderio is a recognized figure, both nationally and internationally, in the field of mass spectrometry. He has also done extensive research work in chemistry and lipid research and was co-investigator with L. Cass Terry, M.D. in the U.T. Department of Neurology in an N.I.H.-supported research project to accurately measure quantities of endorphin-like peptides in the growth-inhibiting somatostatin. He came to the University of Tennessee, Memphis in 1978 as a Professor of Neurology and Director of the above-mentioned mass spectrometry laboratory, which was founded at U.T. Memphis in 1971 through private endowment. He also holds a joint appointment as Professor in the U.T. Department of Biochemistry, since 1985. He served as President of the Memphis Neuroscience Society (1984–1985), a member of the Advisory Board for the Rockefeller University Extended Range Mass Spectrometric Research Resource in New York, a member of 11 N.I.H. Site Visit Teams, and has trained 17 postdoctoral fellows.[16, 56]

Another distinguished alumnus of the U.T. College of Dentistry Graduate Program in Pedodontics is Vincent N. Liberto, D.D.S. He took both his college and dental educational training at Loyola University of New Orleans, receiving his D.D.S. degree in 1957. He completed the M.S. Program in Pedodontics at the University of Tennessee, Memphis in 1960. Except for two years of military service (1957–1959) in the U.S. Navy Dental Corps, Dr. Liberto has been in private practice in New Orleans. He is a member of numerous professional organizations and served as President of the New Orleans Dental Association (1976), President of the Southwestern Society of Pedodontics (1973–1974), President of the Louisiana Society of Dentistry for Children (1967–1968), and President of the American Academy of Pediatric Dentistry (1981–1982).[14]

With the retirement of June Montgomery in 1969, William C. Robinson, who had been his assistant, became the Director of Student Affairs for U.T. Memphis. Mr. Montgomery remained Director of Alumni Affairs until his retirement in 1973. In the new administrative reorganization during the 1980's, Mr. Bill Robinson was named Assistant Vice Chancellor, Student Affairs under the Vice Chancellor for Academic and Student Affairs (see Table 14).

Two unexpected, sudden and tragic deaths struck U.T. Memphis in the mid-1980's. Robert A. Crocker, M.D. (Figure 232), who was an Associate Professor in the U.T. Department of Pathology and a faculty member for more than 30 years, died from an acute coronary occlusion on December

25, 1984 at the age of 58. Dr. Crocker obtained his B.S. degree in Chemistry-Biology from Austin Peay State College in Clarksville, Tennessee in 1948. In March of 1953, he received his M.D. degree from the U.T. College of Medicine. His postgraduate training in Pathology was taken at the University of Tennessee Institute of Pathology and the City of Memphis Hospital from 1953–1955; he also served as an Instructor in Pathology, commencing in 1955. In 1966, Dr. Crocker was appointed Assistant Dean for Student Affairs for the U.T. College of Medicine and served in this position until 1969. Dr. Bob Crocker was best known and will be well-remembered for his love of teaching by the many U.T. students and pathology residents who benefited by their association with him. At the time of his death, Robert L. Summitt, M.D., Dean of the U.T. College of Medicine, stated: "Dr. Bob Crocker was a valuable and devoted member of the University community. He will be missed by everyone who knew him, and especially by his many friends and co-workers on the campus." Bob Crocker had a keen interest and a deep appreciation of history, and in the late 1960's, Douglas H. Sprunt, M.D. (Professor and Chairman of the Department from 1944–1968) and he co-authored *The History of the U.T. Pathology Department.*[46]

Mr. Leon D. Hess, who had been Registrar at the University of Tennessee, Memphis since 1974, died suddenly on April 9, 1985 at Baptist Memorial Hospital after collapsing while jogging at the U.T. Student-Alumni Center. Mr. Hess was 51 years old. Prior to his joining U.T. Memphis, he had been Assistant Dean of Men at Middle Tennessee State University. Leon Hess was awarded his Ed.D. degree from Memphis State University posthumously. Mrs. Jean B. Melton, who has served the University in an exemplary fashion since July of 1970 in the Records Office, was named Registrar in 1985.[4]

One of the fine internists in the U.T. Department of Medicine is James Gibb Johnson, M.D. (Figure 233), whose major medical contributions have been in the areas of nephrology and hypertension. His clinical investigations, contributions to the medical literature, and authorship of portions of three books in this area attest to these accomplishments. He was born November 2, 1937 in Knoxville, Tennessee, received his undergraduate education at the University of Tennessee, Knoxville with a B.A. degree in 1959, and completed his M.D. degree at the University of Tennessee, Memphis in March of 1963. In medical school he was a member of Alpha Omega Alpha Honor Fraternity and was the recipient of the C. Riley Houck Award in Physiology during his sophomore year. His internship was taken at the City of Memphis Hospital and the Columbia Division of Bellevue Hospital in New York. His residency in Medicine was taken at the City of Memphis Hospital and was completed in June of 1967. At that time, he received a postdoctoral fellowship in Nephrology from the National Institutes of Health which was taken at the University of Tennessee, Memphis. He completed an additional year at the National Institutes of Health in Bethesda, Maryland, completing this work in June of 1969.[56]

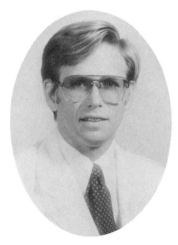

FIGURE 233. *James Gibb Johnson, M.D. (1937–   ) Professor, U.T. Department of Medicine, 1975–present and Associate Dean, Graduate Medical Education, U.T. College of Medicine, 1979–present*

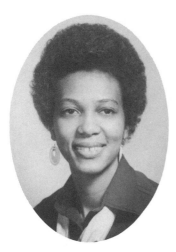

FIGURE 234. *Beverly Jean Williams, M.D. (1943–   ) Associate Professor, U.T. Departments of Medicine and Community Medicine, 1983–present*

He became a Diplomate of the American Board of Internal Medicine in December of 1969 with a subspecialty in nephrology in November of 1972. Dr. Jim Gibb Johnson is a member of numerous professional societies, including the American Federation for Clinical Research, the American Heart Association, the American Society of Nephrology, Memphis Academy of Internal Medicine (Council member 1982-present), and the Tennessee Society of Internal Medicine (Council member 1981-present). He was also elected a Fellow of the American College of Physicians in 1975. He was first appointed in 1966 to the U.T. Memphis faculty as an Instructor in Medicine, and in 1975 he became a Professor of Medicine in the U.T. College of Medicine. Administratively, he served as Associate Dean for Hospital Affairs in the U.T. College of Medicine from July of 1975 through January of 1979. At that time he became Associate Dean for Graduate Medical Education and continues to serve in that capacity. Nationally, he has served as a member on the Council on the Kidney in Cardiovascular Diseases for the American Heart Association, as a member of the State Scientific Advisory Board from 1968–1972 for the Kidney Foundation of Tennessee, and was Clinical Program Director of the Special Center of Research in Hypertension under an N.I.H. grant from 1971 through 1975.[16,56]

Beverly Jean Williams, M.D. (Figure 234) has made specific medical contributions in the areas of diabetes mellitus, thyroid function, and adrenal-ovarian function, plus clinical out-patient care. Dr. Williams was born August 16, 1943 in Mason, Tennessee and was reared in North Memphis. Her premedical education was obtained at Howard University in Washington, D.C. where she obtained a B.A. degree in 1965 with honors in Psychology. In March of 1966 she became the second black woman and the fifth black person to be admitted to the U.T. College of Medicine and graduated in June of 1969 with honors in Psychiatry. Her early interest in mental disorders changed to a preference for General Medicine and is summed up in her own words, "After I was in medical school, I became so involved and fascinated with Medicine in general, I gave up the idea of Psychiatry as a separate discipline. I felt I could incorporate my psychiatric interests in the comprehensive approach in Internal Medicine, so I chose that specialty, with a subspecialty in Endocrinology."[25]

She completed her internship in straight Medicine and took a year of Internal Medicine residency at Beth Israel Hospital in Boston. From July of 1971 through July of 1972 she continued her postgraduate education with an Endocrinology Fellowship at the Massachusetts General Hospital. She became a Diplomate of the American Board of Internal Medicine in 1974, a Fellow of the American College of Physicians, a member of the American Society of Internal Medicine, and President of the Mid-South Health Care Professionals. After leaving the Harvard-affiliated hospitals in Boston in 1972, she next joined a group practice in San Francisco and remained there until the spring of 1975. She had intended to return to Memphis eventually, and after conversations with Dr. Stollerman and Dr. Runyan, she joined the

U.T. Memphis faculty with appointments in Medicine and Community Medicine in 1975. She is currently an Associate Professor in both of these Departments and is Medical Director of the Gailor Medical Clinic in the City of Memphis Hospital. There, her interests have been in health care systems, community health education, and self-help programs, as well as a special three-year study for the American College of Physicians to develop a preventive medicine checklist of ten procedures that is affixed to the back of patients' clinic cards. Dr. Beverly Williams' goal can be stated as follows: "For my first area of interest and my abiding concern—the Medical Clinics—I have this goal: that we can make them a demonstration of organized, quality health care for an inner-city population. This is really close to my heart—partly for old times' sake, I guess, but even more for the sake of the future."[25,56]

In January of 1982, Charles W. Mercer, M.D. (Figure 235) returned to the University of Tennessee, Memphis to become Director of the U.T. Medical Center, Associate Dean for Clinical Affairs, and Associate Professor in the Department of Medicine in the College of Medicine. From 1969–1970 he was a Fellow in Cardiology at the University of Tennessee College of Medicine. In 1970 he first joined the faculty as Director of the Intensive Circulatory Care Unit for the City of Memphis Hospitals and as an Assistant Professor of Medicine. He was promoted to Associate Professor of Medicine in 1972 and left U.T. Memphis in 1973 to become Chief of Cardiology and Director, Coronary Care Unit, Cooper Green Hospital of Birmingham, Alabama. Dr. Charlie Mercer was born January 30, 1935 in Murray, Kentucky, obtained his B.A. degree from Murray State University in 1956, and earned his M.D. degree from the University of Louisville, Kentucky in 1960. After two years of training in Medicine in Florida, he served as a Captain (MC) U.S. Air Force from 1962–1963. He continued his training in Medicine at the University of Kentucky in Lexington, completing his residency and a Fellowship in Cardiology at the same institution in 1966. After several years of private practice, he served another year's Fellowship in Cardiology at the University of Tennessee, Memphis. He holds professional membership in many societies related to Internal Medicine and Cardiology. In 1971 he became a Diplomate of the American Board of Internal Medicine, and in 1974 he was certified in the subspecialty of Cardiology. The following year he became a Fellow of the American College of Cardiology. Dr. Mercer has made significant contributions in the areas of control and treatment of heart disease and also in hospital management. In 1985, he was awarded membership in the American College of Physician Executives, which is a select group of physicians who have been recognized for achieving excellence in the clinical practice of medicine, as well as demonstrating advanced management and leadership ability.[16,56]

Andrew H. Kang, M.D. (Figure 236), who is a major figure in research at the University of Tennessee, Memphis and the Veterans Administration Medical Center, was named Chairman of the U.T. Department of Medicine on July 1, 1982 by Dean Robert L. Summitt. Dr. Andy Kang possesses an

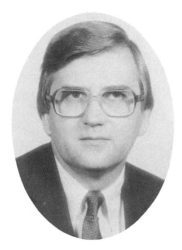

FIGURE 235. *Charles Wayne Mercer, M.D. (1935–) Associate Professor of Medicine, 1982–present, Associate Dean for Clinical Affairs, 1982–present, and Director, U.T. Medical Center 1982–present*

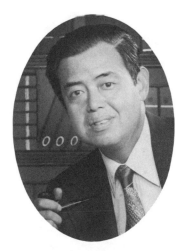

FIGURE 236. *Andrew H. Kang, M.D. (1934–) Professor and Chairman, U.T. Department of Medicine, 1982–present; Professor of Biochemistry, 1978–present*

international reputation for his research into the nature of collagen, having published in excess of 150 papers in the scientific literature, representing original work in this field. His research may be divided into three major categories: (a) the determination of the covalent structure of the various genetic types of collagens and their behavior in various fibrotic disorders, (b) the mechanism of modulation of fibroblast functions by the products of inflammatory cells and the biological effects of collagen on these cells, and (c) experimental polyarthritis induced by immunization with type II (cartilage-type) collagen and the immunopathogenesis of the experimental and human arthritides. For his research he has been honored as the recipient of the Russell L. Cecil Award from the Arthritis Foundation (1971) and the Philip Hench Award from the Association of U.S. Military Surgeons (1977).[16]

Dr. Andy Kang was born December 16, 1934 in Seoul, Korea and became a naturalized American citizen in 1964. His undergraduate education was taken at Wofford College in Spartanburg, South Carolina, where he received his B.S. degree in 1957 summa cum laude. He received his M.D. degree in 1962 from Harvard Medical School, also with highest honors. As a student he was a member of Phi Beta Kappa and Alpha Omega Alpha Honor Fraternities. From 1962 through 1964, he spent a year of straight Medicine internship and began a medical residency at the Peter Bent Brigham Hospital in Boston. Next, he spent two years under the tutelage of the distinguished collagen biochemist, Carl Piez, Ph.D., at the National Institute of Dental Research at the N.I.H. in Bethesda, Maryland. He returned to Boston and completed his medical residency and also served as a Clinical and Research Fellow at the Massachusetts General Hospital through 1969. While serving as a Senior Investigator for the Arthritis Foundation in New York, he was also an Assistant Professor of Medicine at the Harvard Medical School until 1972, when he joined the faculty of U.T. Memphis as a Professor of Medicine, an Associate Professor of Biochemistry, and a Medical Investigator for the Veterans Administration Medical Center in Memphis. From 1972–1977 Dr. Kang was Chief of the Rheumatology Section at the VA Medical Center, and from 1973 through the present he has been Associate Chief-of-Staff for Research for the VA Medical Center. He was promoted to Professor of Biochemistry in 1978 and also Director of the Division of Connective Tissue Diseases at the University of Tennessee, Memphis. Then, in July of 1982 he became Professor and Chairman of the U.T. Department of Medicine.[56]

Dr. Kang holds membership in numerous professional societies, including the American Society for Clinical Investigation, the American Society of Biological Chemists, the American Rheumatism Association, and Sigma Xi. He is a Fellow of the American College of Physicians, a Diplomate of the American Board of Internal Medicine, and a Diplomate of the American Board of Medical Examiners. In addition to his many clinical, teaching, and research accomplishments, Dr. Kang has also served as a member of the Editorial Board for the *Journal of Laboratory and Clinical Medicine*. The medical accomplishments of his wife, Ellen Kang, M.D., who is an Associate Professor in the U.T. Department of Pediatrics, have been described previously.[16,56]

Effective February 1, 1986, E. Eric Muirhead, M.D. retired as Chairman of the U.T. Department of Pathology and was sincerely thanked by Dean Robert L. Summitt for his outstanding leadership in the Department over the last five years. Concurrently, James Allison Pitcock, M.D. was appointed Acting Chairman of the U.T. Department of Pathology, and on March 1, 1986 his Clinical Professorship was changed to permanent Professor of Pathology. Dr. Pitcock (Figure 237) is an outstanding pathologist and a widely-published and recognized researcher. His extensive work includes 57 abstracts, significant contributions to 15 textbooks (including the tumor pathology portion of the Sixth Edition of *Campbell's Operative Orthopaedics*), and 68 papers in scientific journals. Much of his pertinent research has been in the area of hypertension, neoplasia, and prostaglandins.[56]

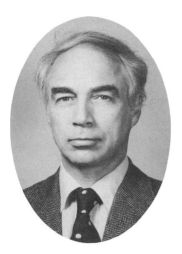

FIGURE 237. *James Allison Pitcock, M.D. (1929–   ) Professor and Acting Chairman, U.T. Department of Pathology, 1986–present*

His B.S. degree in Chemical Engineering was earned at the Massachusetts Institute of Technology in 1952; his graduate training was taken at the Washington University School of Medicine in St. Louis, receiving his M.D. degree with honors in 1955. He is a member of Alpha Omega Alpha and Sigma Xi. After a year of surgical internship at the Vanderbilt University Hospital, he began his residency in Pathology at Barnes Hospital in St. Louis, serving as a National Cancer Institute Fellow in Pathology (1957–1958), an American Cancer Society Fellow in Hematology (1959–1960), and an American Cancer Society Fellow in Surgical Pathology (1961–1962), also at Barnes Hospital. His military service (1959–1961) was taken as a Captain with the U.S. Air Force Medical Corps attached to the School of Aerospace Medicine at Brooks Air Force Base in San Antonio, Texas. He is American Board certified in both Anatomic Pathology (1962) and Clinical Pathology (1976). He is a member of the American Society of Clinical Pathologists, a Fellow of the College of American Pathologists, the International Academy of Pathologists, the American Association of Pathologists, and the Arthur Purdy Stout Society of Surgical Pathologists.[16,56]

In the summer of 1985, an interesting series of events resulted in a fascinating, collaborative research project between U.T. Memphis and Memphis State University. Dr. Rita Freed, an Egyptologist and Director of the Institute of Egyptian Art and Archaeology at M.S.U., acquired an extremely well-preserved Egyptian mummy head from the family of Mr. and Mrs. Donald G. Austin of Memphis. This relic (which is displayed at M.S.U.) had been in the Austin family since it had been brought back to the United States in the mid-1850's by Mr. Austin's uncle, who was an explorer. Dr. Freed contacted Hugh E. Berryman, Ph.D., a forensic anthropologist in the U.T. Department of Pathology, to inquire if modern medical diagnostic tools could be used to examine the mummy to learn more about it. A special team of more than a dozen doctors, composed chiefly of pathologists, radiologists, toxicologists, and forensic anthropologists from the University

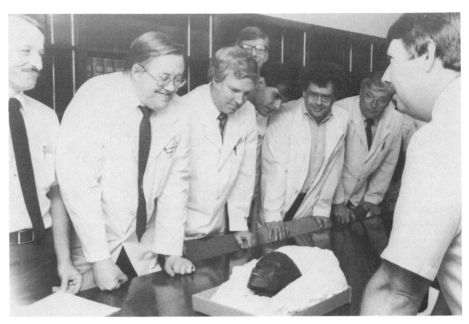

FIGURE 238. *"U.T. Mummy Team", 1985*

of Tennessee, Memphis, studied this relic extensively. The "U.T. Mummy Team" (Figure 238) is composed of : Raoul A. Arreola, Ph.D.; Richard W. Babin, M.D.; James S. Bell, M.D.; Hugh E. Berryman, Ph.D.; F. Curtis Dohan, Jr., M.D.; Jerry T. Francisco, M.D.; Elizabeth A. Fowler, M.T.; James E. Hamner, III, D.D.S., Ph.D.; Joel Kahane, Ph.D.; Craig H. Lahren, M.A.; James W. Langston, M.D.; Harry H. Mincer, D.D.S., Ph.D.; Steven Payne, M.D.; Jeno I Sebes, M.D.; Thomas A. Singarella, Ph.D.; David T. Stafford, Ph.D.; James E. Turner, D.D.S.; and Jack L. Wilson, Ph.D. Using x-rays and other techniques that did not destroy any part of the mummy head, the team is hoping to discover more about the life of the mummy, including questions about her health, diet, embalming methods, and cause of death. A monograph describing the historical, anthropological, and medical aspects of this mummy head—named "Se-Ankh" by Dr. Rita Freed, which means "brought to life"—will be published as a joint U.T.-M.S.U. effort in late 1986 under the editorship of Dr. James Hamner. It will become an important part of the national Ramses II Exhibition, which will be shown in Memphis from August 15-August 31, 1987.[49]

In 1984 an Epilepsy Center (Epicare) was established as a joint venture between the University of Tennessee, Memphis, Baptist Memorial Hospital, and the Semmes-Murphey Clinic. The U.T. Departments of Neurology and Neurosurgery are involved in this Center, which is another rare example of a private institution, a State institution, and private practice physicians working together to provide a clinically-needed service in the community.[11]

On October 15, 1984 the 12-story, 300-room East Pavilion of the University of Tennessee Medical Research Center and Hospital in Knoxville, Tennessee was officially dedicated. The East Pavilion increases total floor space at UTMRCH by 350,000 square feet which, with a total bed capacity of 602 beds, makes UTMRCH the largest health care facility in East Tennessee. Including ancillary improvements, it was constructed at a cost of $44,000,000 which makes it the largest, most expensive single building project in the history of the University of Tennessee.[16]

The University of Tennessee Medical Center and the Baptist Memorial Hospital joined cooperative hands again to establish the joint Baptist-U.T. Nuclear Magnetic Resonance Facility at 10 North Pauline Street. This effort represents one of the largest joint ventures in the United States, and it will be managed by radiologists from the University of Tennessee, Memphis.[11]

The first Program on Human Values and Ethics began in the College of Community and Allied Health Professions under the direction of Dr. David Thomasma in 1973. It became an Interdisciplinary Program, which reported to the Vice Chancellor, Academic Affairs, in 1976. The Program was finally located in the U.T. College of Medicine in 1981 under the new Directorship of Terrence F. Ackerman, Ph.D. It is scheduled to become the Department of Human Values and Ethics with Dr. Ackerman as Chairman in 1986, when the U.T. Board of Trustees grants formal approval.[16]

Some of the most unique medical contributions made by a U.T. Memphis alumna are the aerospace accomplishments attributed to Rhea Seddon, M.D. (Figure 239), who is a 1973 graduate of the University of Tennessee College of Medicine. Dr. Seddon, a 37 year old native of Murfreesboro,

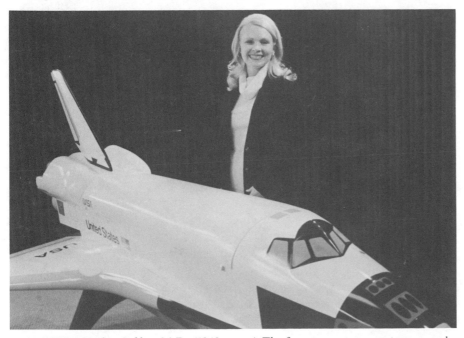

FIGURE 239. M. Rhea Seddon, M.D. (1948–   ) The first astronaut surgeon in space and graduate of the U.T. College of Medicine, 1973 (courtesy of NASA)

Tennessee, was selected as an astronaut by NASA in 1978.[32]

After graduation from medical school, she completed a straight Surgery internship at Baptist Memorial Hospital, then three years of surgical residency at the University of Tennessee, Memphis. During this time she served as an emergency room physician at a number of hospitals in Tennessee and Mississippi, and she performed research into the effects of radiation therapy on nutrition and cancer patients. In the words of Dr. James Pate, Professor and Chairman of the U.T. Department of Surgery, "Rhea Seddon, with other physicians at U.T., introduced the concept of hyperalimentation to the world. When she was selected for the space program, NASA was concerned about the astronauts' diet and feeding. Dr. Seddon's expertise in the nutrition of the stressed individual was of major interest to the program. We are extremely proud of her as a physician and as an astronaut."[32] Dr. Rhea Seddon was selected to be on the crew of space shuttle "Discovery" in April of 1985. During that flight she performed certain medical experiments, vis-a-vis taping of echocardiograph soundings, hand/eye coordination experiments, and observations of the relationship between bowel sounds and space sickness. As a true Volunteer, Rhea Seddon will long be remembered as the astronaut who pasted a Tennessee bumper sticker to the space shuttle cabin wall for all the world to see. She carried samples of the U.T. Memphis letterhead, copies of the U.T. College of Medicine seal, and an original of the Surgery Gold Medal in the space shuttle cargo hold. This "stationery from outer space" will be used during the University's 75th Anniversary in 1986, and the Surgery Medal was presented to Dr. James Pate during Dr. Seddon's campus visit in May of 1985. She was slated to accompany a second space shuttle flight in late 1986 that would be dedicated to life science experiments, but the unfortunate tragedy in the explosion and loss of space shuttle "Challenger" on January 28, 1986 has delayed this program. The medical experiments proposed will be ones on why osteoporosis increases during space travel, the changes that occur in body fluids when the body is at zero gravity, and how the lungs function in weightlessness. The results of these studies will have implications for earth-bound patients as well as space travelers. The entire University can well be proud of Dr. Rhea Seddon for being the first surgeon in space.[32]

After months of extremely arduous work by City, County, State, and University leaders, a positive decision was rendered on February 6, 1986 by the St. Jude Board of Governors which met in Miami, Florida—they voted definitely to keep all of their clinical and research activities in Memphis and not to relocate and affiliate with Washington University of St. Louis. James C. Hunt, M.D., Chancellor of U.T. Memphis, summarized the Memphis medical community's feelings on this matter, as follows: "The news that St. Jude is staying is warmly welcomed throughout the Memphis Medical Center and the U.T. Memphis community. We are delighted that the St. Jude Board of Governors has elected to decline the invitation to move to St. Louis."[55]

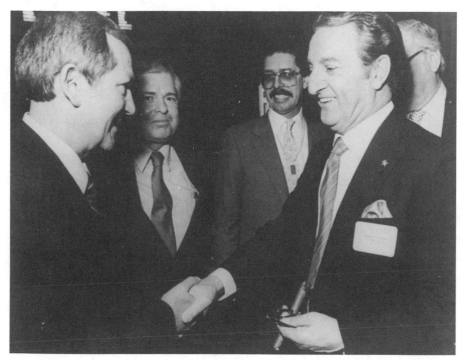

FIGURE 240. *U.T. Chancellor James C. Hunt (left) and Danny Thomas, founder of St. Jude Children's Research Hospital, 1986 (courtesy of the State of Tennessee)*

In a unanimous gesture of support and approval, the Tennessee General Assembly set aside February 19, 1986 to honor Danny Thomas, St. Jude Children's Research Hospital, its Board of Governors, and Arab-Americans across the State and to celebrate the successful efforts of the Memphis civic, business, and health professional communities and the elected officials of Memphis to convince St. Jude that their brightest future lay in remaining here (Figure 240). Danny Thomas, the founder of St. Jude, responded to this spontaneous acclaim and outpouring of support and affection with the proud admission that Tennessee is his adopted State, and he plans to be buried in Memphis. Dr. Ed Boling, President of the University of Tennessee, echoed the previous rejoicing sentiments of other speakers at the news conference in Nashville: "U.T. Memphis welcomes the opportunity to join with St. Jude in a research effort that we anticipate will achieve even greater national and international stature. We pledge that the University will not let up in its role as a vital partner in that commitment."[55]

Governor Lamar Alexander reiterated his previous commitment to strengthening the University of Tennessee, Memphis and its research facilities. He again pledged his earlier commitment of a $50,000,000 overall proposal to the General Assembly, including 20 additional Chairs of Excellence endowed at $1,000,000 each at U.T. Memphis. He also requested $25,000,000 for renovation of current facilities and the addition of new research space for U.T. Memphis. Chancellor James Hunt promised an even closer working relationship with St. Jude, having Dr. Joseph Simone, the

Director of St. Jude Children's Research Hospital, become a member of the Chancellor's Administrative Council. Dr. Simone is already involved as a Trustee for the Crippled Children's Hospital Foundation Forum on Child Health, which is administered by the University of Tennessee, Memphis. Many of the physicians and scientists at St. Jude also hold academic appointments at U.T. Memphis. The Chancellor reiterated his commitment of five of the next 20 Chairs of Excellence to be devoted to Pediatric Medicine.[52,55]

As U.T. Memphis heads toward the final years of the 1980's decade, several important developments and contributions, which will affect its life and future, are nearing fruition. Dr. Al Mauer has worked diligently to build the clinical and basic science health professional staff to demonstrate academic strength in cancer research in Memphis. Next, he will apply for a core grant from the National Cancer Institute to establish a Comprehensive Cancer Center, which will be concerned with adult cancer, similar to St. Jude's expertise in childhood cancer. The newly-funded support from the Dorothy Snider Foundation to create a national Forum on Cancer Research at U.T. Memphis, coupled with the adult cancer research commitments of Governor Alexander and the Tennessee General Assembly, and the support of the American Cancer Society and private endowments should gel to make the U.T. Comprehensive Cancer Center a functioning reality.

With the naming of its new Board of Directors in the near future, the Biomedical Research Zone should gather even greater momentum. With a permanent manager appointed and the ongoing construction of new buildings within the BRZ, its potential in the revitalization of the part of Memphis that it encompasses will be a boon to Memphis and Shelby County.

More than $13,000,000 has been appropriated by the Tennessee General Assembly, and bids are planned to be let in September of 1986, to commence construction of an addition to the Nash Building to house the Consolidated Animal Laboratory and to provide some 40,000 square feet of new research laboratory space, which will be housed in the upper floors of the new addition. Another $14,000,000 in funding has also been approved for the continuing renovation of the Pathology Institute Building, completion of the Health Science Library Building, and renovation of the Wittenborg Building for the Neuroscience Center.

The third Center of Excellence at U.T. Memphis has been approved by the Tennessee Higher Education Commission and will be announced in the near future. This Center for Pediatric Pharmacokinetics and Therapeutics will be located in the Le Bonheur Children's Medical Center, and it will be administered jointly by John F. Griffith, M.D., Professor and Chairman of the U.T. Department of Pediatrics, and William E. Evans, Pharm.D., Professor and Chairman of the U.T. Department of Clinical Pharmacy and Chief of Pharmacy at St. Jude Children's Research Hospital.

Dr. Martha Howe, Professor of Bacteriology at the University of Wisconsin, Madison, has accepted the appointment as the Van Vleet Professor of

Virology in the Department of Microbiology and Immunology. A nation-wide search is nearing completion for the appointment of a distinguished individual to occupy the Van Vleet Chair of Excellence in Pharmacology. These distinguished scientist appointments will be announced during the forthcoming year.

Dr. James Hamner chairs the U.T. Pathology Relocation Committee, charged by Chancellor Hunt and Dean Summitt, to merge the U.T. Department of Pathology and the Baptist Memorial Hospital Pathology Department into a joint U.T.-Baptist Pathology Department, which will be physically located within leased space in the Baptist Madison West (Physicians and Surgeons) Building. Once this move is completed in 1987, a concurrent search committee will seek an appropriate individual to be the Department Chairman, who would fill the Muirhead Chair of Excellence in Pathology.

In addition to the current five U.T. Distinguished Visiting Professorship Lectures, two other ones are proposed for the immediate future. Bland W. Cannon, M.D., Special Advisor to the Chancellor and a noted Memphis neurosurgeon, will fund the Cannon Distinguished Visiting Professorship in Neuroscience. The second such new Lectureship will be established in the U.T. College of Nursing to honor Emeritus Dean Ruth Neil Murry and will be known as the Ruth Neil Murry Distinguished Visiting Professorship in Nursing. It will be funded by Dr. Michael A. Carter, Dean of the U.T. College of Nursing, and his wife, Dr. Sarah A. Carter, Assistant Professor, U.T. Department of Medicine.

On recommendation from Governor Alexander, the Tennessee General Assembly has continued the Chairs of Excellence Program through funding for ten additional Chairs for the U.T. System during the 1986–1987 fiscal year. Several of these Chairs will be established on the U.T. Memphis campus and will include a Crippled Children's Hospital Foundation Chair of Excellence in Biomedical Engineering. In addition, five Chairs of Excellence in Pediatrics have been approved and funded as part of the St. Jude Accord. In expressing appreciation to the Governor and General Assembly, Chancellor James Hunt emphasized that the Memphis Medical Center, St. Jude, and U.T. Memphis look forward to a bright future and ever closer working relationship.

In 1985, the U.T. College of Medicine launched its Alumni Endowment Campaign, "New Perspective." It will make possible two endowed professorships: the Lemuel W. Diggs Professorship in Medicine and the Harwell Wilson Professorship in Surgery. Also, a student merit scholarship program and a medical student loan program are planned.

The University of Tennessee has completed 75 tremendous years as a medical center in Memphis since its launching in 1911, and it has grown from the infant stage of one building (Lindsley Hall) to the massive complex seen in Map #2. It has weathered many storms during its rise to maturity. Its reputation has been justifiably earned as a school that graduated extremely well-trained clinicians (dentists, nurses, pharmacists, physicians,

"All's well that ends well."

William Shakespeare

283

surgeons, and technicians)—and as a school closely allied with quality clinical care for its catchment area patients. Recently, emphasis has changed to strengthen the third vital support of the balanced academic chair—research. Three basic elements are essential for a quality health science university: education, clinical care, and research. A debt of gratitude is owed the early faculty who laid the groundwork for research, because in the early days, what research that was done had to be performed on the faculty's own time.

As the University of Tennessee, Memphis sails into the uncharted waters of the next 75 years, it enters a fast-paced course in which medical accomplishments, scientific breakthroughs, and modes of health care delivery change quite rapidly. At times, the individual seems diminished and lost, yet we must not forget our roots which stretch back to the University of Nashville Medical Department in 1850. We must remember that precious balance between education, patient care, and research—and we must remember our most important responsibility—the students of today and the health care professionals of the future.

It is essential that we seek the best possible facilities, stimulating, dedicated teachers, the most skilled clinicians, excellent, responsible researchers, and motivated students. Yet above all, we must profess belief and confidence in ourselves. Thomas Watson, Jr., of International Business Machines (IBM), is quoted in the book, *In Search of Excellence*, as saying that "the most important factor in corporate success is faithful adherence to beliefs." An organization, institution, or university can, and sometimes must, change everything except those beliefs. Many things weigh heavily in the success of an organization, but all else is "transcended by how strongly the people in the organization believe in its basic precepts and how faithfully they carry them out."

We, who are fortunate enough to be in this calling, are walking daily in the footsteps of many famous, dedicated men and women who have lived the life of the University of Tennessee, Memphis—good people, who have made many varied medical contributions for us and to mankind. The next 75 years promise to be even more exciting and productive for the University of Tennessee, Memphis as it strides forward under competent, concerned leadership. The three so-termed "learned professions," Medicine, Law, and Theology, have a common thread that runs through each of them—seeking and serving the interest of others, rather than one's self.

In closing this moment in our history, we can go forward with great confidence and with great expectations, if we remember the four major ethical precepts in Medicine:

(1) To be professionally competent
(2) To save life, wherever possible
(3) To relieve pain and suffering
(4) And above all, to do no harm.

REFERENCES

1. *ADA News:* November 18, 1985 (Dr. Overbey).

2. Babin, R.W. and Tag, A.R.; "The University of Tennessee Otolaryngology Training Program", *Amer. J. of Otology* 6:521–523, 1985.

3. *Biomedical Research Zone Brochure,* 1985.

4. *Commercial Appeal:* April 10, 1985 (Dr. Hess).

5. *Commercial Appeal:* Editorial—June 11, 1985.

6. *Commercial Appeal* Mid-South Magazine: January 12, 1986.

7. *Dental Alumni News:* Spring, 1984.

8. Hamner, James E., III: "Report on the U.T. Memphis International Programs to President Boling", 1985.

9. Hughes, James G.: *Department of Pediatrics—UTCHS: 1910–1985,* 1985.

10. Hunt, James C.: Personal Communication, 1985.

11. Jacobs, Barbara S.: "U.T. Memphis Annual Report", 1985.

12. Lollar, Michael: *Commercial Appeal* Mid-South Magazine, May, 1984.

13. Martin, Jess A.: Personal Communication, 1985.

14. McKnight, James P.: Personal Communication, 1985.

15. Medical Accomplishments: U.T. College of Dentistry.

16. Medical Accomplishments: U.T. College of Medicine.

17. Medical Accomplishments: U.T. College of Nursing.

18. Medical Accomplishments: U.T. College of Pharmacy.

19. *Memphis Center for Stone Disease Brochure,* 1986.

20. Pate, James W.: Personal Communication, 1986.

21. Pigott, Jack: Personal Communication, 1986.

22. Reynolds, Richard J.: Personal Communication, 1985.

23. Simmons, Heber, Jr.: Personal Communication, 1985.

24. Summitt, Robert L.: Personal Communication, 1985.

25. *Tennessee Medical Alumnus:* Spring, 1980 (Coleman Building; Dr. Beverly J. Williams).

26. *Tennessee Medical Alumnus:* Fall, 1980 (Dr. Mayberry).

27. *Tennessee Medical Alumnus:* Winter, 1981 (General Vorder Bruegge).

28. *Tennessee Medical Alumnus:* Spring, 1981 (Dr. James Hunt; Dr. Robert Summitt).

29. *Tennessee Medical Alumnus:* Summer, 1982 (Liver Transplant Program).

30. *Tennessee Medical Alumnus:* Summer, 1983 (Transplant Program).

31. *Tennessee Medical Alumnus:* Winter, 1984 (Dr. Dismuke—Wellness Program; Drs. Tooms, Summitt, Verstandig, Duckworth).

32. *Tennessee Medical Alumnus:* Fall, 1985 (Dr. Rhea Seddon).

33. *U.T. Record:* December 1, 1980 (Dr. Hunt).

34. *U.T. Record:* March 15, 1982 (Dr. Slagle).

35. *U.T. Record:* June 15, 1982 (Dr. Bruesch).

36. *U.T. Record:* July 15, 1982 (Dr. Autian).

37. *U.T. Record:* September 15, 1982 (Hirosaki University agreement).

38. *U.T. Record:* February 1, 1983 (Dr. James Hamner).

39. *U.T. Record:* March 1, 1983: (Dr. Michael Ryan).

40. *U.T. Record:* October 1, 1983 (Forum on Child Health).

41. *U.T. Record:* June 27, 1984 (Drs. Freeman, Carman, Huffman).

42. *U.T. Record:* October 1, 1984 (Dr. Hinkle; Dr. Dismuke—Wellness Program).

43. *U.T. Record:* November 1, 1984 (Department of Education).

44. *U.T. Record:* November 15, 1984 (Van Vleet gift).

45. *U.T. Record:* December 6, 1984 (Comprehensive Cancer Center; Dr. Mauer).

46. *U.T. Record:* January 18, 1985 (Dr. Bob Crocker).

47. *U.T. Record:* March 1, 1985 (Minority Program).

48. *U.T. Record:* May 1, 1985 (Dr. Terrance Cooper).

49. *U.T. Record:* July 15, 1985 ("Mummy Team").

50. *U.T. Record:* August 28, 1985 (Computers).

51. *U.T. Record:* September 20, 1985 (Methodist Hospitals Neuroscience Program).

52. *U.T. Record:* October 1, 1985 (Library; Chairs of Excellence).

53. *U.T. Record:* October 18, 1985 (Dr. Pate; Heart Transplant Program).
54. *U.T. Record:* December 11, 1985 (Dr. Fain; Muirhead Chair of Excellence).
55. *U.T. Record:* March 17, 1986 (Forum on Cancer Research; St. Jude).
56. University of Tennessee, Memphis: Personnel Records.

APPENDIX

Appendix A

Chancellors or Chief Administrative Officers of The University of Tennessee, Memphis

1911–1919
Brown Ayres, Ph.D., LL.D., D.C.L., President of the University of Tennessee

1920–1921
Harcourt A. Morgan, B.S., LL.D., President of the University of Tennessee

1921–1925
Orren Williams Hyman, A.B., M.A., Ph.D., Business Manager of the Medical Units, Memphis

1926–1942
Orren Williams Hyman, A.B., M.A., Ph.D., Administrative Officer of the Colleges in Memphis

1943–1948
Orren Williams Hyman, A.B., M.A., Ph.D., Dean of Administration of the U.T. Health Units in Memphis

1949–1961
Orren Williams Hyman, A.B., M.A., Ph.D., Vice President in Charge of the U.T. Medical Units

1961–1970
Homer F. Marsh, B.S., M.S., Ph.D., Vice President and Chancellor, U.T. Medical Units

1970 (February–October)
Jack K. Williams, Ph.D., Chancellor *pro tem*, U.T. Medical Units

1970 (November)
Roland H. Alden, A.B., Ph.D., Chancellor *pro tem*, U.T. Medical Units

1970 (December)–1971 (October)
Joseph E. Johnson, A.B., A.M., Ed.D., Interim Chancellor, U.T. Medical Units

1971 (October)–1973 (October)
Joseph E. Johnson, A.B., A.M., Ed.D., Chancellor, U.T. Medical Units, and Vice President for Health Affairs, The University of Tennessee

1973 (October)–1974
Edmund D. Pellegrino, B.S., M.D., Chancellor, The University of Tennessee Center for the Health Sciences, and Vice President for Health Affairs, The University of Tennessee

1975–1980
T. Albert Farmer, Jr., B.S., M.D., Chancellor, The University of Tennessee Center for the Health Sciences, and Vice President for Health Affairs, The University of Tennessee

1980 (November)–Present
James Calvin Hunt, A.B., M.S., M.D., Chancellor, The University of Tennessee, Memphis and Vice President for Health Affairs, The University of Tennessee

Appendix B

Deans and Acting Deans of The University of Tennessee College of Medicine

1911–1912	Edward Coleman Ellett, B.A., M.D.
1912–1919 (on leave 1917–1919 due to illness)	Herbert Thomas Brooks, B.A., M.D.
1917	Lucius Junius Desha, B.A., Ph.D., Acting Dean
1917–1919, 1920, 1921	August Hermsmeier Wittenborg, A.B., M.D., Acting Dean
1919 (12 Days)	Leverett Dale Bristol, M.D.
1920–1921	McIver Woody, A.B., M.D.
1921–1923	James Bassett McElroy, B.S., M.D., Acting Dean
1923–1957	Orren Williams Hyman, A.B., M.A., Ph.D.
1957–1970	Maston Kennerly Callison, B.S., M.D.
1970–1972	Richard Roll Overman, A.B., M.A., Ph.D., Acting Dean
1972–1974	T. Albert Farmer, Jr., B.S., M.D.
1975, 1977–1978	E. William Rosenberg, B.S., M.D., Acting Dean
1975–1977	Charles Barnard McCall, A.B., M.D.
1978–1980	James Calvin Hunt, A.B., M.S., M.D.
1981–Present	Robert Layman Summitt, M.S., M.D.

Appendix C

Deans and Acting Deans of the University of Tennessee College of Dentistry

1911–1923	Joseph Archibald Gardner, D.D.S.
1924–1932	Robert Sherman Vinsant, A.B., D.D.S.
1933–1942	Edgar Dupree Rose, D.D.S.
1943–1949	Richard Doggett Dean, B.S., D.D.S., M.D.
1950–1959	James Theda Ginn, B.S., D.D.S., F.A.C.D.
1959 (October)– 1961 (July)	William Herbert Jolley, D.D.S., F.A.C.D., Acting Dean
1961–1969 (February)	Shailer A. Peterson, B.A., M.A., Ph.D., F.A.C.D.
1969 (February)– 1970 (August)	William Herbert Jolley, D.D.S., F.A.C.D., Acting Dean
1970 (August)–1981	Jack Edward Wells, D.D.S., M.S., F.A.C.D.
1981 (March)–1982 (March)	William F. Slagle, B.S., D.D.S., M.Ed., F.A.C.D., Acting Dean
1982 (March)–Present	William F. Slagle, B.S., D.D.S., M.Ed., F.A.C.D.

Appendix D

Deans and Acting Deans of the University of Tennessee College of Pharmacy

1911–1928	William Krauss, PH.C., M.D., Chief Administrative Officer, School of Pharmacy, College of Medicine	1959–1975	Seldon D. Feurt, B.S., M.S., Ph.D., Dean, College of Pharmacy
1928–1933	Andrew Richard Bliss, Jr., A.M., PHM.D., M.D., Dean, School of Pharmacy	1975	Martin E. Hamner, B.S., M.S., Ph.D., Acting Dean, College of Pharmacy
1933–1936	Orren Williams Hyman, A.B., M.A., Ph.D., Acting Dean, School of Pharmacy	1975–1982	John Autian, B.S., M.S., Ph.D., Dean, College of Pharmacy
1936–1953	Robert Latta Crowe, PH.C., Dean, School of Pharmacy	1982–1983	Michael R. Ryan, B.S., M.S., Ph.D., Executive Associate Dean, College of Pharmacy
1953–1959	Karl John Goldner, B.S., M.S., Ph.D., Dean, School of Pharmacy	1983–Present	Michael R. Ryan, B.S., M.S., Ph.D., Dean, College of Pharmacy

Appendix E

Deans and Acting Deans of the University of Tennessee College of Nursing

1927–1944	Ella George Hinton, G.N., R.N., Acting Director, U.T. School of Nursing	1978–1979	Norma J. Long, B.S.N., M.S.N., D.N.Sc., Acting Dean
1945–1949	Ruth Neil Murry, B.S.N., M.A., Director, U.T. School of Nursing	1979–1981	Marie C. Josberger, Ed.D., Dean
1949–1977	Ruth Neil Murry, B.S.N., M.A., Dean, U.T. College of Nursing	1981–1982	E. Dianne Greenhill, B.S.N., M.S., Ed.D., Interim Dean
		1982–Present	Michael A. Carter, B.S.N., M.N.Sc., D.N.Sc., Dean

Appendix F

Deans and Acting Deans of the University of Tennessee College of Allied Health Sciences

1972–1982	Lee Holder, B.S., M.P.H., Ph.D.	1984–Present	William G. Hinkle, B.S., M.S., Ph.D.
1982–1984	Ralph A. Hyde, B.S., M.A., Ed.D., Acting Dean		

Appendix G

Deans and Acting Deans of the University of Tennessee School of Biological Sciences or Graduate School of Medical Sciences

1928–1960	Thomas Palmer Nash, Jr., A.B., A.M., Ph.D.	James Calvin Hunt, A.B., M.S., M.D., Acting Dean
1961–1979	Roland Herrick Alden, A.B., Ph.D.	
1979–1980	John L. Wood, B.S., Ph.D., Acting Dean	1982–1985 John Autian, B.S., M.S., Ph.D.
1980–1981	John A. Shively, A.B., M.D., Acting Dean	1985–Present Bob A. Freeman, B.A., M.S., Ph.D., Vice Chancellor for Academic Affairs
1981–1982	Robert E. Taylor, B.S., M.S., Ph.D., Associate Dean-in-Charge	

Appendix H

The University of Tennessee, Memphis Alumni or Faculty Who Have Reached Flag Rank in the U.S. Armed Forces

1. Rear Admiral Frank H. Anderson, (DC) U.S. Naval Reserve
2. Rear Admiral Paul R. Caudill, Jr., (MC) U.S. Navy
3. Lieutenant General Murphy A. Chesney, Jr., (MC) U.S. Air Force
4. Rear Admiral James A. Crabtree, U.S. Public Health Service
5. Rear Admiral James D. Enoch, (DC) U.S. Navy
6. Brigadier General Marinus Flux, (MC) U.S. Air Force
7. Major General Carl W. Hughes, (MC) U.S. Army
8. Brigadier General James G. Hughes, (MC) U.S. Army Reserve
9. Brigadier General Bill B. Lefler, (DC) U.S. Army
10. Brigadier General Albert Gallatin Love, (MC) U.S. Army
11. Rear Admiral Joseph H. Miller, (MC) U.S. Naval Reserve
12. Rear Admiral Moore Moore, Jr., (MC) U.S. Naval Reserve
13. Brigadier General Robert Malcolm Overbey, (DC) U.S. Army Reserve
14. Rear Admiral James K. Summitt, (MC) U.S. Navy
15. Rear Admiral Robert L. Summitt, (MC) U.S. Naval Reserve
16. Rear Admiral Morton J. Tendler, (MC) U.S. Naval Reserve
17. Rear Admiral Julian J. Thomas, Jr., (DC) U.S. Navy
18. Major General Colin F. Vorder Bruegge, (MC) U.S. Army
19. Brigadier General Frank E. Wilson, (MC) U.S. Army

Appendix I

The University of Tennessee, Memphis Alumni or Faculty Who Have Sacrificed Their Lives in the Service of Their Country

World War I:

1. Grover Carter, M.D.
   Captain, 121st. Brigade, Royal Field Artillery, British Army.
   He received his M.D. degree from the University of Tennessee in 1917 and was killed in action in France on October 16, 1918 in World War I.

2. Norwin Batte Norris, M.D.
   Lieutenant (j.g.), (MC) U.S. Navy.
   He received his M.D. degree from the University of Tennessee in 1917 and was killed in action in October, 1918 while serving aboard the U.S.S. Ticonderoga in World War I.

3. Robert Boyden Underwood, M.D.
   Captain, (MC) U.S. Army.
   He received his M.D. degree from the University of Nebraska in 1904, was a member of the University of Tennessee medical faculty 1914–1917, and died from pneumonia at Rouen, France while serving as an Army physician in World War I.

World War II:

4. Everett Benjamin Archer, M.D.
   Major, (MC) U.S. Army.
   He received his M.D. degree from the University of Tennessee in 1920 and died January 18, 1945 while serving as an Army physician in New Guinea during World War II.

5. Alton Coleman Bookout, M.D.
   Lieutenant, (MC) U.S. Navy.
   He received his M.D. degree from the University of Tennessee in 1938 and was killed in Manila Bay on December 7, 1941 when the destroyer on which he was serving was sunk by Japanese aircraft, at the commencement of World War II.

6. Newton Alexander Cannon, M.D.
   1st Lieutenant, (MC) U.S. Army.
   He received his M.D. degree from the University of Tennessee in 1941 and was killed in action on March 31, 1945 on Luzon, Philippines.

7. James Allison Fannin, D.D.S.
   1st Lieutenant, U.S. Army Air Corps.
   He received his D.D.S. degree from the University of Tennessee in 1935 and was killed in an airplane crash into the Atlantic, while flying at night off Cape Charles, Virginia on January 14, 1942.

8. Earl O'Dell Henry, D.D.S.
   Lt. Commander, (DC) U.S. Navy.
   He received his D.D.S. degree from the University of Tennessee in 1935 and lost his life when the cruiser Indianapolis was sunk by a Japanese submarine on June 30, 1945 in the Pacific.

9. John Gilbert Hudgins, D.D.S.
   Captain, (DC) U.S. Army.
   He received his D.D.S. degree from the University of Tennessee in 1940 and died on January 22, 1945, following injuries which were received aboard a prison ship while being transported as a prisoner of war from the Philippines to Japan.

10. Claude Raymond Huffman, M.D.
    Lieutenant, (MC) U.S. Navy.
    He received his M.D. degree from the University of Tennessee in 1936 and died October 10, 1943 from chest wounds caused by shrapnel received aboard a destroyer under attack in the South Pacific.

11. Lee New Minor, B.S. (Pharmacy)
    1st Lieutenant, U.S. Army Air Corps.
    He received his B.S. degree in Pharmacy from the University of Tennessee in 1940, volunteered for flight school in the U.S. Army Air Corps, and was killed on August 6, 1942 while serving with General Clare Chenault's "Flying Tigers".

12. David Edward Nolte, B.S. (Pharmacy)
    Chief Pharmacist Mate, U.S. Navy.
    He received his B.S. degree in Pharmacy from the University of Tennessee in 1927 and was killed in action on December 11, 1944 when his destroyer was hit by Japanese bombs and sank off the coast of Leyte.

13. Lewis Cowan Ramsay, M.D.
    He received his M.D. degree from the University of Tennessee in 1936 and was killed on November 4, 1944 in an airplane accident during World War II.

14. Robert Henry Robbins, M.D.
    Captain, (MC) U.S. Army
    He received his M.D. degree from the University of Tennessee in 1937 and died June 5, 1943 from a fractured skull in the North African theatre.

15. Wendell F. Swanson, M.D.
    Major, (MC) U.S. Army.
    He received his M.D. degree from the University of Tennessee in 1932, was taken prisoner after the fall of Bataan and Corregidor, and lost his life when the Japanese prison ship on which he was being taken to Japan was sunk December 13, 1944.

16. Jehu Creed Walker, M.D.
    Major, (MC) U.S. Army.
    He received his M.D. degree from the University of Tennessee in 1936 and was killed April 12, 1945 in an airplane crash in England, while serving as a flight surgeon with the Eighth Air Force during late World War II.

Korean War:

17. Ralph Lee Borum, B.S. (Pharmacy)
    1st Lieutenant, U.S. Air Force.
    He received his B.S. degree in Pharmacy from the University of Tennessee in 1949, flew 50 missions over Europe as a Flying Fortress navigator during World War II, and was killed October 14, 1951 in a B-29 crash landing near Tokyo, as his plane came in from a raid over Korea.
18. Bert Nelson Coers, M.D.
    Lt. Colonel, (MC) U.S. Army.
    He received his M.D. degree from the University of Tennessee in 1937, was wounded by artillery fire and captured December 1, 1950, and died on August 22, 1953 in a North Korean prisoner of war camp.

19. William Lindsey Wallace, Jr., M.D.
    Baptist Medical Missionary in China.
    He received his M.D. degree from the University of Tennessee in 1932, was jailed by the Chinese Communists after World War II on a fake charge, and was killed by them in his cell on February 9, 1951.
20. James M. Thayer, Jr., M.D.
    Captain, (MC) U.S. Air Force.
    He received his M.D. degree from the University of Tennessee in 1954 and was killed on February 15, 1958 when his troop transport plane crashed into Mt. Vesuvius, Italy.

Viet Nam Conflict:

21. Karl Edmond Shenep, M.D.
    Captain, (MC) U.S. Army.
    He received his M.D. degree from the University of Tennessee in 1964 and was killed on April 16, 1967 by ground fire while flying on a rescue helicopter mission in Viet Nam.

Appendix J

The University of Tennessee, Memphis Alumni or Faculty Who Have Authored or Edited Scientific/Professional Textbooks

The Wallace Collection*

William L. Wallace, M.D. was a 1932 graduate of the University of Tennessee College of Medicine. His outstanding, dedicated career as a Christian medical missionary ended in his death in a Chinese Communist prison camp on February 9, 1951. The Memorial Book Collection was begun by his classmates as a tribute to his life and courage.

The William L. Wallace Memorial Book Collection in The University of Tennessee, Memphis Library is a collection of scientific books that have been written, compiled, or edited by alumni or faculty of U.T. Memphis.

1. Adams, John Quincy:
   Chemistry and therapy of diseases of pregnancy, (Springfield, IL.: Thomas), 1962.
2. Akers, Michael J.:
   Sterile preparation for the hospital pharmacist: an illustrated manual of procedures, (Ann Arbor, MI.: Ann Arbor Science Publishers), 1981.

3. Akiskal, Hagop S.,
   co-editor:
   Psychiatric diagnosis: exploration of biological predictors, (New York, NY.: SP Medical and Scientific Books), 1978.
4. Alden, Roland Herrick:
   A laboratory atlas of the mouse embryo, (Memphis, TN.: University of Tennessee. Medical Units, Division of Anatomy), 1957.
5. Andersen, Richard N.,
   associate editor:
   Clinical use of sex steroids: based on the proceedings of the Fourth Annual Symposium on Gynecologic Endocrinology, held May 7–9, 1979 at The University of Tennessee, Memphis, Tennessee, (Chicago, IL.: Year Book Publishers), 1980.
6. Andersen, Richard M.:
   Manual of gynecologic endocrinology and infertility, (Baltimore, MD.: Williams and Wilkins), 1979.

7. Anderson, Garland D.:
Endocrinology of pregnancy: based on the proceedings of the Fifth Annual Symposium on Gynecologic Endocrinology held March 3–5, 1980 at The University of Tennessee, Memphis, Tennessee, (Chicago, IL.: Year Book Pub.), 1981.

8. Anthony, Courtney L.:
Pediatric cardiology, (Garden City, NY.: Medical Examination Pub. Co.), 1979.

9. Arnon, Rica G.:
Pediatric cardiology, (Garden City, NY.: Medical Examination Pub. Co.), 1979.

10. Autian, John:
Toxicity and health threats of phthalate esters: review of the literature, (Oak Ridge, TN.: Toxicology Information Response Center), 1972.

11. Avis, Kenneth Edward:
Parenteral dosage forms; annotated bibliography for the period 1959 through 1973, (Philadelphia, PA.: Parenteral Drug Association), 1969–1975.

12. Avis, Kenneth Edward, editor:
Pharmaceutical dosage forms: parenteral medications, (New York, NY.: Dekker), 1984.

13. Avis, Kenneth Edward:
Sterile preparation for the hospital pharmacist: an illustrated manual of procedures, (Ann Arbor, MI.: Ann Arbor Science Publishers), 1981.

14. Bell, Ann:
The morphology of blood cells in Wright stained smears of peripheral blood and bone marrow, (North Chicago, IL.: Abbott Laboratories), 1954.

15. Bell, Ann:
The morphology of human blood cells, (Philadelphia, PA.: Saunders), 1956.

16. Bell, Ann:
The morphology of human blood cells in Wright stained smears of peripheral blood and bone marrow. Revised edition, (North Chicago, IL.: Abbott Laboratories), 1970.

17. Bell, Ann:
The morphology of human blood cells in Wright stained smears of peripheral blood and bone marrow. 3rd edition, (North Chicago, IL.: Abbott Laboratories), 1975.

18. Bell, Ann:
The morphology of human blood cells in Wright stained smears of peripheral blood and bone marrow. 4th edition, (North Chicago, IL.: Abbott Laboratories), 1978.

19. Bisno, Alan L., editor:
Treatment of infective endocarditis, (New York, NY.: Grune & Stratton), 1981.

20. Black, William T., Jr., editor:
History of medicine in Memphis, (Jackson, TN.: McCowst-Mercer), 1971.

21. Bourgoyne, Julius Roy:
Surgery of the mouth and jaws, (Brooklyn, NY.: Dental Items of Interest Pub. Co.), 1949.

22. Bowers, Margaretta K.:
Counseling the dying, (New York, NY.: Thomas Nelson), 1964.

23. Brown, Fountaine Christine:
Hallucinogenic drugs, (Springfield, IL.: Thomas), 1972.

24. Bruesch, Simon Rulin, compiler:
History of anatomy: the rise of modern anatomy; bibliography, (Memphis, TN.: Private Printing), 1962.

25. Bruesch, Simon Rulin, compiler:
History of anatomy seminar: development of modern anatomy, (Memphis, TN.: Private Printing), 1966.

26. Bursten, Ben:
Beyond psychiatric expertise, (Springfield, IL.: Thomas), 1984.

27. Byrne, William L.:
Molecular approaches to learning and memory, (New York, NY.: Academic), 1970.

28. Campbell, Willis Cohoon:
Operative orthopaedics, (St. Louis, MO.: Mosby), 1939.

29. Campbell, Willis Cohoon:
Textbook on orthopaedic surgery, (Philadelphia, PA.: Saunders), 1930.

30. Clark, James W.:
Diet and the periodontal patient, (Springfield, IL.: Thomas), 1970.

31. Coffey, Kitty R.:
Fun foods for fat folks, (Memphis, TN.: Child Development Center of The University of Tennessee), 1974.

32. Cohen, Brian M., associate editor:
Clinical use of sex steroids: based on the proceedings of the Fourth Annual Symposium on Gynecologic Endocrinology, held May 7–9, 1979 at The University of Tennessee, Memphis, Tennessee, (Chicago, IL.: Year Book Publishers), 1980.

33. Cohen, Brian M.:
Manual of gynecologic endocrinology and infertility, (Baltimore, MD.: Williams and Wilkins), 1979.

34. Cohn, Sidney A.:
Anatomy review; 2003 multiple choice questions and referenced explanatory answers. 5th edition, (Flushing, NY.: Medical Examination Pub. Co.), 1975.

35. Cohn, Sidney A.:
Head and neck anatomy review; 1550 multiple choice questions and referenced explanatory answers, (Flushing, NY.: Medical Examination Pub. Co.), 1976.

36. Connolly, Barbara,
joint editor:
A comprehensive handbook for management of children with developmental disabilities, (Memphis, TN.: University of Tennessee Center for the Health Sciences), 1977.

37. Corliss, Clark Edward:
Patten's human embryology; elements of clinical development, (New York, NY.: McGraw-Hill), 1976.

38. Corliss, Clark Edward:
Embriologia humana de Patten: fundamentos del desarrollo clinica, (Buenos Aires, Argentina: Libreria "El Ateneo" editorial), 1979.

39. Corliss, Clark Edward:
Embiologia umana di Patten. Edizione Italiana, (Bologna, Italy: Editoriale Grasso), 1981.

40. Coury, Victor M.:
PreTest preparation for the dental admission test, (New York, NY.: McGraw-Hill), 1980.

41. Coury, Victor M.:
Review of basic science and clinical dentistry, (Hagerstown, MD.: Harper and Row), 1980.

42. Crawford, Lloyd V.:
Pediatric allergic diseases; focus on clinical diagnosis, (Flushing, NY.: Medical Examination Pub. Co.), 1977.

43. Crawford, Lloyd V.:
Pediatric allergic diseases; focus on clinical diagnosis, (Garden City, NY.: Medical Examination Pub. Co.), 1982.

44. Crenshaw, Andrew H.,
editor:
Campbell's operative orthopaedics. 4th edition, (St. Louis, MO.: Mosby), 1963.

45. Crenshaw, Andrew H.,
editor:
Campbell's operative orthopaedics. 5th edition, (St. Louis, MO.: Mosby), 1971.

46. Crocker, Robert:
A history of the Department of Pathology, 1944–1964, (Memphis, TN.: University of Tennessee Medical Units), 1965.

47. Cruse, Julius M.:
Immunology examination review book, (Flushing, NY.: Medical Examination Pub. Co.), 1971.

48. Davies, Dean F.:
Clinical cytology and the pathologist: papers and recommendations of the Workshop on Cytology, (New York, NY.: The American Cancer Society, Inc.), 1962.

49. Davies, Dean F.,
editor:
Health evaluation: an entry to the health care system, (New York, NY.: Intercontinental Medical Book Corp.), 1973.

50. Dearman, Henry B.:
Not the critic: a novel of psychiatry and the law, (Kingsport, TN.: House of Wingate), 1965.

51. Diggs, Lemuel W.:
Laboratory procedures. 2nd edition revised, (Memphis, TN.: C. A. Davis Printing Co.), 1957.

52. Diggs, Lemuel W.:
Basic medical laboratory procedures. 3rd edition, revised, (Memphis, TN.: C. A. Davis Printing Co.), 1967.

53. Diggs, Lemuel W.:
The morphology of blood cells in Wright stained smears of peripheral blood and bone marrow, (North Chicago, IL.: Abbott Laboratories), 1954.

54. Diggs, Lemuel W.:
The morphology of human blood cells, (Philadelphia, PA.: Saunders), 1956.

55. Diggs, Lemuel W.:
The morphology of human blood cells in Wright stained smears of peripheral blood and bone marrow. Revised edition, (North Chicago, IL.: Abbott Laboratories), 1970.

56. Diggs, Lemuel W.:
The morphology of human blood cells in Wright stained smears of peripheral blood and bone marrow. 3rd edition, (North Chicago, IL.: Abbott Laboratories), 1975.

57. Diggs, Lemuel W.:
The morphology of human blood cells in Wright stained smears of peripheral blood and bone marrow. 4th edition, (North Chicago, IL.: Abbott Laboratories), 1978.

58. Dilts, Preston Vine:
Core studies in obstetrics and gynecology. 3rd edition, (Baltimore, MD.: Williams and Wilkins), 1981.

59. DiLuzio, Nicholas R.,
editor:
The reticuloendothelial system and atherosclerosis. Proceedings of an international symposium on atherosclerosis and the reticuloendothelial system . . . 1966, (New York, NY.: Plenum), 1967.

60. Dornette, William H. L.:
Anatomy for the anesthesiologist; a stereoscopic atlas, (Springfield, IL.: Thomas), 1963.

61. Dornette, William H. L.:
Hospital planning for the anesthesiologist, (Springfield, IL.: Thomas), 1958.

62. Dornette, William H. L.:
Instrumentation in anesthesiology, (Philadelphia, PA.: Lea), 1959.

63. Duenas, Danilo A.:
Pediatriac neurology handbook, (Flushing, NY.: Medical Examination Pub. Co.), 1973.

64. Ellett, Edward Coleman:
Syllabus of diseases of the eye, prepared for the use of the students of the University of Tennessee, College of Medicine, of Memphis, Tenn., (Memphis, TN.: Privately Printed), 1911.

65. Feit, Marvin D.:
Management and administration of drug and alcohol programs, (Springfield, IL.: Thomas), 1979.

66. Fitch, Charles W.:
Pediatric cardiology, (Garden City, NY.: Medical Examination Pub. Co.), 1979.

67. Fletcher, John L.,
editor:
Effects of noise on wildlife, (New York, NY.: Academic Press), 1978.

68. Fowler, Noble O.:
Physical diagnosis of heart disease, (New York, NY.: Macmillan), 1962.

69. Freeman, Bob W.:
Burrows textbook of microbiology. 21st edition, (Philadelphia, PA.: Saunders), 1979.

70. Freeman, Bob W.:
Burrows textbook of microbiology. 22nd edition, (Philadelphia, PA.: Saunders), 1985.

71. Gay, James R.,
editor:
Competition in the marketplace: health care in the 1980's, (New York, NY.: SP Medical and Scientific Books), 1982.

72. Gay, James R.,
co-editor:
The technology explosion in medical science: implications for the health care industry and the public (1981–2001), (New York, NY.: SP Medical and Scientific Books), 1982.

73. Gilmartin, Richard D.:
Pediatric neurology handbook, (Flushing, NY.: Medical Examination Pub. Co.), 1973.

74. Gilmer, Walter Scott:
Atlas of bone tumors, including tumorlike lesions, (St. Louis, MO.: Mosby), 1963.

75. Ginski, John M.:
History: Department of physiology, 1879–1984, University of Tennessee Medical College, Memphis, Tennessee, (Memphis, TN.: Private Printing), 1984.

76. Givens, James R.,
editor:
Clinical use of sex steroids: based on the proceedings of the Fourth Annual Symposium on Gynecologic Endocrinology, held May 7–9, 1979 at the University of Tennessee, Memphis, Tennessee, (Chicago, IL.: Year Book Publishers), 1980.

77. Givens, James R.,
editor:
Endocrine causes of menstrual disorders: based on the proceedings of the second Annual Symposium on Gynecologic Endocrinology, held March 16–18, 1977 at the University of Tennessee, Memphis, Tennessee, (Chicago, IL.: Year Book Medical Publishers), 1978.

78. Givens, James R.,
editor:
Endocrinology of pregnancy: based on the proceedings of the Fifth Annual Symposium on Gynecologic Endocrinology held March 3–5, 1980 at the University of Tennessee, Memphis, Tennessee, (Chicago, IL.: Year Book Pub.), 1981.

79. Givens, James R.,
editor:
Gynecologic endocrinology: based on the proceedings of the first annual Symposium on Reproductive Medicine, held March 15–17, 1976 at the University of Tennessee, Memphis, Tennessee, (Chicago, IL.: Year Book Medical Publishers), 1977.

80. Givens, James R.,
editor:
The hypothalamus: based on the proceedings of the seventh annual Symposium on Gynecologic Endocrinology, held March 4–6, 1982 at the University of Tennessee, Memphis, Tennessee, (Chicago, IL.: Year Book Medical Publishers), 1984.

81. Givens, James R.:
Manual of gynecologic endocrinology and infertility, (Baltimore, MD.: Williams and Wilkins), 1979.

82. Gorline, Lynne L.:
Common problems in primary care, (St. Louis, MO.: Mosby), 1982.

83. Gotten, Henry Bragg:
Physicians' office attendants manual. Section for office work, (Springfield, IL.: Thomas), 1955.

84. Gotten, Nicholas:
Neurologic nursing, (Philadelphia, PA.: Davis), 1941.

85. Gottlieb, Marvin I.:
Anatomy and physiology; 1500 multiple choice questions and referenced answers. 2nd edition, (Flushing, NY.: Medical Examination Pub. Co.), 1969.

86. Gottlieb, Marvin I.:
Anatomy review; 1500 multiple choice questions and answers completely referenced. 4th edition, (Flushing, NY.: Medical Examination Pub. Co.), 1970.

87. Gottlieb, Marvin I.:
Anatomy review; 2003 multiple choice questions and referenced explanatory answers. 5th edition, (Flushing, NY.: Medical Examination Pub. Co.), 1975.

88. Gottlieb, Marvin I.:
Head and neck anatomy review; 1550 multiple choice questions and referenced explanatory answers, (Flushing, NY.: Medical Examination Pub. Co.), 1976.

89. Gottlieb, Marvin I.:
Pediatric neurology handbook, (Flushing, NY.: Medical Examination Pub. Co.), 1973.

90. Gottlieb, Marvin I.:
Pediatrics; specialty board review; 1235 multiple choice questions and answers referenced to textbooks and journals. 3rd edition, (Flushing, NY.: Medical Examination Pub. Co.), 1971.

91. Hall, Carolyn Gray:
Parenteral dosage forms; annotated bibliography for the period 1959 through 1963. (Philadelphia, PA.: Parenteral Drug Association), 1969.

92. Hamner, James E., III:
Oral cancer and precancerous conditions in India, (Copenhagen, Denmark: Munksgaard), 1971.

93. Hamner, James E., III,
editor:
The distinguished visiting professorship lectures, 1983, (Memphis, TN.: The University of Tennessee Center for the Health Sciences), 1984.

94. Hamner, James E., III:
The management of head and neck cancer, (Heidelberg, West Germany: Springer-Verlag), 1984.

95. Hamner, James E., III,
co-editor:
Marketing and managing health care: health promotion and disease prevention, (Memphis, TN.: The University of Tennessee Center for the Health Sciences), 1983.

96. Hamner, James E., III,
co-editor:
The media, communication, and health policy, (Memphis, TN.: The University of Tennessee Center for the Health Sciences), 1984.

97. Hamner, James E., III,
editor:
The distinguished visiting professorship lectures, 1984, (Memphis, TN.: The University of Tennessee Center for the Health Sciences), 1984.

98. Hamner, James E., III,
co-editor:
How business can control employee health care costs, (Memphis TN.: The University of Tennessee Center for the Health Sciences), 1985.

99. Hamner, James E., III,
co-editor:
Abstracts—The biology of transplantation, (Memphis, TN.: The Crippled Children's Hospital Foundation Forum on Child Health), 1984.

100. Hamner, James E., III,
co-editor:
Abstracts—Brain growth and differentiation, (Memphis, TN.: The Crippled Children's Hospital Foundation Forum on Child Health), 1985.

101. Hamner, James E., III:
75th anniversary medical accomplishments: The University of Tennessee, Memphis, (Memphis, TN.: The University of Tennessee, Memphis), 1986.

102. Hanissian, Aram S.:
Pediatric rheumatology case studies: a compilation of 50 clinical studies, (Garden City, NY.: Medical Examination Pub. Co.), 1979.

103. Hardy, James Daniel:
Fluid therapy, (Philadelphia, PA.: Lea), 1954.

104. Hardy, James Daniel:
Nutrition and the alarm response in cancer patients, and steriod excretion in the presence of an adrenocortical tumor and in adrenocortical hyperplasia, (Memphis, TN.: University of Tennessee), 1953.

105. Hardy, James Daniel:
Surgery and the endocrine system: physiologic response to surgical trauma and operative management of endocrine dysfunction, (Philadelphia, PA.: Saunders), 1952.

106. Harrell, William:
Panama's Gorgas Hospital and staff doctors, (New York, NY.: Carlton Press), 1976.

107. Hay, Floyd B.:
The country doctor, (Cumberland, KY.: Private Printing), 1983.

108. Haynes, Margaret E.:
A nursing study of day care for mentally retarded children, (Memphis, TN.: University of Tennessee. College of Nursing), 1970.

109. Hiatt, Roger L.:
Basic pearls in ophthalmology, (Memphis, TN: University of Tennessee Center for the Health Sciences), 1979.

110. Higley, G. B., Jr.:
Atlas of bone tumors, including tumor-like lesions, (St. Louis, MO.), 1963.

111. Holmes, Marguerite C.,
editor:
Anatomy and physiology; 1500 multiple choice questions and referenced answers. 2nd edition, (Flushing, NY.: Medical Examination Pub. Co.), 1969.

112. Hughes, Carl W.:
Traumatic lesions of peripheral vessels, (Springfield, IL.: Thomas), 1961.

113. Hughes, James Gilliam:
Pediatrics in general practice, (New York, NY.: McGraw-Hill), 1952.

114. Hughes, James Gilliam:
Synopsis of pediatrics (St. Louis, MO.: Mosby), 1963.

115. Hughes, James Gilliam:
Synopsis of pediatrics. 2nd edition, (St. Louis, MO.: Mosby), 1967.

116. Hughes, James Gilliam:
Synopsis of pediatrics. 5th edition, (St. Louis, MO.: Mosby), 1980.

117. Hughes, James Gilliam,
editor:
Synopsis of pediatrics. 6th edition, (St. Louis, Mo.: 1984.

118. Hunt, James C.,
editor:
Hypertension update: mechanisms, epidemiology, evaluation, management, (Bloomfield, NJ.: Health Learning Systems, Inc.), 1980.

119. Hunt, James C.:
Living better: recipes for a healthy heart, (Radnor, PA.: Chilton Book Co.), 1980.

120. Hunt, James C.:
Living with high blood pressure: the hypertension diet cookbook, (Bloomfield, NJ.: HLS Press), 1978.

121. Hunt, James C.:
The Mayo Clinic renal diet cookbook, (New York, NY.: Western Pub.Co.), 1974.

122. Hutchinson, Emma L.:
Pharmacy lectures, compiled from various authors, (Memphis, TN: Leon T. Whitten), 1922.

123. Hyman, Orren W.:
Early Development of the Medical Units, University of Tennessee, (Privately typed manuscript bound by Miss Kate A. Stanley, Registrar, University of Tennessee Medical Units: Memphis, TN.), 1970.

124. Jabbour, J. T.:
Atlas of C.T. scans in pediatric neurology, (Flushing, NY.: Medical Examination Pub. Co.), 1977.

125. Jabbour, J.T.:
Pediatric neurology handbook, (Flushing, NY.: Medical Examination Pub. Co.), 1973.

126. Jacobs, Barbara J. Sax,
co-editor:
Competition in the marketplace: health care in the 1980's, (New York, NY.: SP Medical and Scientific Books), 1982.

127. Jacobs, Barbara J. Sax,
co-editor:
Marketing and managing health care: health promotion and disease prevention, (Memphis, TN.: University of Tennessee Center for the Health Sciences), 1983.

128. Jacobs, Barbara J. Sax,
co-editor:
The media, communication, and health policy, (Memphis, TN.: University of Tennessee Center for the Health Sciences), 1984.

129. Jacobs, Barbara J. Sax,
co-editor:
The technology explosion in medical science: implications for the health care industry and the public (1981–2001), (New York, NY.: SP Medical and Scientific Books), 1982.

130. Jacobs, Barbara J. Sax,
co-editor:
How business can control employee health care costs, (Memphis, TN.: The University of Tennessee Center for the Health Sciences), 1985.

131. Jacobs, Barbara J. Sax,
co-editor:
Abstracts — The biology of transplantation, (Memphis, TN.: The Crippled Children's Hospital Foundation Forum on Child Health), 1984.

132. Jacobs, Barbara J. Sax,
co-editor:
Abstracts — Brain growth and differentiation, (Memphis, TN.: The Crippled Children's Hospital Foundation Forum on Child Health), 1985.

133. Johnson, Thomas W.,
editor:
Family practice, (Philadelphia, PA.: Saunders), 1973.

134. Jones, Ellen Whiteman:
Maternity care in two counties: Gibson County, Tennessee, Pike County, Mississippi 1940–41, 1943–44, (New York, NY.: Commonwealth Fund), 1950.

135. Khanna, J. L.,
editor:
Brain damage and mental retardation; a psychological evaluation, (Springfield, IL.: Thomas), 1967.

136. Khanna, J. L.,
editor:
Brain damage and mental retardation; a psychological evaluation. 2nd edition, (Springfield, IL.: Thomas), 1973.

137. Khanna, J. L.,
editor:
New treatment approaches to juvenile delinquency, (Springfield, IL.: Thomas), 1975.

138. Kilgore, W. E.:
Atlas of tumors, including tumor-like lesions, (St. Louis, MO.: Mosby), 1963.

139. Kitabchi, Abbas E.,
associate editor:
The hypothalamus: based on the proceedings of the seventh annual Symposium on Gynecologic Endocrinology, held March 4–6, 1982 at the Univeristy of Tennessee, Memphis, Tennessee, (Chicago, IL.: Year Book Medical Publishers), 1984.

140. Knight, Robert A.,
associate editor:
Campbell's operative orthopaedics. 3rd edition, (St. Louis, MO.: Mosby), 1956.

141. Korones, Sheldon B.:
High-risk newborn infants; the basis for intensive nursing care, (St. Louis, MO.: Mosby) 1972.

142. Korones, Sheldon B.:
High-risk newborn infants; the basis for intensive nursing care. 2nd edition, (St. Louis, MO.: Mosby), 1976.

143. Korones, Sheldon B.:
High-risk newborn infants; the basis for intensive nursing care. 3rd edition, (St. Louis, MO.: Mosby), 1981.

144. Lancaster, Jean:
High-risk newborn infants; the basis for intensive nursing care, (St. Louis, MO.: Mosby), 1972.

145. Lancaster, Jean:
High-risk newborn infants; the basis for intensive nursing care. 2nd edition, (St. Louis, MO.: Mosby), 1976.

146. Lancaster, Jean:
High-risk newborn infants; the basis for intensive nursing care. 3rd edition, (St. Louis, MO.: Mosby), 1981.

147. Lasslo, Andrew,
Symposium Chairman:
Contemporary trends in the training of pharmacologists; IUPHAR satellite symposium in conjunction with the VI International Congress of Pharmacology, Helsinki, Finland, 1975, (Helsinki, Finland: International Union of Pharmacology), 1976.

148. Lasslo, Andrew,
editor:
Surface chemistry and dental integuments, (Springfield, IL.: Thomas), 1973.

149. Levinson, Michael,
co-editor:
Gastroenterology, 1,000 multiple choice questions and referenced explanatory answers. 3rd edition, (Flushing, NY.: Medical Examination Pub. Co.) 1977.

150. Lewis, Myron,
co-editor:
Gastroenterology, 1,000 multiple choice questions and referenced explanatory answers. 2nd edition, (Flushing, NY.: Medical Examination Pub. Co.), 1973.

151. Lewis, Myron,
co-editor:
Gastroenterology, 1,000 multiple choice questions and referenced explanatory answers. 3rd edition, (Flushing, NY.: Medical Examination Pub. Co.), 1977.

152. Livermore, George Robertson:
Gonorrhea and kindred affections: gonorrhea in the male, chancroid and verruca acuminata, (New York, NY.: Appleton), 1929.

153. Love, Albert Gallatin:
Tabulating equipment and Army medical statistics, (Washington, DC.: Office of the Surgeon General), 1958.

154. Lynch, Malcolm A.,
editor:
Burket's Oral Medicine, (Philadelphia, PA: J.B. Lippincott Co.), 1977.

155. McKinney, Richmond:
Syllabus of diseases of the nose, throat and ear, (Memphis, TN.: Private Printing). 190–.

156. McKinney, Richmond:
Syllabus of the diseases of the nose, throat and ear for junior and senior students. 3rd edition, (Memphis, TN.: E. H. Clarke Press), 191–.

157. McKinney, Richmond:
Syllabus of the diseases of the nose, throat and ear. 4th edition, (Memphis, TN.: S. C. Toof Printers), 192–.

158. Milford, Lee W.:
The hand: from the sixth edition of Campbell's operative orthopaedics. 2nd edition, (St. Louis, MO.: Mosby), 1982.

159. Milford, Lee W.:
The hand: from the fifth edition of Campbell's operative orthopaedics, (St. Louis, MO.: Mosby), 1971.

160. Miller, William A.,
co-editor:
The practice of pharmacy: institutional and ambulatory pharmaceutical services, (Cincinnati, OH.: Harvey Whitney Books), 1981.

161. Minor, Jane Wilson,
joint editor:
A comprehensive handbook for management of children with developmental disabilities, (Memphis, TN.: University of Tennessee Center for the Health Sciences), 1977.

162. Murry, Ruth Neil,
Director:
Training in mental retardation for a baccalaureate nursing program (1967–1971), (Memphis, TN.: University of Tennessee, College of Nursing), 1972.

163. Nash, Clinton B.,
co-editor:
Heart and vascular systems basic sciences; 1500 multiple choice questions and referenced answers, (Flushing, NY.: Medical Examination Pub. Co.), 1970.

164. Nash, Clinton B.,
co-editor:
Pharmacology review; 1350 multiple choice questions and answers completely referenced. 2nd edition, (Flushing, NY.: Medical Examination Pub. Co.), 1966.

165. Nash, Clinton B.,
co-editor:
Pharmacology review; 1565 multiple choice questions and answers completely referenced. 3rd edition, (Flushing, NY.: Medical Examination Pub. Co.), 1972.

166. Overman, Richard R.,
co-editor:
Bone marrow therapy and chemotherapy prophylaxis in irradiated primates, (Rijswijk, The Netherlands: Krips), 1962.

167. Partridge, Lloyd D.:
A glossary of neurophysiology terms, (Memphis, TN.: University of Tennessee), 1973.

168. Pate, James W.:
The science of surgery, (New York, NY.: McGraw-Hill), 1964.

169.. Peterson, Shailer Alvarey:
Clinical dental hygiene. 2nd edition, (St. Louis, MO.: Mosby), 1963.

170. Peterson, Shailer Alvarey:
Clinical dental hygiene. 3rd edition, (St. Louis, MO.: Mosby), 1968.

171. Peterson, Shailer Alvarey,
editor:
Comprehensive review for dental hygienists, (St. Louis, MO.: Mosby), 1965.

172. Peterson, Shailer Alvarey,
editor:
Comprehensive review for dental hygienists. 2nd edition, (St. Louis, MO.: Mosby), 1969.

173. Peterson, Shailer Alvarey:
The dentist and his assistant, (St. Louis, MO.: C.V. Mosby), 1961.

174. Peterson, Shailer Alvarey:
The dentist and his assistant, (St. Louis, MO.: C.V. Mosby), 1967.

175. Purcell, William P.:
Strategy of drug design: a guide to biological activity, (New York, NY.: Wiley), 1973.

176. Quintana, Ronald P.:
Surface chemistry and dental integuments, (Springfield, IL.: Thomas), 1973.

177. Rabinowitz, Jack G.:
Pediatric radiology, (Philadelphia, PA.: Lippincott), 1978.

178. Reed, Gretchen Mayo:
Basic structures of the head and neck: a programmed instruction in clinical anatomy for dental professionals, (Philadelphia, PA.: Saunders), 1976.

179. Reed, Gretchen Mayo:
Regulation of fluid and electrolyte balance: a programmed instruction in clinical physiology. 2nd edition, (Philadelphia, PA.: Saunders), 1977.

180. Richmond, Sara Grace:
A history of the Department of Pathology, 1944–1964, (Memphis, TN.: University of Tennessee, Medical Units), 1965.

181. Riggs, Webster:
Pediatric chest roentgenology: recognizing the abnormal, (St. Louis, MO.: Green), 1979.

182. Robbins, Morris L.:
Atlas of oral pathology, (St. Louis, MO.: Mosby), 1981.

183. Roberts, Florence Bright:
High-risk newborn infants; the basis for intensive nursing care, (St. Louis, MO.: Mosby), 1972.

184. Robertson, James T.,
associate editor:
The hypothalamus: based on the proceedings of the seventh annual Symposium on Gynecologic Endocrinology, held March 4–6, 1982, at the University of Tennessee, Memphis, Tennessee, (Chicago, IL.: Year Book Medical Pub.), 1984.

185. Rosenthal, Ted L.:
Social learning and cognition, (New York, NY.: Academic Press), 1978.

186. Roy, Frederick Hampton:
Ocular differential diagnosis, (Philadelphia, PA.: Lea & Febiger), 1972.

187. Roy, Frederick Hampton:
Ocular differential diagnosis. 2nd edition, (Philadelphia, PA.: Lea & Febiger), 1975.

188. Roy, Frederick Hampton:
Practical management of eye problems: glaucoma, strabismus, visual fields, (Philadelphia, PA.: Lea & Febiger), 1975.

189. Russell, Fay F.,
editor:
Identification and management of selected developmental disabilities: a guide for nurses, (Memphis, TN.: University of Tennessee Center for the Health Sciences Child Development Center), 1973.

190. Russell, Fay F.,
editor:
Identification and management of selected developmental disabilities: a guide for nurses, (Rockville, MD.: U.S. Dept. of Health, Education, and Welfare), 1978.

191. Russell, Fay F.:
A nursing study of day care for mentally retarded children, (Memphis, TN.: University of Tennessee, College of Nursing), 1970.

192. Said, Margaret:
A history of the Department of Pathology, 1944–1964, (Memphis, TN.: University of Tennessee, Medical Units), 1965.

193. Sanders, Sam H.,
co-author:
The lung and paranasal sinuses, (Springfield, IL.: Thomas), 1969.

194. Semmes, Raphael Eustace:
Ruptures of the lumbar intervertebral disc, their mechanism, diagnosis, and treatment, (Springfield, IL.: Thomas), 1964.

195. Sharma, Rameshwar K.,
co-editor:
Endocrine control in neoplasia, (New York, NY.: Raven Press), 1978.

196. Sheppard, Charles Wilcox:
Basic principles of the tracer method; introduction to mathematical tracer kinetics, (New York, NY: Wiley), 1962.

197. Sherman, R. T.:
The science of surgery, (New York, NY.: McGraw-Hill), 1964.

198. Siskin, Milton,
editor:
The biology of the human dental pulp; proceedings of the Conference on Biology of the Human Dental Pulp held in Memphis, Tennessee, September 16–19, 1970 and the Workshop on the Biologic Basis of Modern Endodontic Practice held in Chicago, Illinois, November 19–21, 1971, (St. Louis, MO.: Mosby), 1973.

199. Sklaire, Harris:
A compend of electrocardiography. 4th edition, (Dansville, NY.: F.A. Owen Pub.), 1955.

200. Sklaire, Harris:
Pictorial handbook of electrocardiography. 5th edition, (Rouses Point, NY.: Northern Pub. Co.), 1959.

201. Skoutakis, Vasilios A.,
editor:
Clinical toxicology of drugs: principles and practice, (Philadelphia, PA.: Lea and Febiger), 1982.

202. Sloane, Nathan H.:
Review of biochemistry, (New York, NY.: MacMillan), 1969.

203. Smith, Hugh,
associate editor:
Operative orthopaedics. 2nd edition, (St. Louis, MO.: Mosby), 1949.

204. Smith, James Floyd:
Histopathology of salivary gland lesions, (Philadelphia, PA.: Lippincott), 1966.

205. Smith, Mary Ann Harvey:
Feeding management of a child with a handicap: a guide for professionals, (Memphis, TN.: University of Tennessee Center for the Health Sciences, Child Development Center), 1982.

206. Smith, Mary Ann Harvey,
editor:
Feeding the handicapped child. Compilation of papers from Nutrition Workshops, (Memphis, TN.: University of Tennessee Center for the Health Sciences, Child Development Center), 1971.

207. Smith, Mary Ann Harvey,
editor:
Feeding the handicapped child. Compilation of papers from Nutrition Workshops given at the Child Development Center, (Memphis, TN.: University of Tennessee Center for the Health Sciences, Child Development Center), 1977.

208. Smith, Mary Ann Harvey,
editor:
Proceedings of Third National Nutrition Workshop for Nutritionists from University Affiliated Facilities, The Child Development Center, University of Tennessee Center for the Health Sciences, Memphis, Tennessee, April 4–9, 1976, (Memphis, TN.: The University of Tennessee Center for the Health Sciences, Child Development Center), 1976.

209. Smith, Roy M.:
Atlas of oral pathology, (St. Louis, MO.: Mosby), 1981.

210. Sparer, Phineas Jack:
Personality, stress, and tuberculosis, (New York, NY.: International University Press), 1956.

211. Speed, J.S.,
editor:
Campbell's operative orthopaedics. 2nd edition, (St. Louis, MO.: Mosby), 1949.

212. Speed, J.S.,
editor:
Campbell's operative orthopaedics. 3rd edition, (St. Louis, MO.: Mosby), 1956.

213. Sprunt, Douglas H.:
A history of the Department of Pathology, 1944–1964, (Memphis, TN.: University of Tennessee Medical Units), 1965.

214. Sprunt, Douglas H.:
Physicians office attendant's manual: Section for laboratory work, (Springfield, IL.: Thomas), 1955.

215. Stegbauer, Cheryl Cummings:
Common problems in primary care, (St. Louis, MO.: Mosby), 1982.

216. Stern, Neuton Samuel:
The bases of treatment, (Springfield, IL.: Thomas), 1957.

217. Stern, Neuton Samuel:
Clinical diagnosis, physical and differential, (New York, NY.: MacMillan), 1933.

218. Stern, Neuton Samuel,
editor:
Rare diseases in internal medicine, (Springfield, IL.: Thomas), 1966.

219. Stern, Neuton Samuel:
Understanding sexual behavior, (Memphis, TN.: Davis Printing Co.), 1968.

220. Stern, Thomas Neuton:
Clinical examination; a textbook of physical diagnosis, (Chicago, IL.: Year Book Medical Pub.), 1964.

221. Stewart, Marcus Jefferson,
editor:
History of medicine in Memphis, (Jackson, TN.: McCowat-Mercer), 1971.

222. Sticht, Frank D.,
co-editor:
Heart and vascular systems, basic sciences: 1,500 multiple questions and referenced answers, (Flushing, NY.: Medical Examination Pub. Co.), 1977.

223. Stollerman, Gene H.:
Rheumatic fever and streptococcal infection, (New York, NY.: Grune & Stratton), 1975.

224. Storer, Edward H.:
The science of surgery, (New York, NY.: McGraw-Hill), 1964.

225. Storer, Edward H.,
associate editor:
Principles of surgery, (New York, NY.: McGraw-Hill), 1969.

226. Strain, Samuel Frederick:
From the Nolichucky to Memphis: reminiscences of a Tennessee doctor, (Memphis, TN.: Memphis State University Press), 1979.

227. Swafford, William B.:
Pharmacy and the law; a manual for practicing pharmacists, (Memphis, TN.: Private Printing), 1969.

228. Swafford, William B.:
Tennessee pharmacy law handbook, (Memphis, TN.: University of Tennessee Center for the Health Sciences), 1980.

229. Taylor, Rachel,
associate editor:
The five school consortium nursing core curriculum: design, objectives, content, and process, (Memphis, TN.: The University of Tennessee Center for the Health Sciences), 1977.

230. Tchobanoff, James B.,
assistant editor:
Health evaluation: an entry to the health care system, (New York, NY.: Intercontinental Medical Book Corp.), 1973.

231. Terrell, Margaret Anne:
Fun foods for fat folks, (Memphis, TN.: Child Development Center of the University of Tennessee), 1974.

232. Trefler, Elaine,
compiler and editor:
Seating for children with cerebral palsy: a resource manual, (The University of Tennessee Center for the Health Sciences Rehabilitation Engineering Program), 1984.

233. Turner, James E.:
Atlas of oral pathology, (St. Louis, MO.: Mosby), 1981.

234. Walker, Virginia H.:
Nursing and ritualistic practice, (New York, NY: Macmillan), 1967.

235. Wall, Hershel P.:
Pediatrics; specialty board review; 1,235 multiple choice questions and answers referenced to textbooks and journals. 3rd edition, (Flushing, NY.: Medical Examination Pub. Co.), 1971.

236. Walter, Charles:
Enzyme kinetics; open and closed systems, (New York, NY.: Ronald Press), 1966.

237. Walter, Charles:
Steady-state applications in enzyme kinetics, (New York, NY.: Ronald Press), 1965.

238. Webb, William L.,
co-editor:
Psychiatric diagnosis: exploration of biological predictors, (New York, NY.: SP Medical and Scientific Books), 1978.

239. Wells, Gerre Givens:
Manual of histologic technics. 3rd edition, (Memphis, TN.: University of Tennessee, Institute of Pathology), 1966.

240. Wells, Jack E.:
PreTest preparation for the dental admission test, (New York, NY.: McGraw-Hill), 1980.

241. Wells, Jack E.:
Review of basic science and clinical dentistry, (Hagerstown, MD.: Harper and Row), 1980.

242. Wentz, Anne Colston,
associate editor:
Clinical use of sex steriods: based on the proceedings of the Fourth Annual Symposium on Gynecologic Endocrinology, held May 7–9, 1979 at the University of Tennessee, Memphis, Tennessee, (Chicago, IL.: Year Book Medical Publishers), 1980.

243. Wentz, Anne Colston:
Manual of gynecologic endocrinology and infertility, (Baltimore, MD.: Williams and Wilkins), 1979.

244. Wessels, Kenneth E.,
editor:
Dentistry and the handicapped patient, (Littleton, MA.: PSG Pub. Co.), 1979.

245. Whitacre, Frank E.:
Maternity care in two counties; Gibson County, Tennessee, Pike County, Mississippi 1940–41, 1943–44, (New York, NY.: Commonwealth Fund), 1950.

246. White, Carol Sue:
A comprehensive handbook for management of children with developmental disabilities, (Memphis, TN.: University of Tennessee Center for the Health Sciences), 1977.

247. Wittenborg, August Hermsmeier:
Outline plan for the study of physiology, (Memphis, TN.: Paul & Douglas), 1907.

248. Wood, William B.,
co-editor:
Heart and vascular systems, basic sciences: 1500 multiple choice questions and referenced answers, (Flushing, NY.: Medical Examination Pub. Co.), 1977.

249. Woodbury, Robert A.:
Heart and vascular systems, basic sciences: 1500 multiple choice questions and referenced answers, (Flushing, NY.: Medical Examination Pub. Co.), 1970.

250. Woodbury, Robert A.,
co-editor:
Pharmacology review, 1350 multiple choice questions and answers completely referenced. 2nd edition, (Flushing, NY.: Medical Examination Pub. Co.), 1966.

251. Woodbury, Robert A.,
co-editor:
Pharmacology review, 1565 multiple choice questions and answers completely referenced. 3rd edition, (Flushing, NY.: Medical Examination Pub. Co.), 1972.

252. Wruble, Lawrence D.:
Gastroenterology, 1000 multiple choice questions and referenced answers, (Flushing, NY.: Medical Examination Pub. Co.), 1970.

253. Wruble, Lawrence D.:
Gastroenterology, 1000 multiple choice questions and referenced answers. 2nd edition, (Flushing, NY.: Medical Examination Pub. Co.), 1973.

254. Wruble, Lawrence D.:
Gastroenterology, 1000 multiple choice questions and referenced answers. 3rd edition, (Flushing, NY.: Medical Examination Pub. Co.), 1977.

255. Zurhellen, Joan H.:
The five school consortium nursing core curriculum: design, objectives, content, and process, (Memphis, TN.: University of Tennessee Center for the Health Sciences), 1977.

Appendix K

List of the University of Tennessee, Memphis Buildings

This listing of the buildings at the University of Tennessee, Memphis gives details, if known, regarding the name, the date of construction, the name of the principal architects, the insured value, and the date of destruction. Certain facts and details, especially with respect to the earlier buildings, are no longer available. Cost figures, when known, are insurable replacement value as of 1985, or in the case of demolished buildings, 1971.

For teaching, clinical clerkships, and residency programs the University of Tennessee, Memphis faculty and students utilize many nearby medical institutions through collateral agreements. These include: Le Bonheur Children's Medical Center, the V.A. Hospital, the Regional Medical Center at Memphis, the Newborn Center, the Trauma Center, the Crump Maternity Hospital, the Memphis Mental Health Institute, Campbell's Clinic (Orthopedics), and the Baptist Memorial Hospital. However, U.T. Memphis does not own these buildings. It also has affiliate agreements with the University of Tennessee Memorial Hospital in Knoxville, Baroness Erlanger Hospital in Chattanooga, and a special Family Practice Program in Jackson, Tennessee.

1. Y.M.CA. Building (College of Dentistry); 1900; destroyed by fire in 1943.
2. Rogers Hall (College of Dentistry); 1902; demolished in 1952.
3. Lindsley Hall (College of Medicine); 1906; demolished in 1974.
4. Eve Hall (College of Medicine); 1912; demolished in 1974.
5. University Center; 1906; this building was called the Rex Club and was then renamed and remodeled as the University Center in 1933; demolished in 1974.
6. Institute of Pathology; 1921 (vacated in 1951 and then occupied by the Institute of Clinical Investigations); demolished in 1980.
7. Wittenborg Anatomy Building; 1926; Jones and Furbringer; ($5,812,100).
8. Goodman House Dormitory; 1926; (was named the Forrest Park Apartments and was acquired by U.T. Memphis in 1948); Hander and Cairns; ($2,847,400).
9. Mooney Library; 1928; ($2,709,200).
10. Crowe Pharmacy Building; 1928; ($6,714,000).
11. Kraus Warehouse; 1930; ($339,600), demolished in 1983.
12. University Dormitory for men; 1939; demolished in 1974.
13. Bishop Gailor Clinics; 1944; Walk C. Jones; ($8,788,600).
14. Polyclinic Dormitory; 1943; demolished 1960.
15. M.U.S. Building Dormitory; 1946; demolished 1965.
16. Faculty Building (former Dental College); 1949; Walk C. Jones, Sr. and Jr.; ($6,941,000).
17. Institute of Pathology Building; 1951; Walk C. Jones, Sr. and Jr.; ($10,232,400).

303

18. Van Vleet Memorial Cancer Center; 1951; Walk C. Jones, Sr. and Jr.; Thorne, Howe, Stratton, & Strong; ($5,375,700).

19. U.T. Memorial Hospital and Research Center (Knoxville); 1956; (original funding = $6,000,000 with later additions).

20. T.P. Nash Chemistry-Physiology Building; 1955; Walk C. Jones, Sr. and Jr.; ($5,874,00).

21. O.W. Hyman Administration Building; 1955; Furbringer and Ehrman; ($3,107,000).

22. Medical-Surgical Building (Gailor Annex); 1955.

23. Chandler Clinical Services Center; 1962; Walk C. Jones, Jr.; (jointly owned by U.T. Memphis and Regional Medical Center at Memphis).

24. Seldon D. Feurt Pharmacy Building; 1962; Hanker and Heyer; ($2,640,400).

25. Belz-Kriger Cancer Clinic (incorporated into the Van Vleet Cancer Center); 1964; ($496,000).

26. James K. Dobbs Research Institute; 1965; Eason, Anthony, McKinney, and Cox; ($6,571,100).

27. William F. Bowld Hospital; 1965; Eason, Anthony, McKinney, and Cox; ($2,026,400).

28. Wassell Randolph Student-Alumni Center; 1969; Gassner, Nathan, and Browne; ($7,666,100).

29. Randolph Dormitory; 1969; Gassner, Nathan, and Browne; ($3,575,200).

30. Child Development Center; 1969; Roy P. Harrover & Associates; ($9,856,400).

31. Chancellor's Residence; 1972; ($232,500).

32. Purchasing and Physical Plant Building; 1975; ($1,193,500).

33. Doctors' Office Building; 1976; Haglund and Venable; ($5,810,900).

34. Winfield Dunn Dental Clinical Building; 1977; Gassner, Nathan, and Browne; ($10,608,400).

35. Cecil C. Humphreys General Education Building; 1977; Roy P. Harrover & Associates; ($21,486,400).

36. Coleman College of Medicine Building; 1980; O'Brien Associates; ($12,378,300).

37. Off-Campus Animal Care Facility; 1981; McGhee, Nicholson, and Burke; ($1,285,500).

38. Library-Nursing Building; 1985; Gassner, Nathan, & Associates; ($7,264,600).

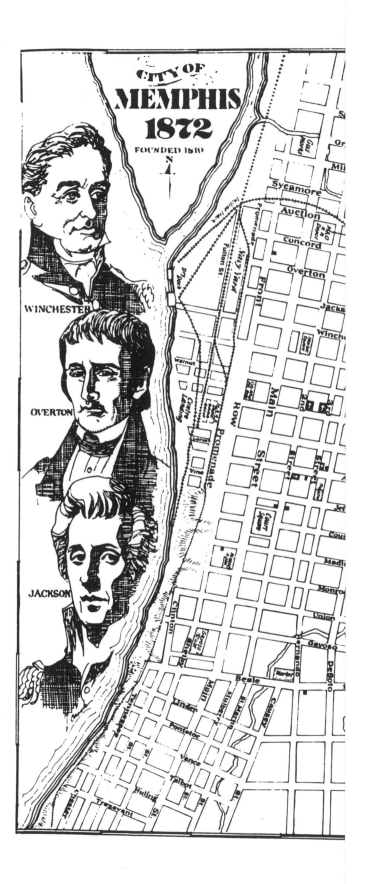

Campus Map

THE UNIVERSITY OF TENNESSEE, MEMPHIS
The Health Science Center

Baptist Memorial Hospital   (29)

William F. Bowld Hospital   (16)

Campbell Clinic   (31)

Child Development Center   (26)

The Regional Medical Center   (27)

Coleman College of Medicine Building   (14)

Crowe Research Building   (6)

Dobbs Medical Research Institute   (15)

Doctors Office Building   (13)

Dunn Building College of Dentistry   (1)

Faculty Building   (4)

Feurt Building   (9)

Gailor Clinic   (30)

Goodman House   (25)

Humphreys General Education Building   (10)

Hyman Administration Building   (3)

Le Bonheur Children's Medical Center   (18)

Les Passees Rehabilitation Center   (20)

Library/Nursing Building   (12)

Memphis Mental Health Institute   (19)

Mooney Memorial Library   (7)

Nash Research Building   (8)

Newborn Center   (17)

Pathology Institute Building   (11)

Physical Plant Purchasing Building   (2)

Randolph Student-Alumni Center   (22)

Randolph Residence Hall   (23)

UT Doctors Field   (24)

UT Medical Center   (13), (15), (16), (21)

Van Vleet Memorial Cancer Center   (21)

Veterans Administration Medical Center   (28)

Wittenborg Anatomy Building   (5)

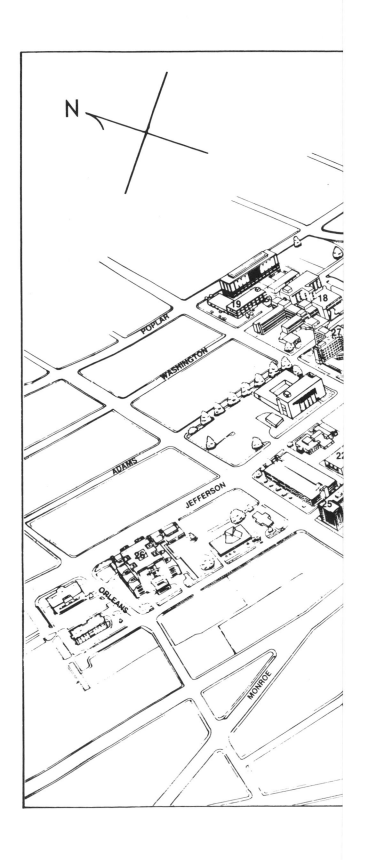

Index

305